Eating For Life
COOKBOOK

———— ❧ ————

TERI SECREST

*Bringing healthy food and fun
back into the kitchen!*

ISBN: 978-0-9979721-5-3
Eating for Life: Bringing healthy food and fun back into the kitchen!
Copyright © 2024 by Joy of Living Publishers
All rights reserved.

Joy of Living Publishers
3140 Pinnacle Club Dr
Kerrville, TX 78028

ISBN: 978-0-9979721-5-3
Cover Design: Lisa Trenary
Cover and Interior Photos: Lisa Trenary
Printed in the United States of America
First Edition: 2024

This book is intended to provide helpful and informative material on the subject matter. It is not intended to replace medical advice or guidance, and readers should consult a professional for advice regarding individual circumstances. The publisher and author are not liable for any actions taken based on the information provided.

Ordering Information:
Visit TeriSecrest.com
Call 830-355-3578

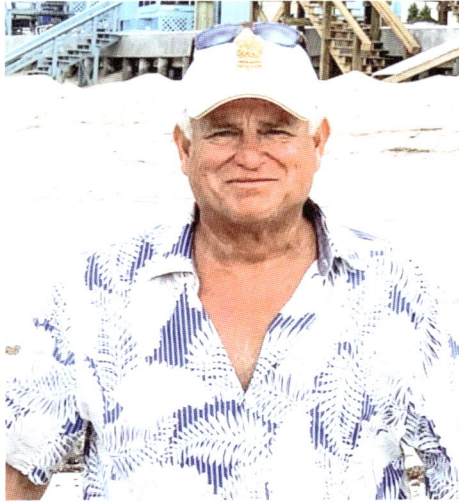

REED GRAFKE

This book is dedicated to my loving husband, the late Reed Grafke. Reed was a kind, thoughtful and gentle person. He also had a little mischievous side, which was endearing to all his friends.

Reed was a magnificent home chef. In fact, he was so talented he could have opened his own 5-star restaurant. Not only was he a purveyor of fine foods, but his core life message centered around loving people through exquisite food, hospitality and good, deep conversation.

Reed and I loved gourmet cooking and entertaining guests together. He was such a passionate grocery shopper until there was no such thing as a hum drum trip to the grocery store. Every shopping experience was a grand adventure!

Reed mentored me in so many areas including the timing of each course. He challenged me to expand the use of essential oils in my recipes to further the flavors even more. The most important lesson I learned from Reed is to make every recipe with love. For this, I am forever grateful and because of this, Reed is deeply missed by all who were blessed to sit at his table.

TABLE OF CONTENTS

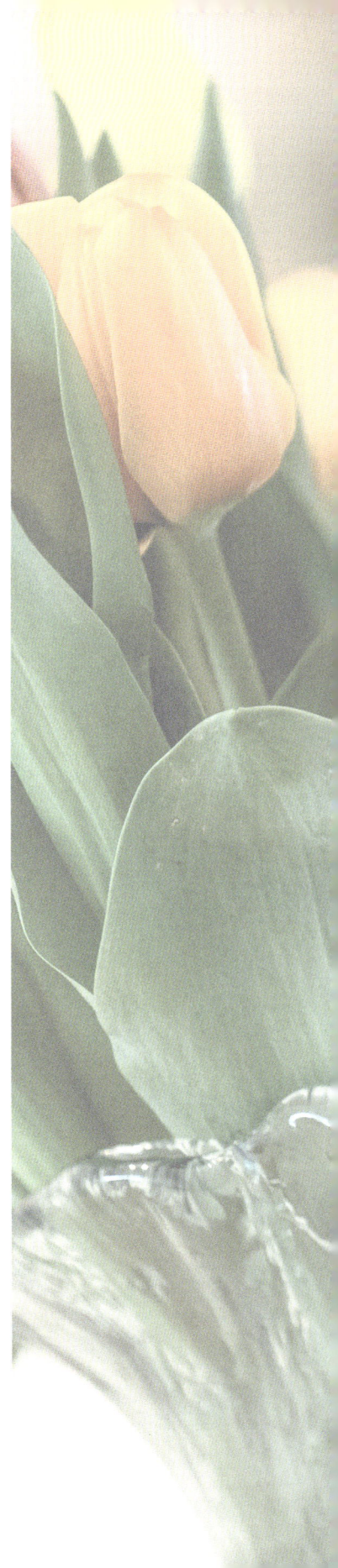

FOREWARD

From Teri's loving children

Some of my favorite memories with our mom, Teri Secrest, include food and hospitality. We have traveled to many countries together and enjoyed some delicious meals, however, nothing compares to a homemade masterpiece from mom's kitchen.

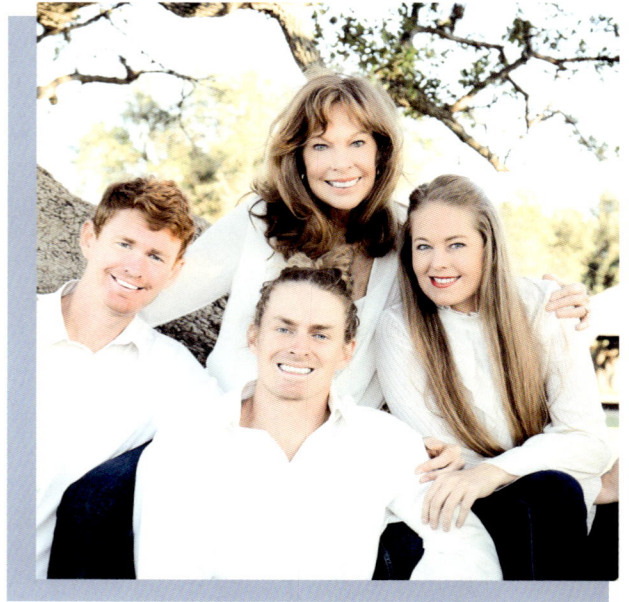

When Mom was writing her very first cookbook, guess who got to sample all her new creations…me! It was wonderful. Years later our mother still adds just as much love into every recipe. I truly believe that you will enjoy the life-giving journey that "Eating For Life" will take you on. Let your family legacy include fun in the kitchen, while getting back to the simplistic nature of food.

Mother taught my brothers and me that food is fuel, and to this day my body craves homemade meals cooked with love! I hope you enjoy your best years ever, as your body says "Thank You" for giving it the fuel it needs! Appreciation for the art of cooking, and the joy of sharing delicious home cooked creations is the making of a good life! *love, Elizabeth Rose*

My mother, Teri Secrest, has always had a love for vibrant, healthy eating. From the home cooked meals, she prepared when we children were young, to the extravagant meals she prepares at her home today, each meal is crafted with a sense of life to it. She never ceases to let anyone leave her table feeling any less than revived. As a wonderful mother of three, our mom is over-qualified to teach on healthy eating because she has spent much of her life studying nutrition. Growing up I can remember she would make us three healthy meals every day. Whether it was an omelet with lots of eggs and vegetables in it or a gourmet five course dinner, she always made sure our meals were made with live foods. I feel blessed to have a mom like this!

love, Daniel

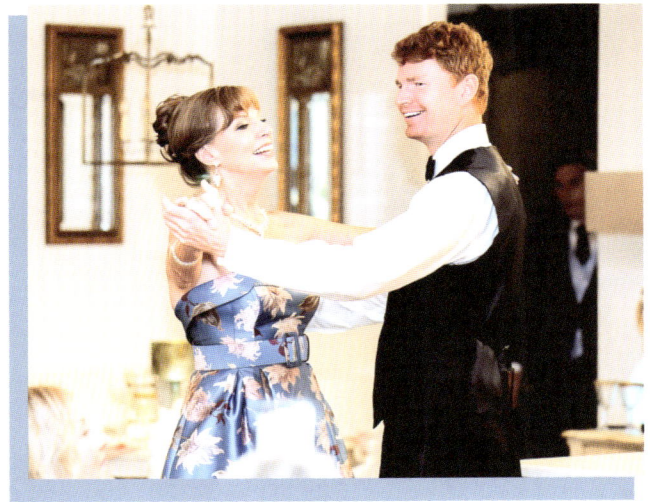

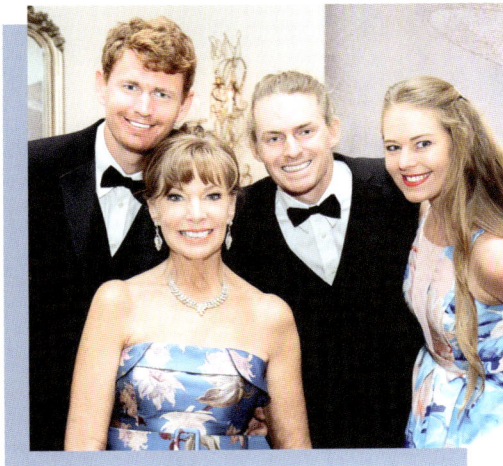

My mom, has spent a lifetime accumulating knowledge and tips to make eating healthy simple. It doesn't have to be hard, or crazy expensive. But being sick is hard and very expensive. Mom makes it easy to have fun while cooking life-giving foods. Throughout high school, Mom would get my friends over to cook with her all the time. If you can imagine a bunch of football players in aprons cooking with my mom... it was quite the scene! That was her secret way of guiding us into lots of healthy homemade foods. I highly recommend this this book for anyone looking to take control of their health, energy and to keep their bodies living abundantly.

love, Joseph

...With Love from all of us!

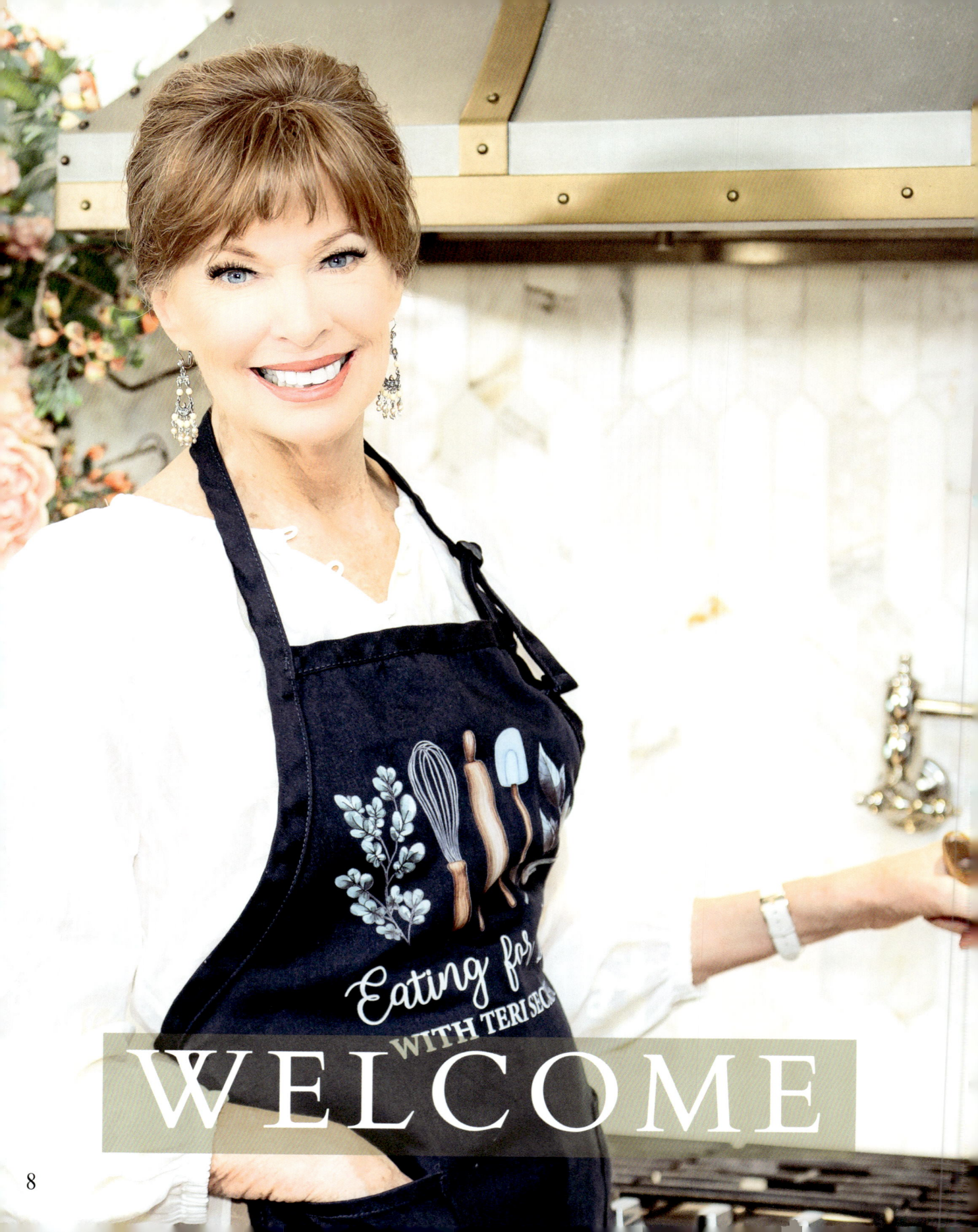

WELCOME

ABOUT THE AUTHOR

Teri Secrest is a certified wellness coach, passionate food lover, best-selling author and international speaker on wellness. As the daughter of a French cooking school founder, Teri discovered the joy of entertaining friends with health foods from a very early age. The addition of food grade essential oils into Teri's recipes in recent years, are taking the flavors from great to extravagant!

In her twenties, Teri suffered from hypoglycemia, a blood sugar imbalance, which lead her on a quest to understand the devastating effects of too much processed white sugar. After changing to natural sugars, all her symptoms disappeared. Today, Teri is dedicated to helping people enjoy their best life at every age. As a sought-after international speaker Teri delivers her message with such enthusiasm and joy she has gained the nickname, "Ambassador of Joy" with her colleagues.

In her free time, Teri loves hiking, swimming, ballroom dancing, horseback riding, the symphony, writing and quality time with family and friends.

Connect with Teri...
TeriSecrest.com
Facebook.com/TeriSecrestInternational
Instagram.com/Teri.Secrest
YouTube.com/TeriLeeSecrest
Info@TeriSecrest.com
(830)355-3578

ESSENTIAL OIL DISCLAIMER

Essential oils like basil, oregano, and rosemary can transform ordinary dishes into extraordinary culinary experiences. Remember, only use Young Living Vitality Essential Oils for ingestion to ensure you get the highest quality essential oils on the market today. Before you begin, it's important to understand a few key points:

❀ **FDA Disclaimer:** The claims made about essential oils in this book and the associated materials have not been evaluated by the Food and Drug Administration (FDA.) Essential oils are not intended to treat, cure, or prevent any disease.

❀ **Educational and Entertainment Purposes Only:** The information provided in this book and the associated materials is for educational and entertainment purposes only. Teri Secrest is not a medical doctor, and the advice given here is not intended to replace professional medical advice, diagnosis, or treatment.

❀ **Quality Matters:** When cooking with essential oils, always use Young Living Vitality high-quality, food-grade oils. Young Living Vitality essential oils are specifically labeled for dietary use and are the only oils recommended for cooking in this book. See where to get them on **Page 21.**

❀ **Proper Usage:** Essential oils are highly concentrated. A little goes a long way, so always start with a very small amount (usually a drop or less) and adjust to taste.

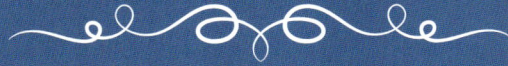

❀ Potential Allergies: Be aware of potential allergies. Just like any other food ingredient, essential oils can cause allergic reactions in some individuals. If you are allergic to the plant, proceed with caution when it comes to the oil. Perform a patch test or start with a very small amount to ensure you do not have an adverse reaction.

❀ Consult Your Healthcare Provider: Before adding any new ingredient to your diet, consider consulting with your healthcare provider. This is particularly important if you are pregnant, nursing, have a medical condition, or are taking medications.

❀ Topical Use Disclaimer: If you choose to use essential oils topically, proceed with caution and do so at your own risk. Always dilute essential oils properly with a carrier oil and perform a patch test before extensive use. Check with your healthcare professional about your specific situation.

It's Time To Enjoy Your Culinary Journey...

Cooking with essential oils can be a wonderful way to add new dimensions to your meals. With proper knowledge and care, you can safely and effectively incorporate these powerful oils into your daily repertoire. Enjoy exploring the vibrant flavors and benefits that essential oils can bring to your table! Remember always to prioritize your health and safety.

HAPPY COOKING!

You are about to embark on a culinary experience of a lifetime!

You're Invited to join my exclusive
7-Week Digital Healthy Cooking Course!

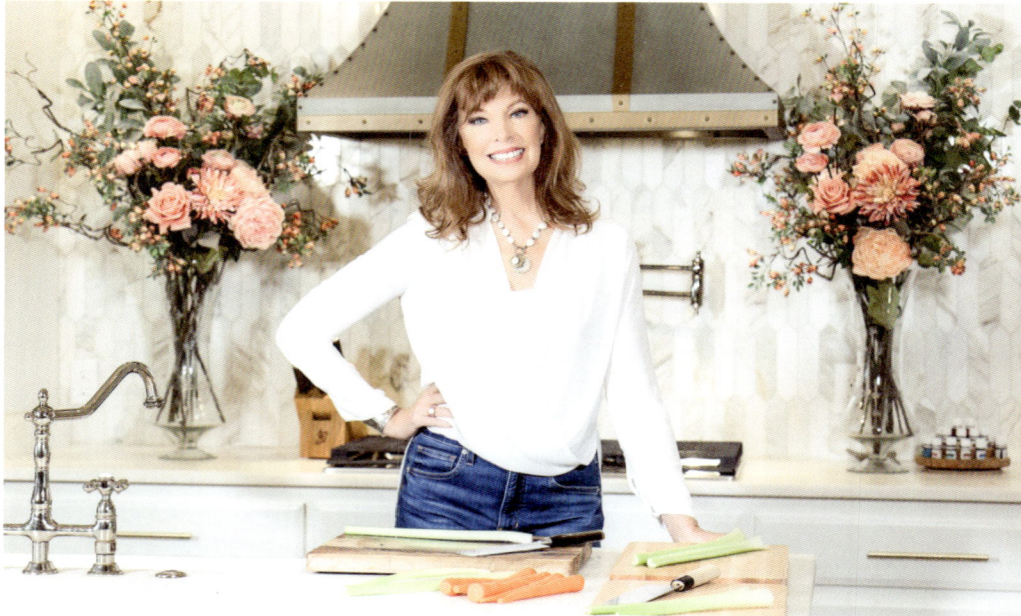

Thank you so much for purchasing my cookbook, If you are a visual learner like me, I'd like to invite you to join me in my complete 7-week online video course! In this digital course, we'll cook side by side together and turn your kitchen into a place of extravagant flavor, and vitality.

What Makes My Digital Course Unique?

⚜ Step-by-Step Video Lessons

In this course, my students and I will show you techniques that will transform your kitchen skills. I'll teach you how to handle a French chef knife with confidence and ease—an essential skill is best learned by video and will make you feel like a true chef!

⚜ Cooking with Essential Oils - Made Easy!

In the videos, I'll show you exactly how to use essential oils in your cooking to add extravagant flavor and wellness benefits to your meals. Once you see how easy it is, you'll wonder why you didn't try it sooner!

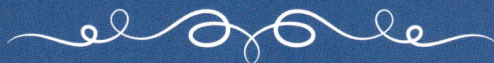

⚜ Interactive Workbook – Track Your Journey

With the downloadable workbook, you'll track your progress, reflect on what you're learning, and stay inspired. From meal planning tools to wellness exercises, this workbook is your personal guide to growing in the kitchen!

⚜ Cook with Others in a Supportive Community

The real beauty happens when we cook together! Join our online community where you can share your cooking adventures, ask questions, and celebrate your wins. It's a space full of encouragement, laughter, and support, because cooking is so much more fun when you're not doing it alone!

⚜ Digital Version of the Cookbook

No need to worry about flipping through pages when you're in the middle of the grocery store! With your digital Eating for Life cookbook, you Just grab your phone, pop open the shopping list and head to the store!

⚜ Exclusive Bonuses – Extras to Keep You Going!

From bonus recipes to spur of the moment live videos, these extras will keep you motivated and keep us connected year after year.

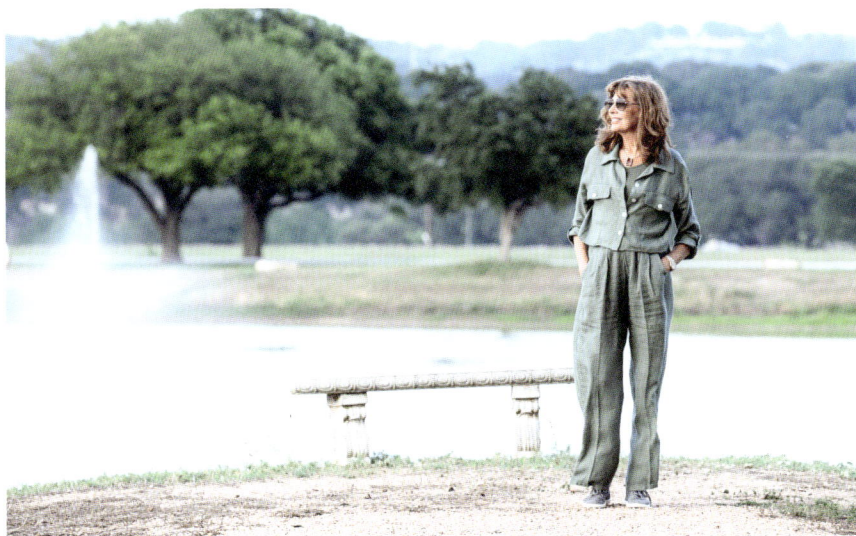

Join me and let's make memories together. To your health with Love! *Teri Secrest*

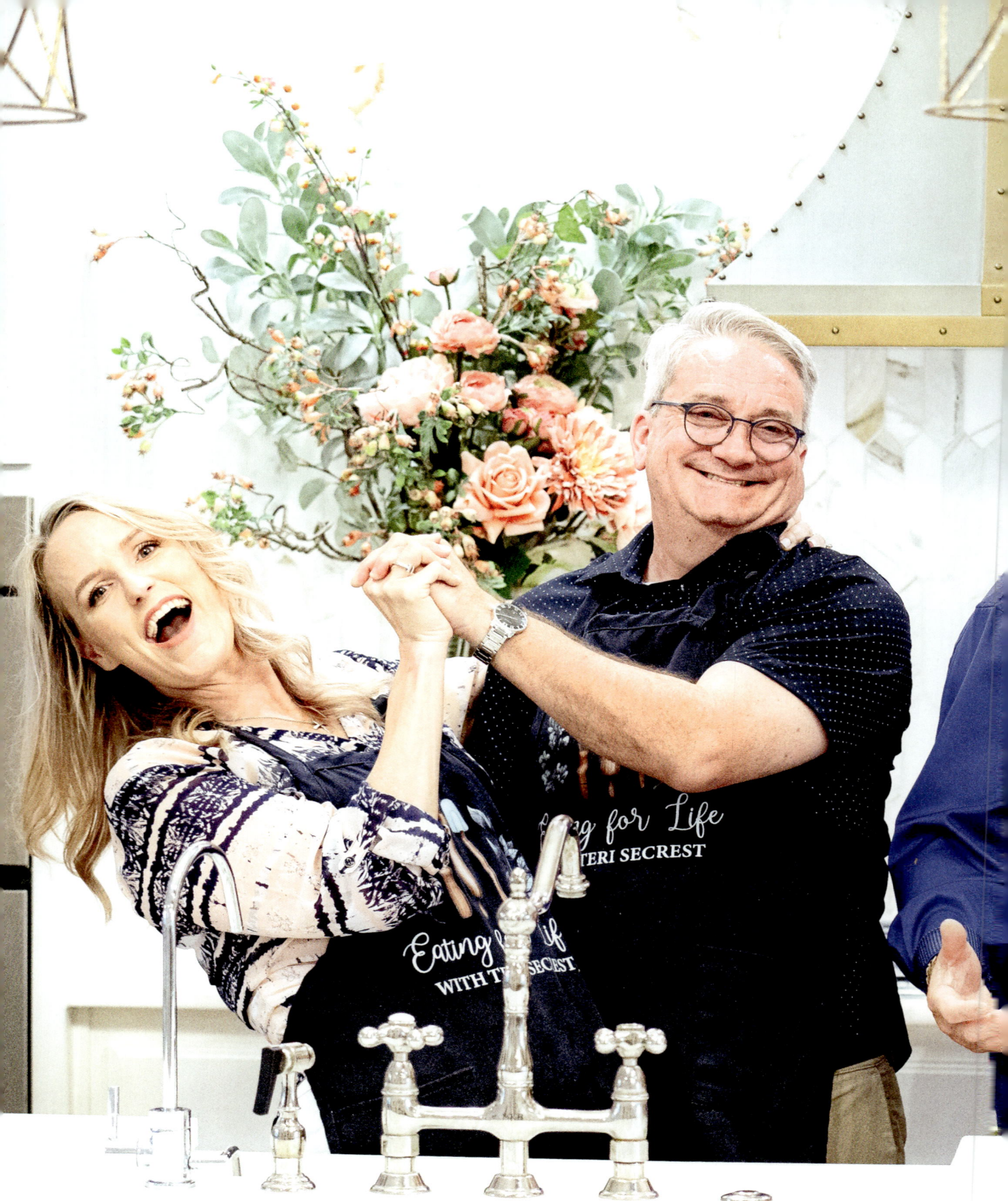

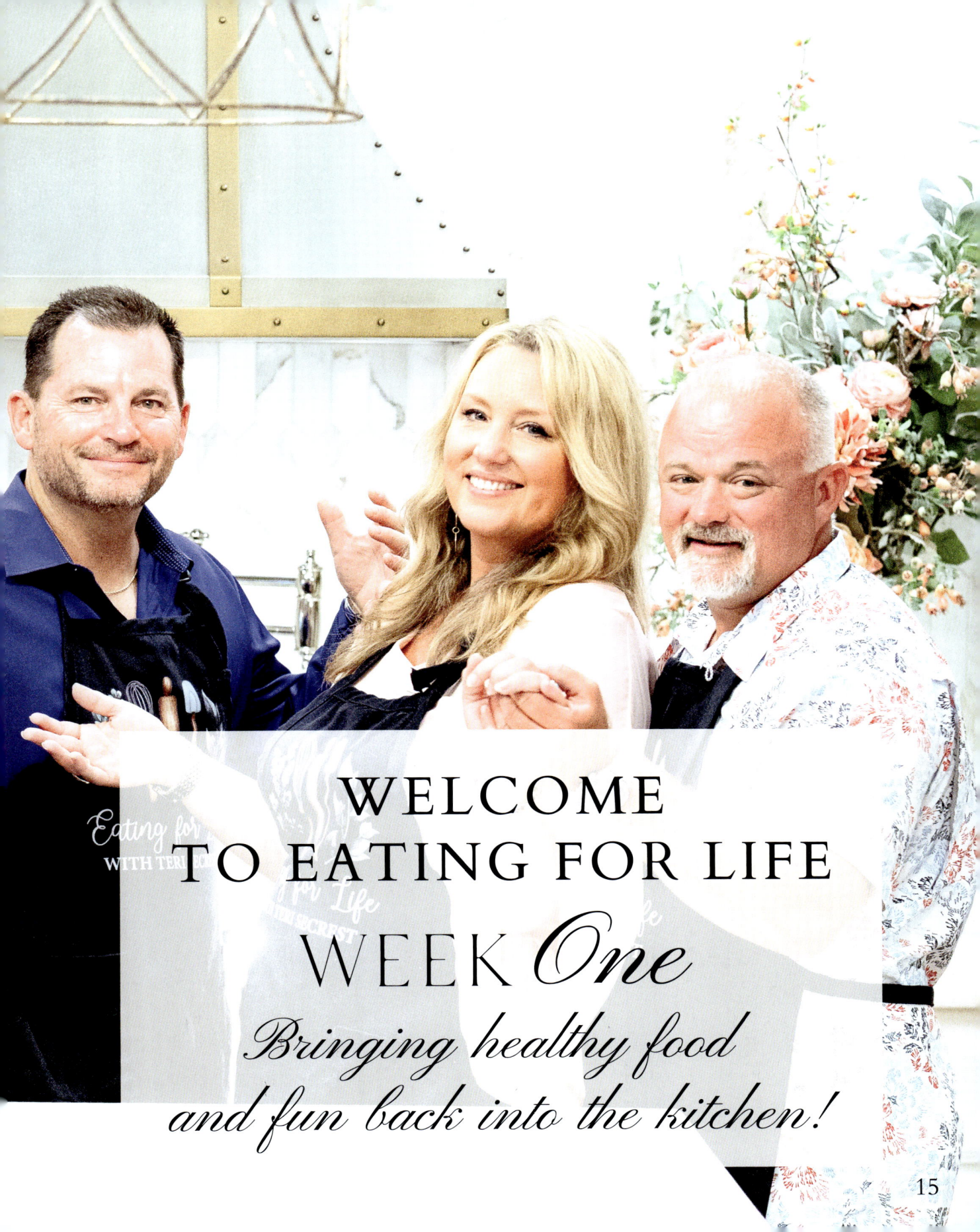

WELCOME
TO EATING FOR LIFE

WEEK *One*

Bringing healthy food
and fun back into the kitchen!

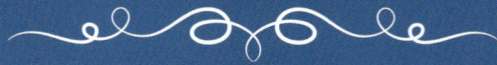

Welcome to Eating For Life....

Imagine stepping into someone's home and feeling as though you've been transported to a place filled with deep love, extravagant hospitality and nurturing care. Now, picture fun music that makes you tap your feet, a curated 5-star menu, and candlelight so soft it seems to melt all your cares away.
Then you sink into your chair for an unforgettable evening of food and fellowship with friends.

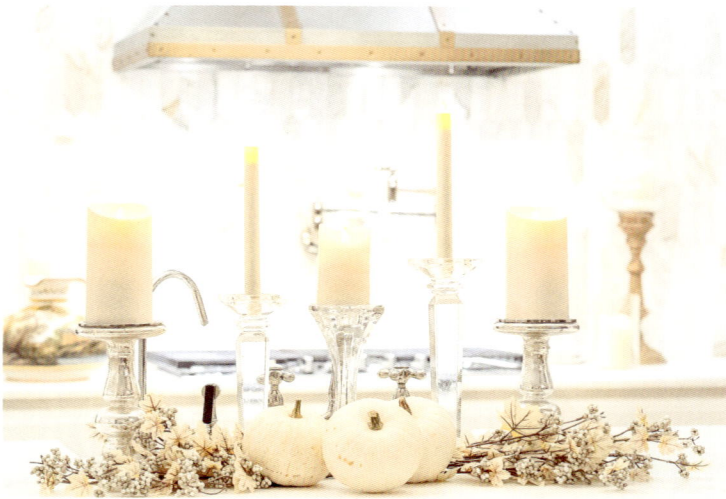

Welcome to "Eating for Life"! It's not just a book; it's a way to gather husbands and wives, parents and children, and friends all together in the kitchen creating 5-Star menus and making memories along the way. Getting messy and making a few mistakes while trying new recipes is half the fun!

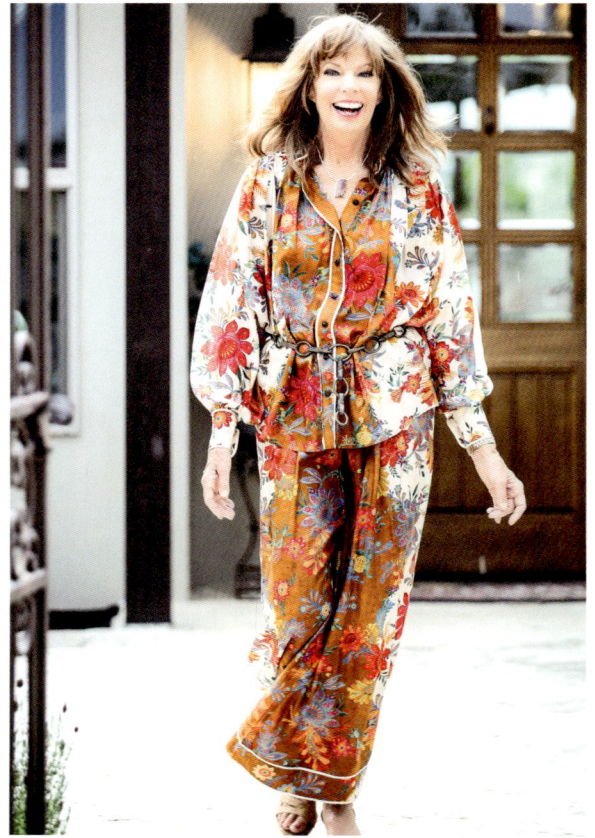

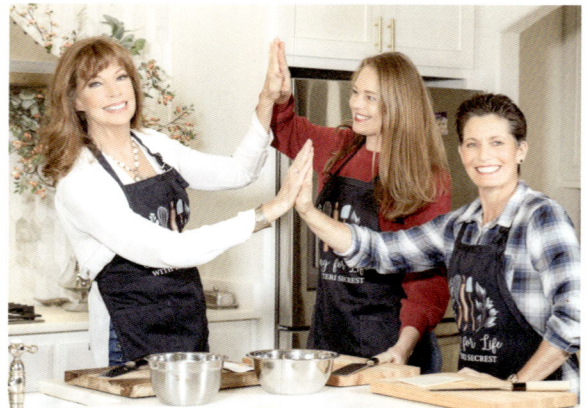

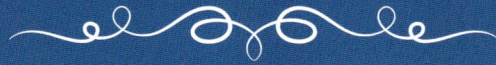

I created *Eating for Life* with three clear goals in mind; first, to help you fall in love with real food; second, to empower you to become a confident home chef; and third, to bring fun back into the kitchen-creating a life filled with vibrant health, meaningful connections, and memorable meals shared with those you love.

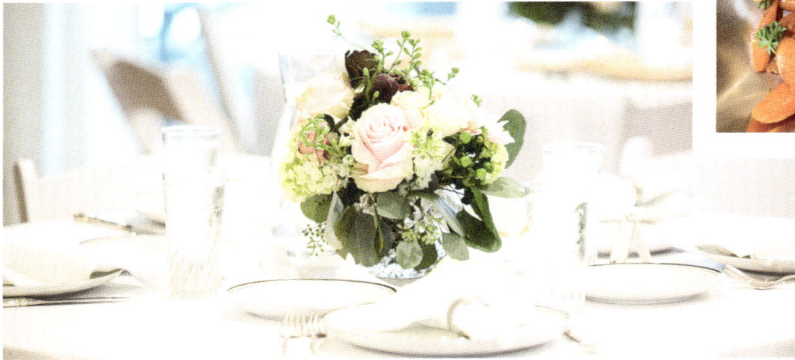

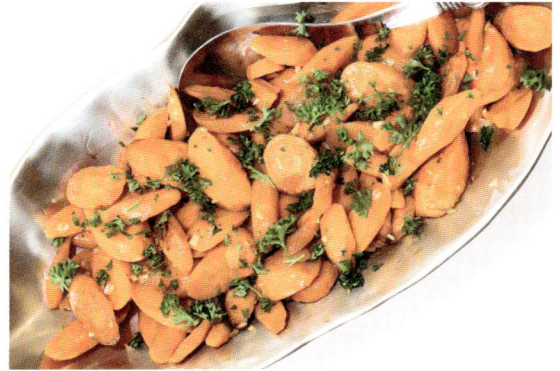

Growing up in the small town of Clear Lake, Iowa, I witnessed first-hand the joy my mother and father brought to others through food and hospitality. My mother, the founder of the French cooking school La Petite Ecole de Cuisine Francaise, turned every meal into a celebration of love and life. Watching her in the kitchen and at the table shaped me in ways I didn't even realize at the time.

I know that for many, the idea of creating beautiful, healthy meals may feel overwhelming. Maybe you're a busy mom thinking, "That's a million miles from my current lifestyle!" Be encouraged, there truly are ways to bring vitality back into your kitchen with ease.

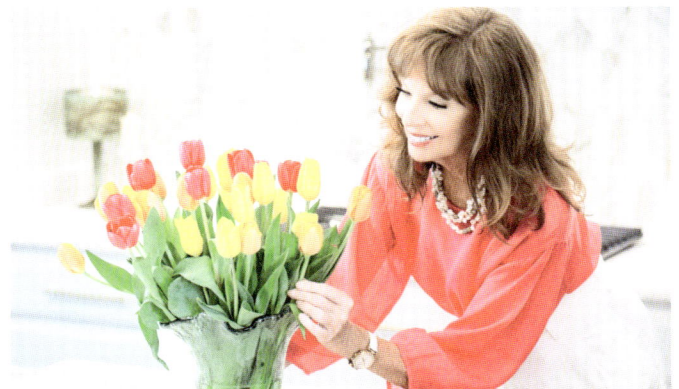

Eating for Life is about embracing the beauty of nourishing food and experiencing that satisfaction that comes from preparing meals with love and intention.

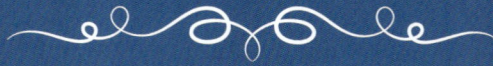

Falling in Love with Real Food

One of the most important parts of living well is learning to love the food that nourishes us. What's my definition of real food? It's doing your best to choose foods that are as close to their original form as possible.

The Importance of Soil

One of my most cherished memories from my childhood was working in our family organic garden. My mother and father would teach us the importance of preparing the soil and making it rich with life. They explained that worms and ladybugs were vital to healthy soil.

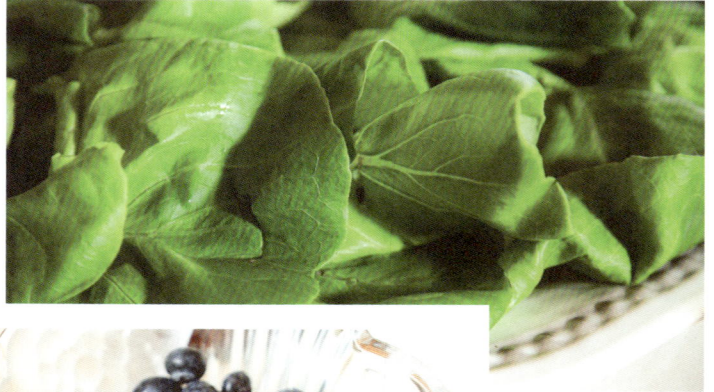

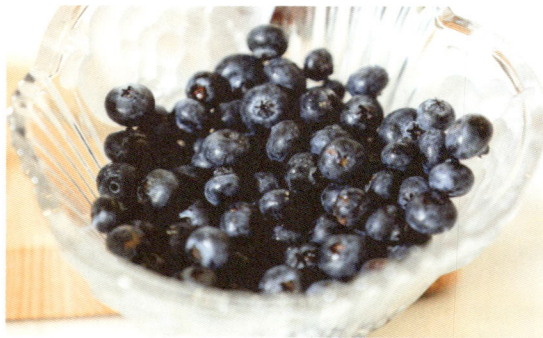

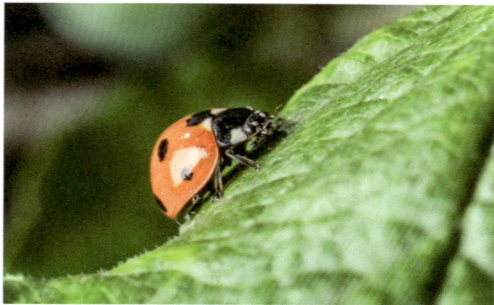

We learned to be grateful for the land, the food it produced, and to pray blessings over the farmers who grew the crops we relied on.

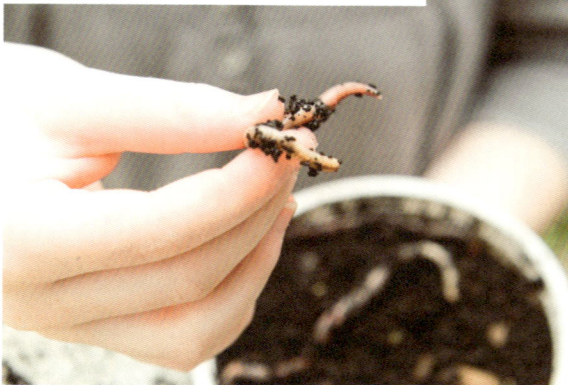

This love for where food comes from and the process of cultivating healthy food stayed with me throughout my life and shaped how I see real food today.

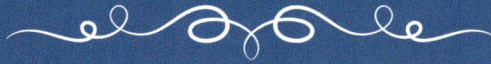

Why do we make poor health choices?

Are you aware that when God created you, He created a masterpiece? You are fearfully and wonderfully made in His image. Your bones, muscles, nerves and organs are intricately made. Each of us have been given a treasured gift, one body to last a lifetime. As we learn to accept God's great love for us and see ourselves as a masterpiece, nourishing and caring for our body will come more naturally our cells will respond!

Beware of long labels!

Award-winning parents are those who care deeply about raising healthy, strong children, and that means reading labels! Foods with labels full of long words we cannot pronounce do not belong in our stomachs or that of our children.

With the rise of diabetes and obesity, particularly in children, we as parents have the opportunity to take back our children's health and stop this cycle! Remember, the good news is that our bodies can heal very quickly if given a fighting chance!

In the pages of Eating for Life, my heart is for you to understand why each specific ingredient is in the recipes. That's why, after each recipe, I list the health benefits of each ingredient and explain why your body loves them!

My hope is that you'll not only fall in love with real food but also pass this knowledge on to your children and grandchildren, bringing joy and health to your family's meals.

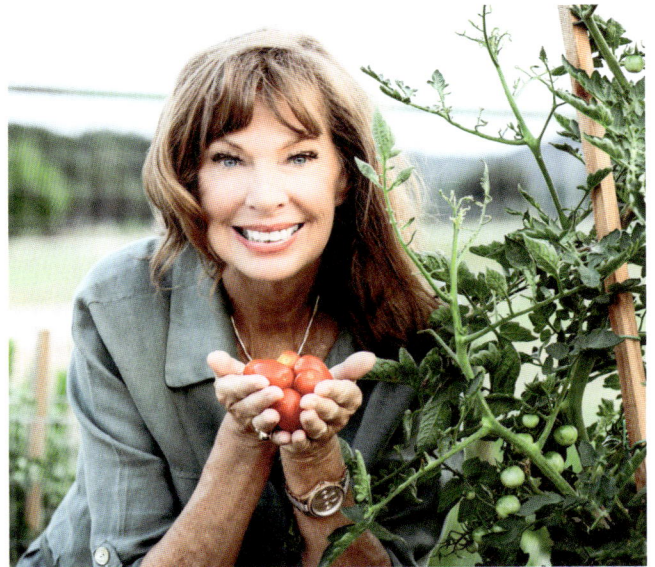

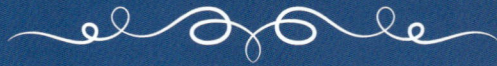

My Health in Crisis *(and the solution that led to JOY)*

Growing up, my mother's culinary talents made every meal an adventure. She was passionate about healthy, wholesome meals that often came straight from our garden, and her lavish desserts were a regular feature of our family meals. At the time, very little was known about the dangers of processed sugar, and it was those indulgent desserts that led to my blood sugar imbalance.

By the time I was in my late teens, I developed a severe blood sugar imbalance. If I ate a candy bar and then got into the car, I was at risk of falling asleep behind the wheel.

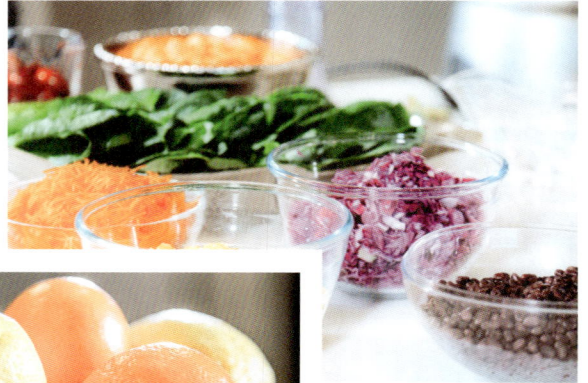

Despite countless doctor's visits and thousands of dollars spent on tests, the doctors insisted the problem was "all in my head." Not one of them asked what I was eating.

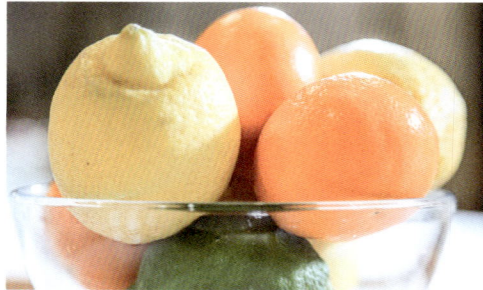

Out of desperation, I decided to take matters into my own hands. I practically parked myself in the local health food store, determined to read every book and article I could find about nutrition and health. I pored over stacks of books, searching for answers.

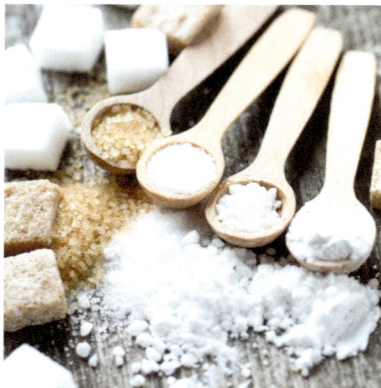

Then, I stumbled upon Sugar Blues by William Duffy. I sat right there in the store and devoured the book in two hours. It was as if the clouds parted—everything finally made sense. This book changed my life.

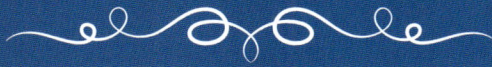

By eliminating white processed sugar from my diet, all my symptoms disappeared in just 30 days. That experience opened my eyes to the power of food and set me on a path to help others understand the connection between what we eat and how we feel—restoring both joy and health.

With all my heart, I believe you can live your best life at every age!

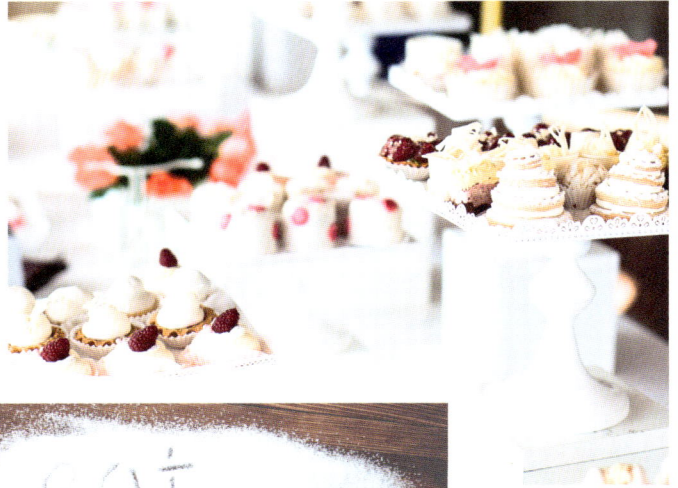

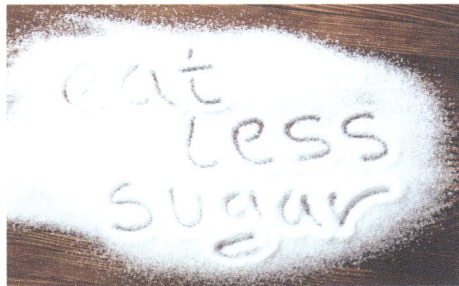

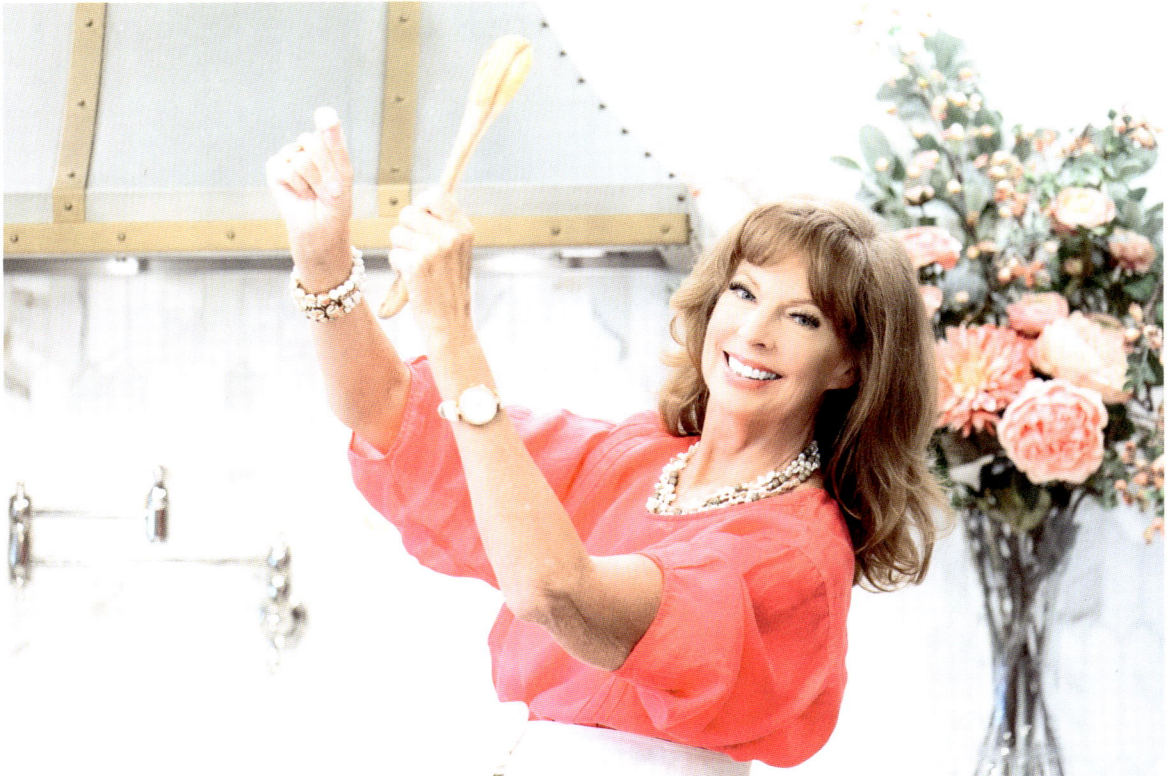

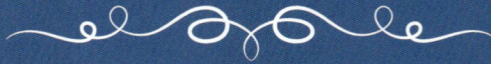

The Mediterranean Way of Eating

Throughout this book, you will see menus that reflect the Mediterranean way of eating. Most people have heard of this, but you may wonder what it means. The Mediterranean diet is based on the traditional foods of four countries that border the Mediterranean Sea: Italy, Greece, Spain, and France. I was blessed to live in two of these countries, Italy and France, between 1975 and 1980.

What I observed in these countries was remarkable. The food was filled with flavor and variety, often including high-quality meat or fish, fresh fruits and vegetables, some pasta or rice, and often a soup. Yet the people in these regions rarely had a weight problem. There was no focus on "low-calorie" diets, and olive oil flowed freely.

More importantly, meals were a time of lighthearted joy. People took the time to embrace those present, share laughter and stories, and savor their food without concern about the clock. The traditions of gathering for meals are part of what I want to bring to your home through Eating for Life—to bring back joy, simplicity, and health to your kitchen.

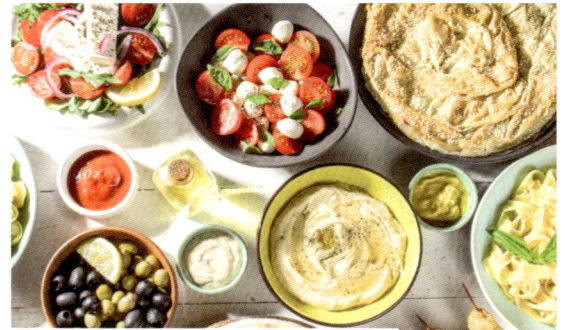

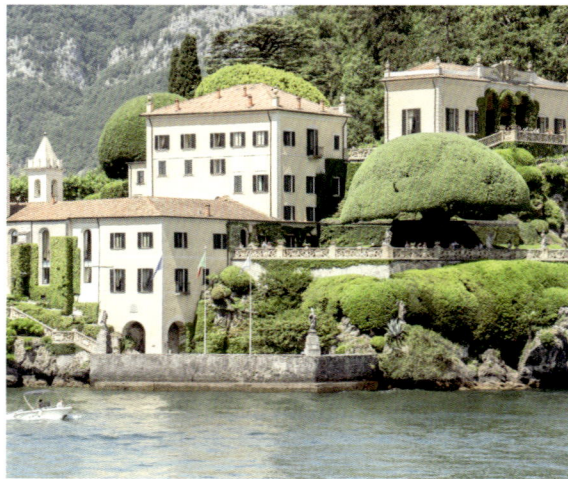

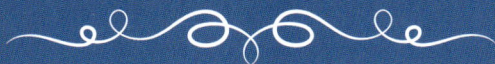

Let me be clear—I'm not a vegetarian. I enjoy high-quality, grass-fed meats and sustainably raised fish. But much of the meat available today is packed with hormones and raised in unhealthy conditions, and that has a direct effect on your hormones too. Fortunately, it's easier than ever to find farmers committed to growing produce and raising meats without chemicals. Many local farmers may not have the official "organic" label but are dedicated to purity and sustainability.

Choosing real food doesn't have to be complicated, but it does require intention. That's why I've made it a point to explain the health benefits of each ingredient in the recipes you'll find in this book. My hope is that you'll fall in love with real food and create happy, healthy traditions that become a lasting legacy for your family for generations to come.

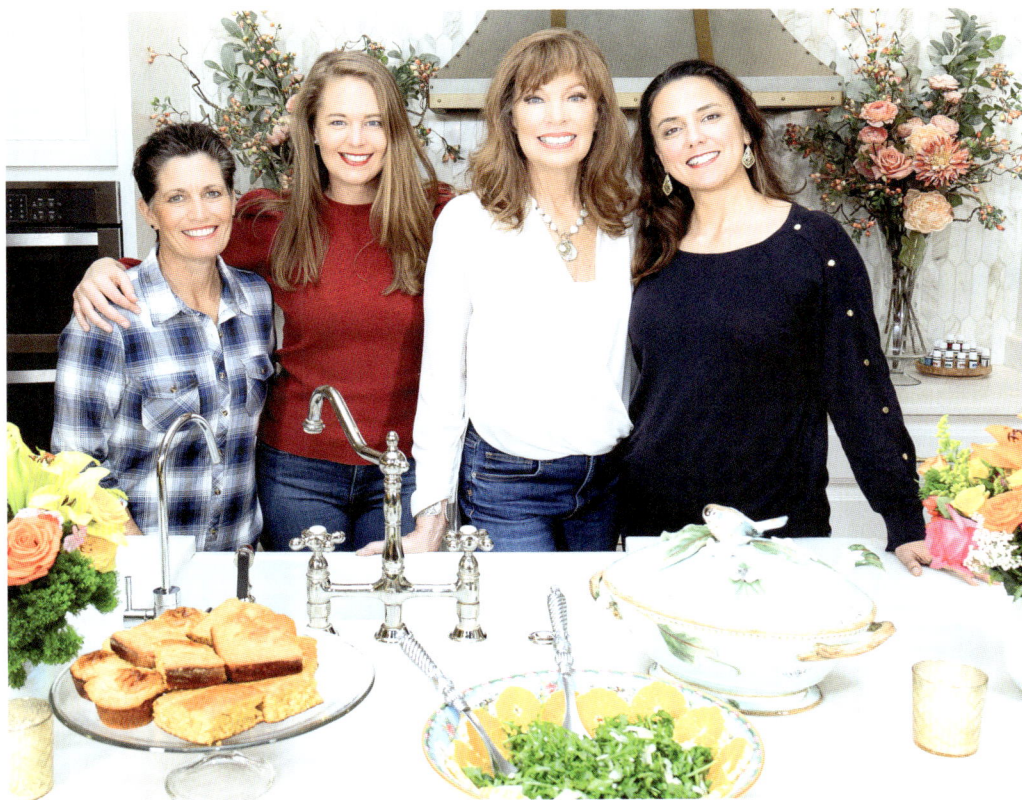

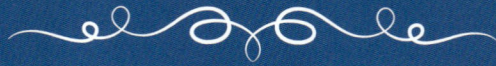

Becoming a Confident Home Chef

Cooking at home can feel intimidating, especially in today's fast-paced world where fewer families take the time to cook from scratch. Believe me, I get it. I remember when my children were young—even though I worked from home, some days I barely had time to take a bath, let alone cook a meal!

I kept having this nagging feeling: my children's health should not suffer because I'm "too busy." So, I went back to what I had learned from my mother in her French cooking school and found ways to make cooking work for my modern life.

If you'd like a boost of confidence in the kitchen, I encourage you to follow along with my step-by-step cooking videos and workbook that complement this cookbook (see page 12 for details.) Imagine being together in the kitchen, walking side by side through each recipe as we cook together and enjoy the process of cooking.

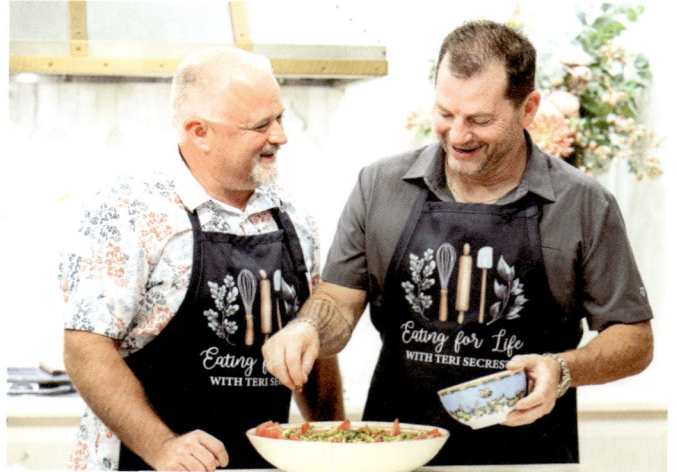

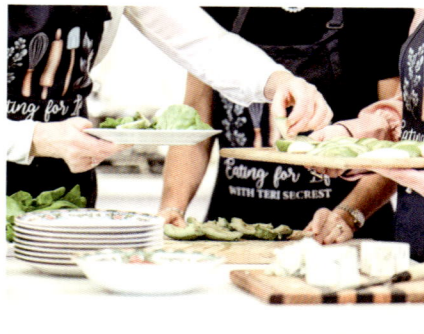

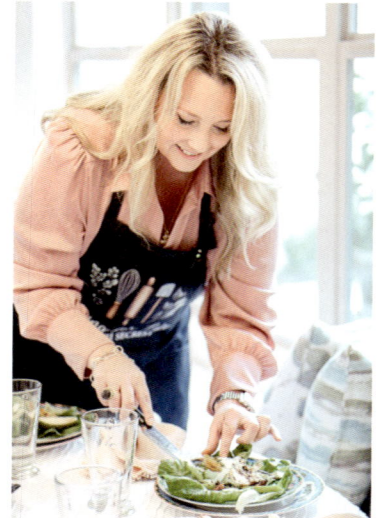

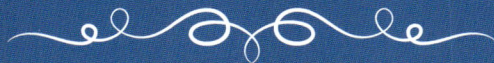

Although my mother was a gourmet chef, trying to get me into the kitchen as a child was like pulling teeth! I loved the outdoors; all I desired to do is ride my horse and go swimming in the lake. I knew how to chop vegetables and set a beautiful table, but it wasn't until I had my first child that I realized, "Oh no, why didn't I listen to Mom?"

I'll never forget my first attempt at making dinner rolls. They were so heavy, my children turned them into bowling balls! Slowly, through trial and error, I became a confident home chef—and so can you.

The recipes in Eating for Life are designed to create a 5-star dining experience in the comfort of your home. Cooking and eating should be an extravagant part of life, not an afterthought. As you follow these recipes, I encourage you to savor the process, invite loved ones to join you, and watch how good food can transform your home, and create life-long memories.

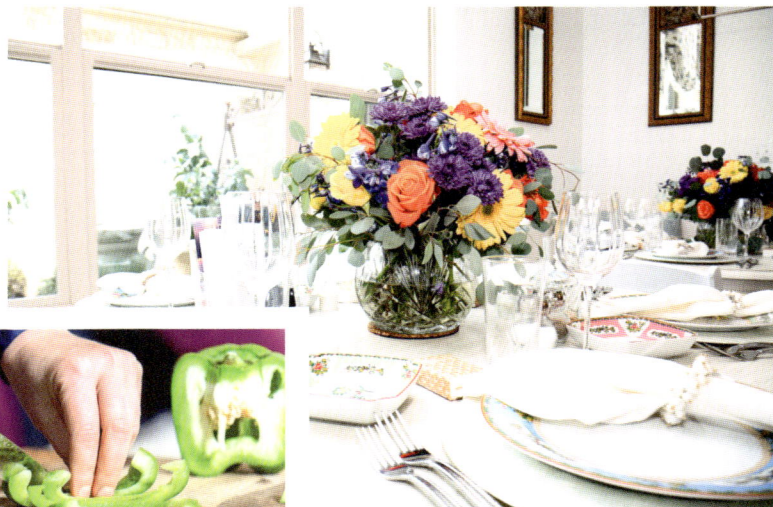

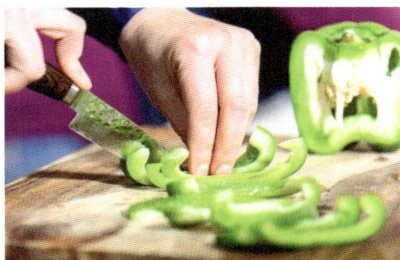

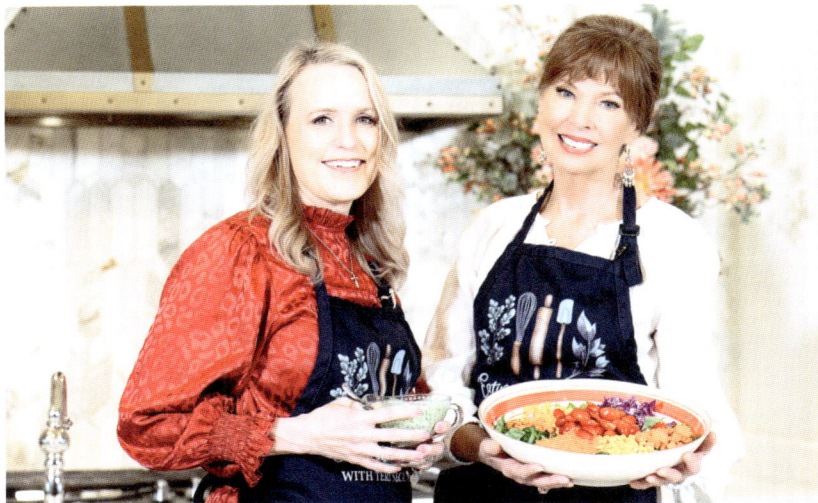

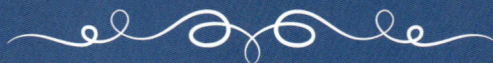

Inspiring Extravagant Hospitality

I was very blessed to grow up in a home where hospitality was a way of life. My parents were always welcoming people—whether it was the sick neighbor, the grumpy priest who couldn't wait to come for brunch, or just casual dinners with friends, hospitality flowed naturally. Hospitality has become a lost art in many parts of the country, but it's a skill that can be learned and nurtured.

Did my mother have a perfectly clean, clutter-free house? Not at all, but she didn't let that stop her. Hospitality isn't about perfection—it's about making people feel loved and cared for. And that can start with something as simple as popcorn.

My father used to fill a soup pot with popcorn, shaking it until every kernel popped, then drizzling it with real butter. He'd hand-squeeze oranges and grapefruits for juice, making us children feel like the most special people in the world.

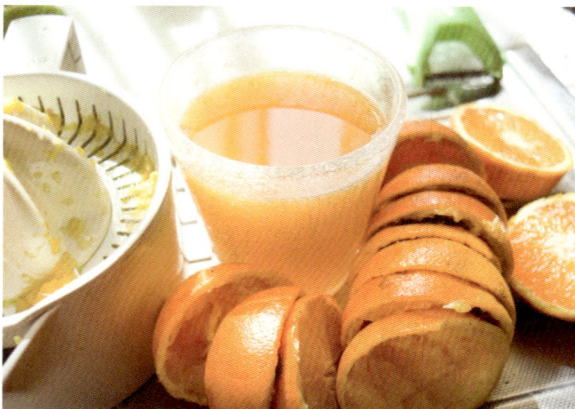

True hospitality isn't about doing all the work yourself. It's about creating memories together, from preparing the meal to enjoying it, to the laughter and the conversation that follows.

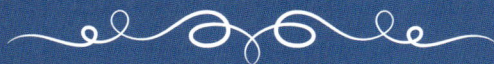

The best part is, you don't need to break the bank to create a delightful evening—consider hosting a cooking party! Send your friends a menu from this book, ask them to choose a few ingredients to bring, and cook the meal together – like an ingredient potluck. Then, put on some music! There's nothing like dancing in the kitchen while a dish bakes in the oven!

In my experience as a health coach, one of the most important elements of wellness is joy. I believe we are created for joy, and when we rediscover joy, our bodies heal faster and we live longer.

As we journey together through Eating for Life, my greatest hope is that you'll not only find better health but also more joy. May this book inspire you to bring 5-star meals, laughter, and extravagant hospitality into your home—bringing joy and healthy cooking back to your kitchen!

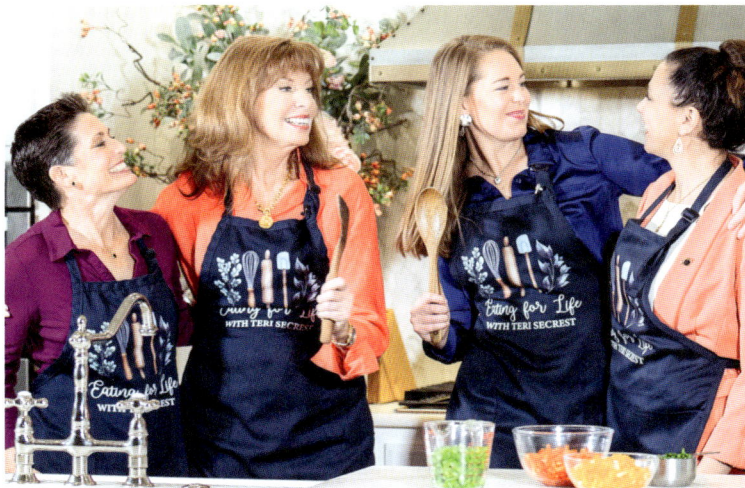

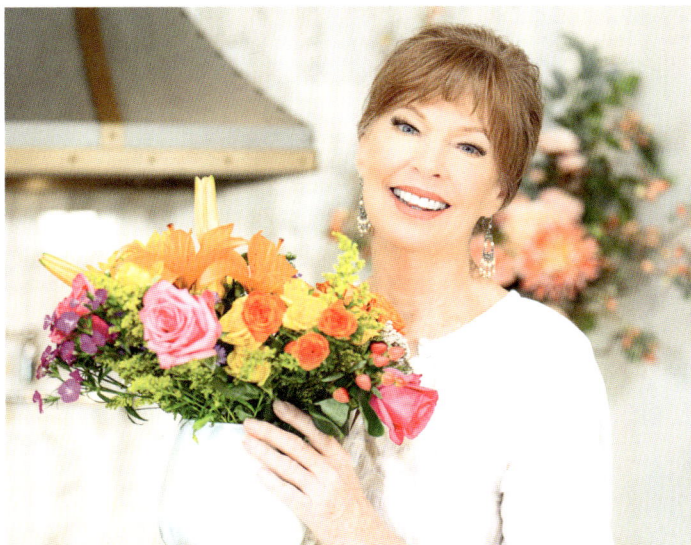

For the love of family, friends, and good food,

Teri Secrest

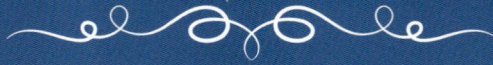

Ten principles for kitchen and pantry success!

"Help, I can't find anything!"

Ever feel like that when you open your pantry door? Mine used to be so stuffed, I would slam the door shut and run the other way! Thanks to some simple three-tiered plastic dividers shown below, I now LOVE my pantry and you will love yours too!

Here are ten simple things you can do to upgrade your pantry and prepare for greater enjoyment around meal preparation. I encourage you to get on this right away so that you are set up for success when we begin cooking in week two. You've got this!

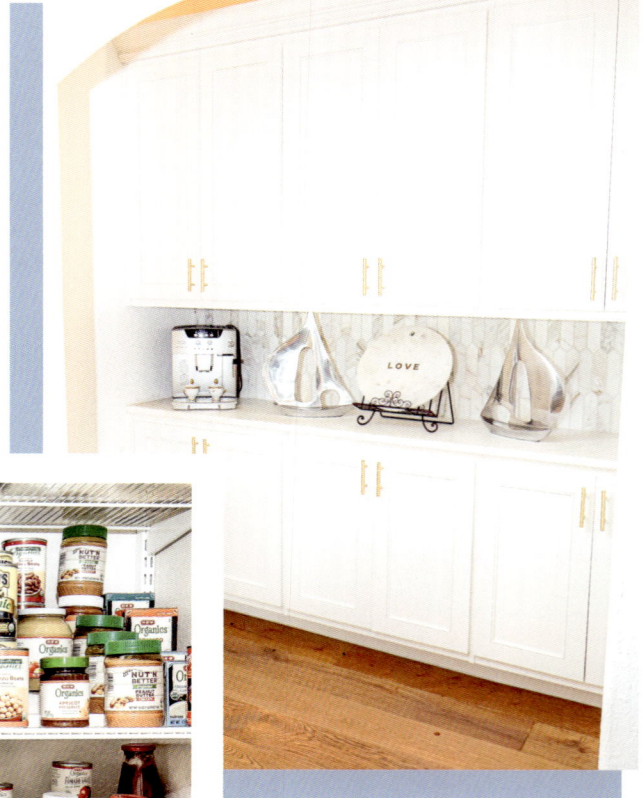

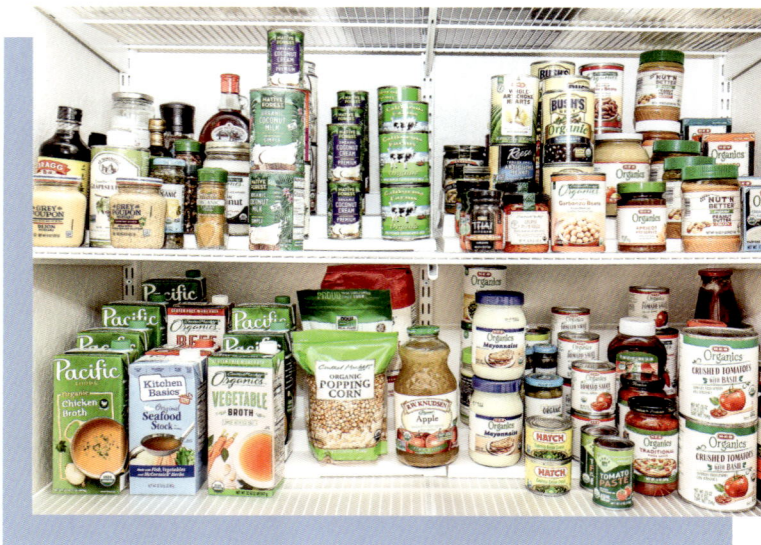

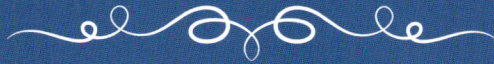

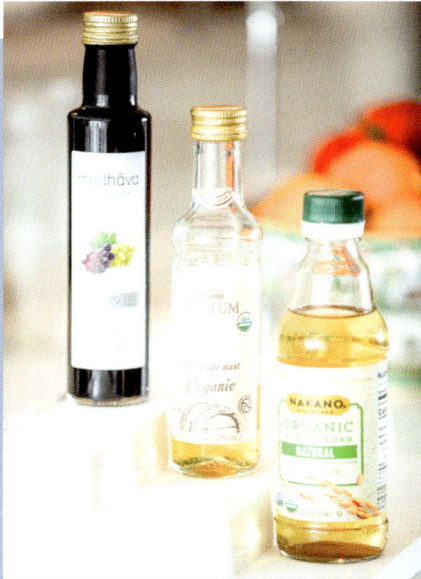

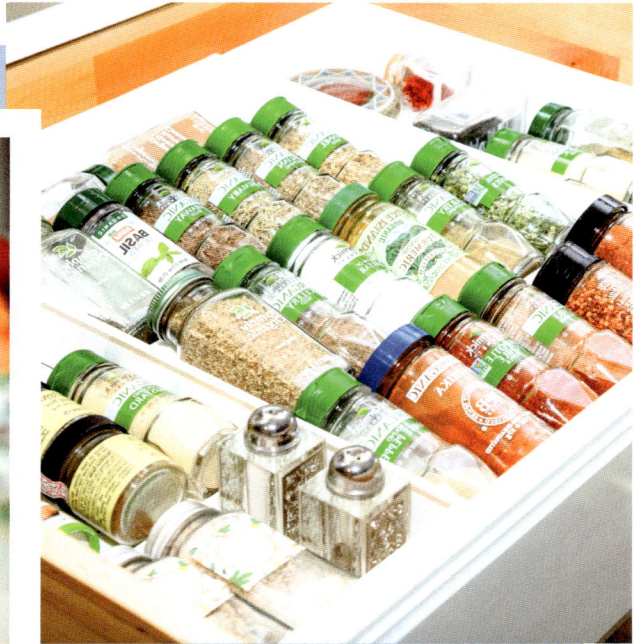

1. Create a space that inspires you when you open the cupboard.
2. Make sure you can easily see and find everything. I love three-tiered organizers!
3. Less is more. Put only in your pantry the things you use on a daily basis. All extra things can be put in a preparedness location.
4. Check expiration date and discard expired items.
5. Discover where your money is going
6. A well thought out pantry allows spontaneous meals.
7. Be aware of your buying needs.
8. Keep a running list of what you are getting low on.
9. Don't shop when you are hungry!
10. Consider organizing your spices by flavor signatures.

Welcome to Essential Oils!

One of the things that makes this book unique, is that we enhance the flavor of our recipes with life-giving essential oils along with dried herbs. Have you ever pondered the power of herbs before they are dried? Twenty-eight years ago, our family began incorporating essential oils into our lives with such profound results, I'd like to introduce you to them.

You may be wondering, "What are essential oils"? Essential oils are the life force of plants. When you tear a leaf, the liquid that drips out of the leaf is the plant's essential oil, vital for its survival and healing.

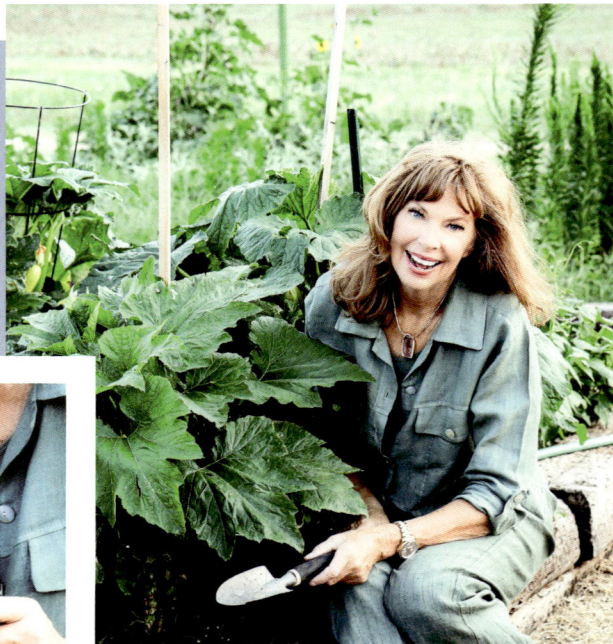

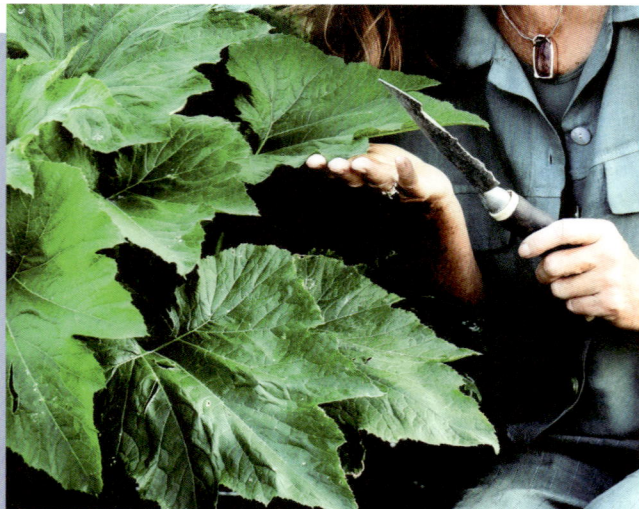

These powerful drops of "liquid gold" are compatible with our bodies, helping to support health and vitality. My favorite essential oil company is Young Living Essential Oils.

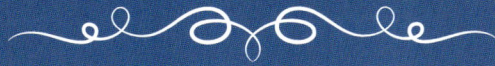

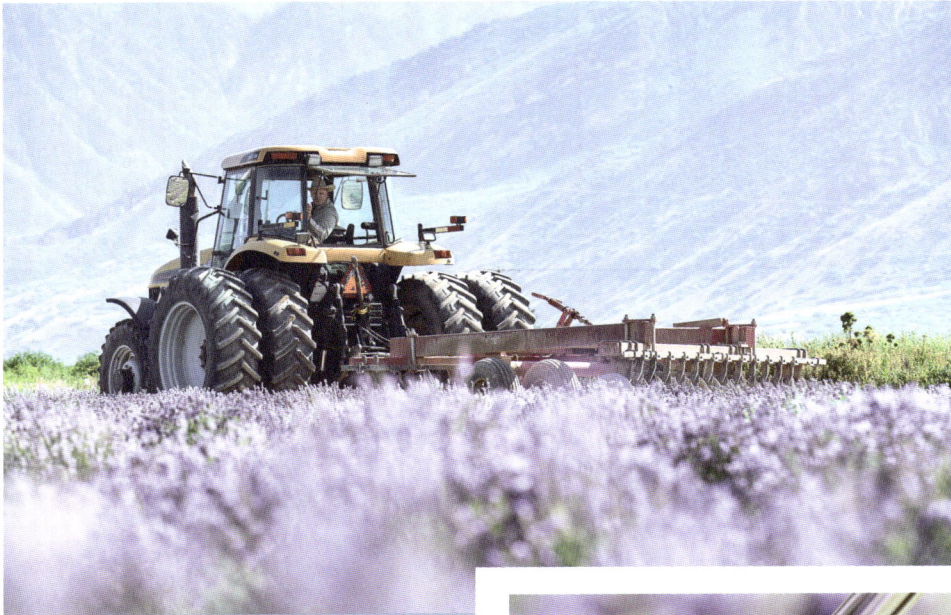

Their unique process called Seed to Seal is what makes cooking with these oils a safe and flavorful experience. Each drop of essential oil captures the pure essence of the plant offering the best quality.

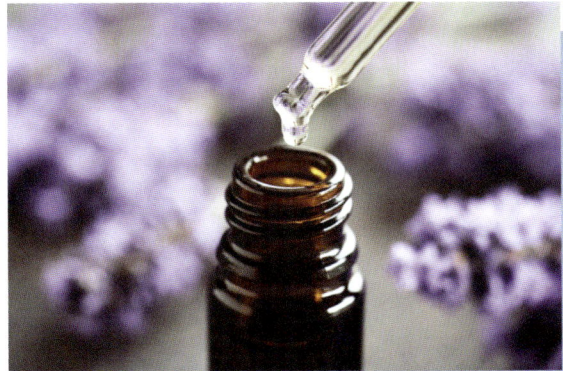

Young Living Vitality Oils are a special category of essential oils approved for food grade use. These oils can be placed in your water and recipes in very small amounts to add flavor and support different body systems.

Spice up your recipes with Essential Oils!

Tired of your humdrum recipes? Get ready to be amazed! The addition of essential oils elevates your recipe flavors from ordinary to extravagant.

Introducing the toothpick method!

The primary principle when using essential oils in your recipes is "less is more". Essential Oils are extremely economical to use because you literally start by dipping a toothpick into your bottle and stirring your recipe with a toothpick (less than one drop of oil.)

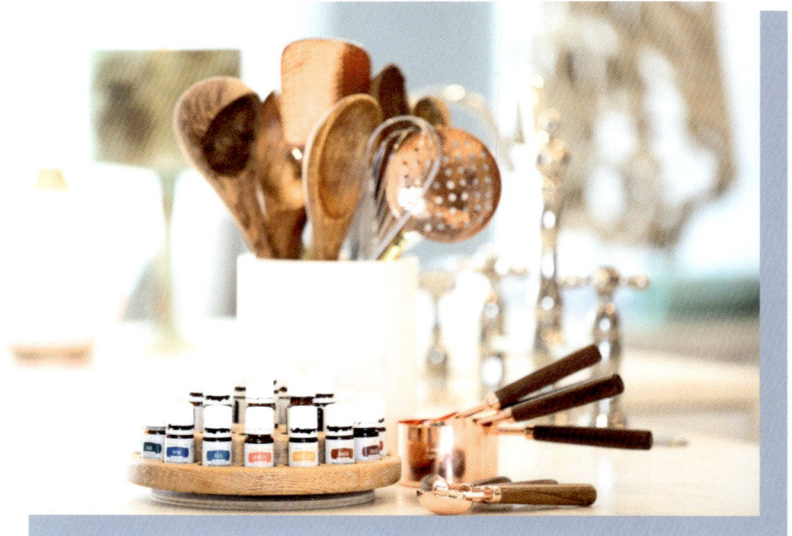

Whenever possible, turn off the heat to the recipe if it is a stove top recipe, let it cool a bit before adding the essential oil. It will retain more of the plant this way.

Savory essential oils are the oils you think of when cooking main dishes and vegetables, such as Mediterranean, Thai, Italian, etc. Just think of every herb you currently use in your cooking and know that "there's an oil for that"! Think of basil, oregano, thyme, black pepper, lemongrass, rosemary, celery seed, marjoram, sage, dill, tarragon etc.

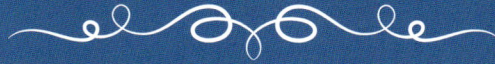

Just like when you throw a pebble into a lake and the pebble creates circles and waves of water, so one drop or one toothpick of oil, rapidly expands out into the entire recipe!

Two teaspoons of dried herbs is similar to one drop of essential oil. One teaspoon of dried herb is similar to one toothpick of essential oil stirred into your recipe. You can always add more but you cannot take it away! Before an herb is dried it is an essential oil. So, using the essential oil gives it a much richer and complex flavor and zest!

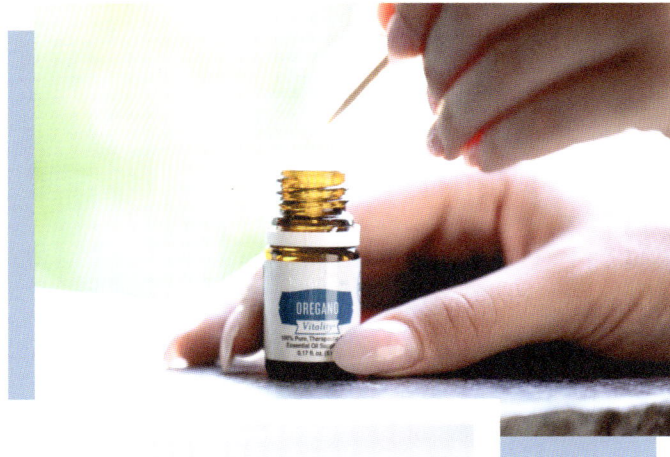

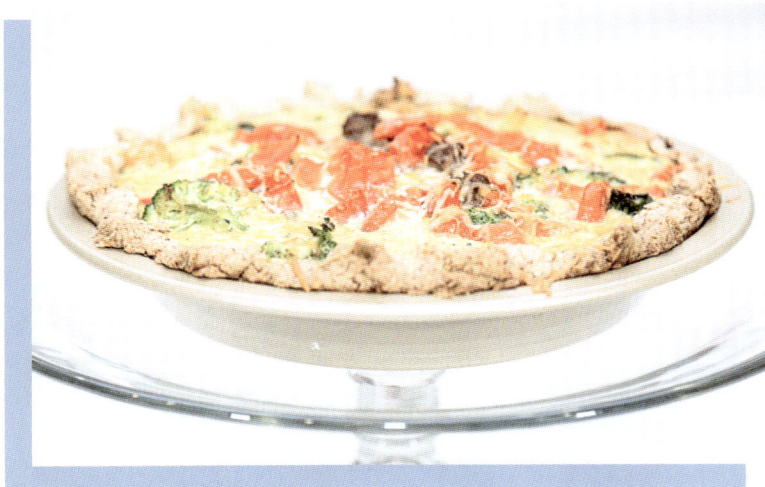

Baking with Essential Oils

What is that glorious smell?

Talk about Heaven on Earth; wait until you start baking with essential oils! When someone walks into your kitchen and you are baking with essential oils like cinnamon, nutmeg, peppermint, orange, lemon, tangerine, clove, ginger, or lavender, they will be happily intoxicated with the smell!

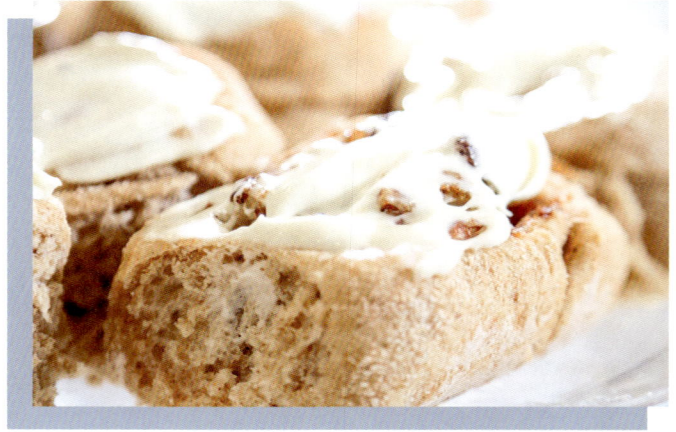

Sometimes, I put a few drops of these in a warm pot of water and keep the heat on simmer, just to enjoy the smell in my kitchen! Because you will be putting your baked goods in the oven, you will lose some of the nutritional benefits of the oil, however, you will win every time in flavor and enjoyment.

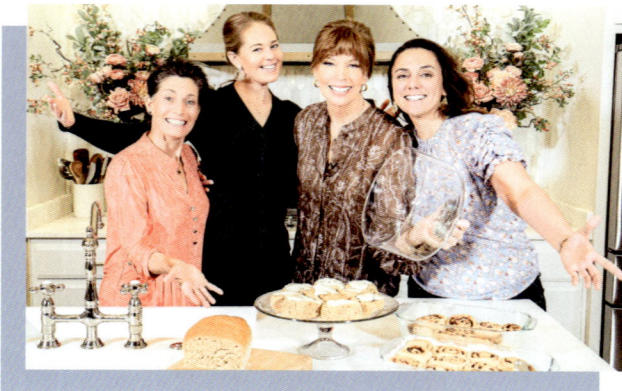

Any opportunity I have to make organic whipping cream or coconut cream for a recipe, I love to flavor it with 3 or 4 drops or orange, lemon or tangerine oil, along with a little bit of agave nectar. You've never had whipping cream like this! You'll learn how to make this in Week 4.

Please check with your doctor before using any new health regime and carefully read labels for any precautions!

Enhancing your water with essential oils

What are the benefits of adding Young Living Vitality essential oils in our water?

Your body is made up of over 50% percent water! Your cells thrive on water! Step one to your health is to drink more pure water! So let's make it delicious. Facinating fact: there are numerous studies which show that citrus essential oils contain high levels of a natural chemical constituent called d-limonene, which offers many health benefits.

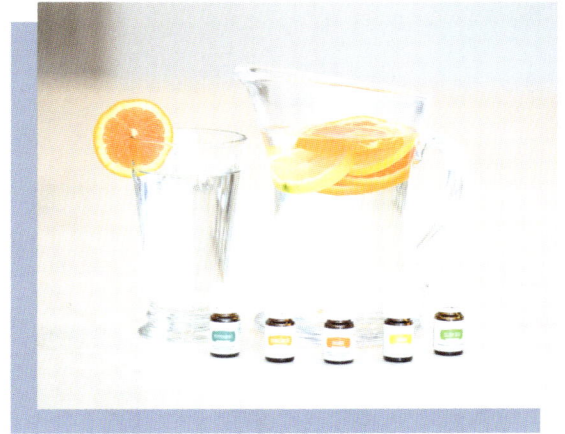

This is because the citrus essential oils, come from the white part of the fruit just under the skin, or the rind of the fruit. Citrus oils add an exciting, surprising element of flavor to your water!

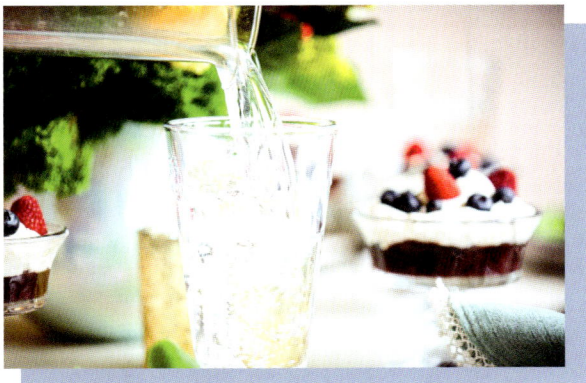

Orange Essential Oil adds a delightful uplifting flavor to your water and has one the highest concentrations of d-limonene. oil is a great support for your healthy liver. Some stellar essential oils you can enjoy in water are Lemon, Lime, Peppermint, Grapefruit, Orange and Tangerine. Peppermint Oil is famous for cooling the body down in the summer.

Try one or two drops of Young Living Vitality essential oils in a glass of water or 5-6 drops in an entire pitcher of water and keep it in your fridge. It's fun to try different ones each day!

Enhance your rest with essential oils!

"After a full day in the kitchen I love to nurture myself with a relaxing essential oil home-spa bath!"

Start with a little Epsom salt and stir in your favorite essential oil scents such as Lavender, Frankincense, or Stress Away. Allow your bathtub to fill half way and then add your epsom salt mixture. Then continue filling the tub. Next, grab your diffuser and add relaxing scents. Turn on some soothing music and be transported to a symphony of revitalization.

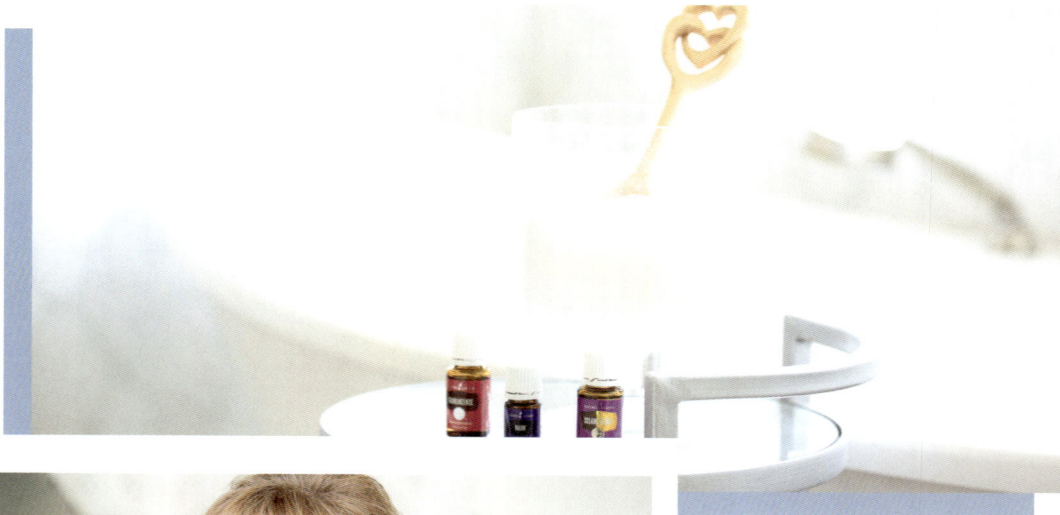

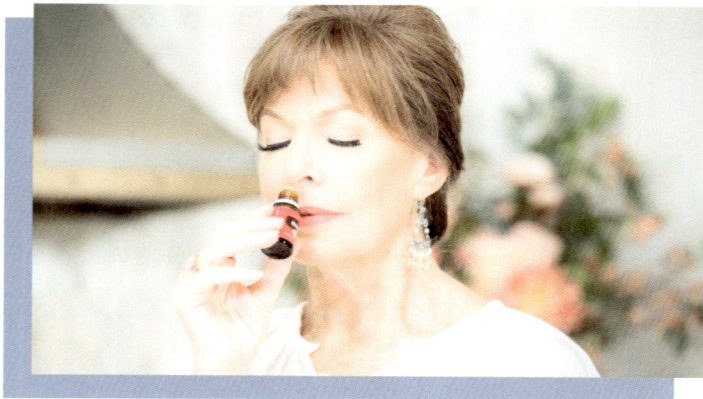

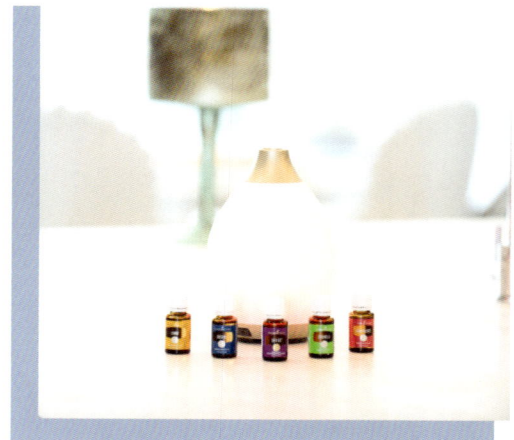

Create an atmosphere of JOY in your home!

*Just like high quality food ingredients give fuel
to your body, a well cared for home fuels love and joy!*

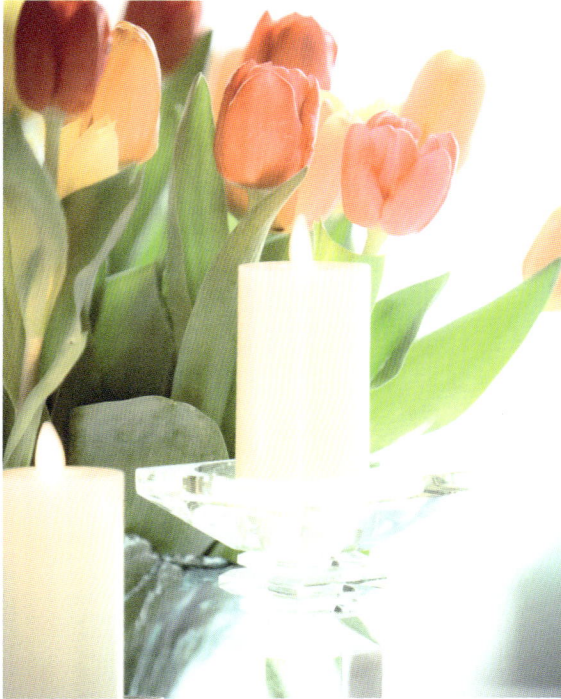

When friends enter your home, what do they see, what do they hear, what do they smell? We are the atmosphere builders in our home. We are the pace-setters and interior designers. We get to choose how people feel in our home. This is our privilege!

When a family works together in this effort to create a lovely home environment, joy and inspiration flourish for the whole family.

My hope is that your community will desire to gather at your home and when the evening is complete, they will feel cared for and cherished!

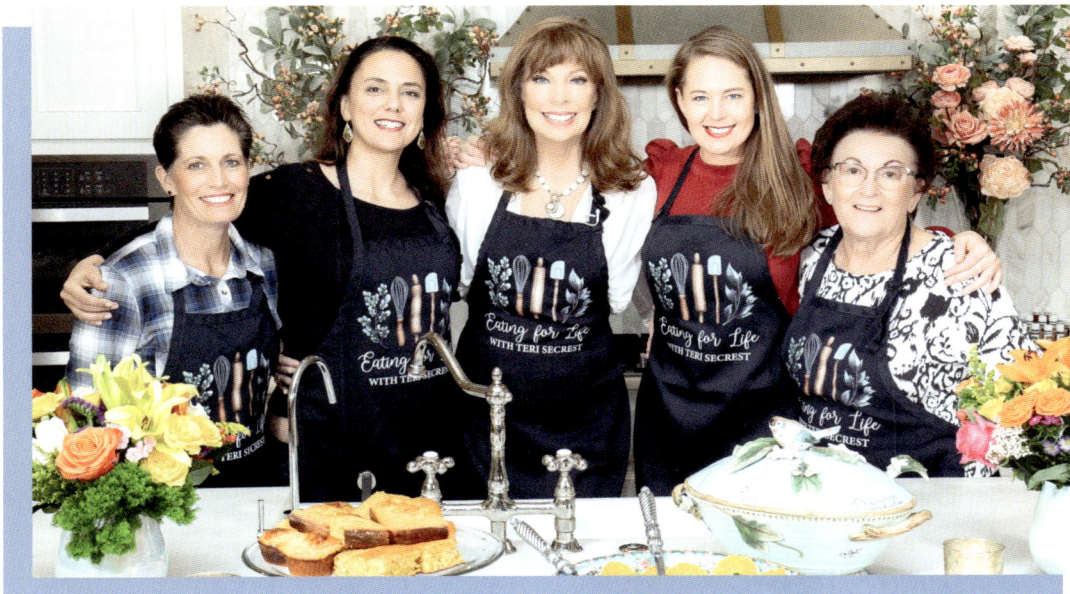

CREATE A FIVE-STAR
DINING EXPERIENCE IN YOUR HOME

To maximize our delicious recipes and innovative cooking techniques, here are the unique ingredients we'll be using throughout this book: Young Living Vitality essential oils, NingXia Red and Einkorn flour.

I encourage you to order these products
today so you can be using them throughout this book.

OILS FOR YOUR WATER
Tangerine
Lime
Orange
Peppermint
Lemon
Citrus Fresh Blend

OILS FOR COOKING
Black Pepper
Celery Seed
Dill
Cinnamon Bark
Thyme
Oregano

RECIPE IN WEEK 4
Young Living
NingXia Red Drink

RECIPES IN WEEK 5 & 6
Young Living
Einkorn Flour

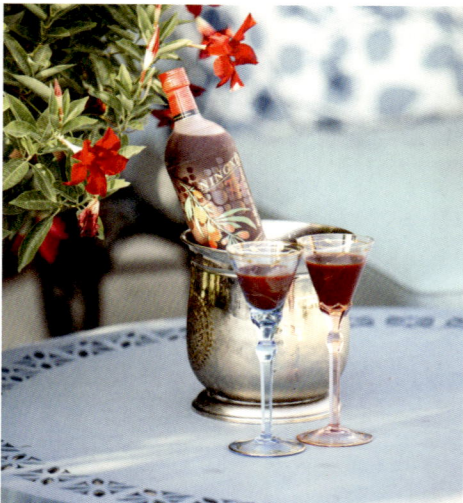

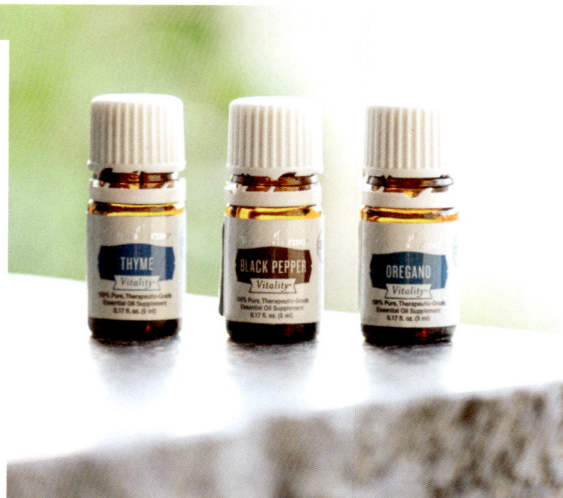

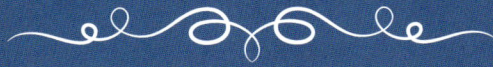

HOW TO PLACE YOUR ORDER

If you're here because of a Young Living Brand Partner, we encourage you to reach out to them for personalized guidance and to place your order. Your amazing Young Living friend is a valuable resource and can help you get the most out of your essential oils experience.

Are you new to Young Living? Here is how you can easily order. Simply scan the QR code and choose the life-giving products you desire to order.

EXCLUSIVE DISCOUNTS FOR NEW CUSTOMERS

If you're a new customer, you will receive 10% off by scanning the QR code and entering the promo code ShareYL into the box at checkout.

Additionally, you will receive an extra 24% off if you spend 100 PV (approximately $100) or more.

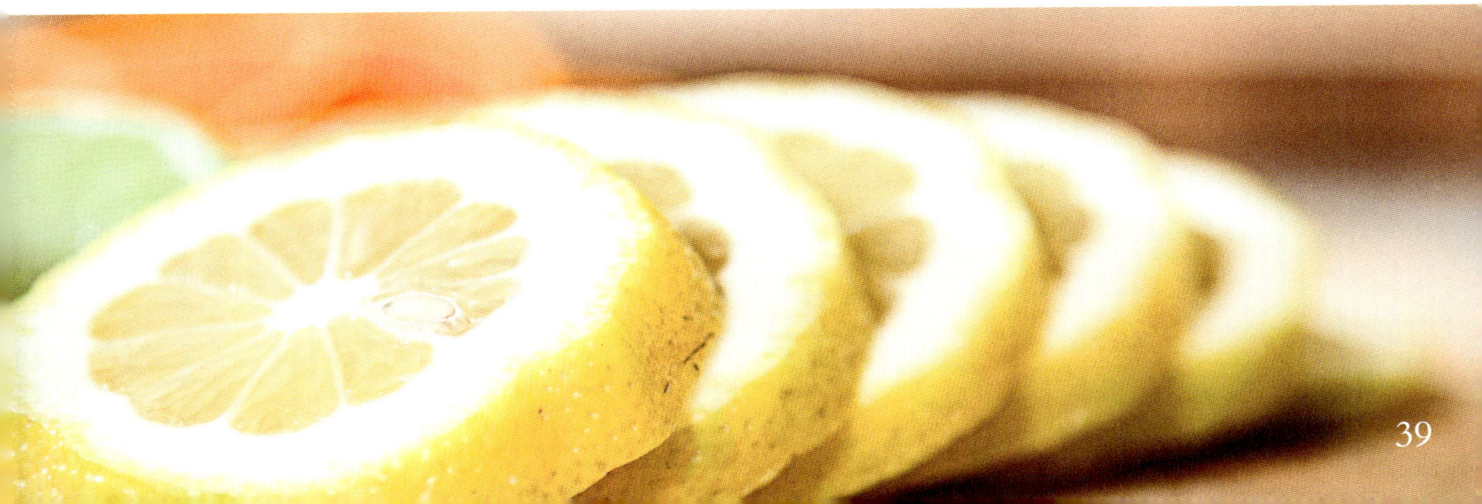

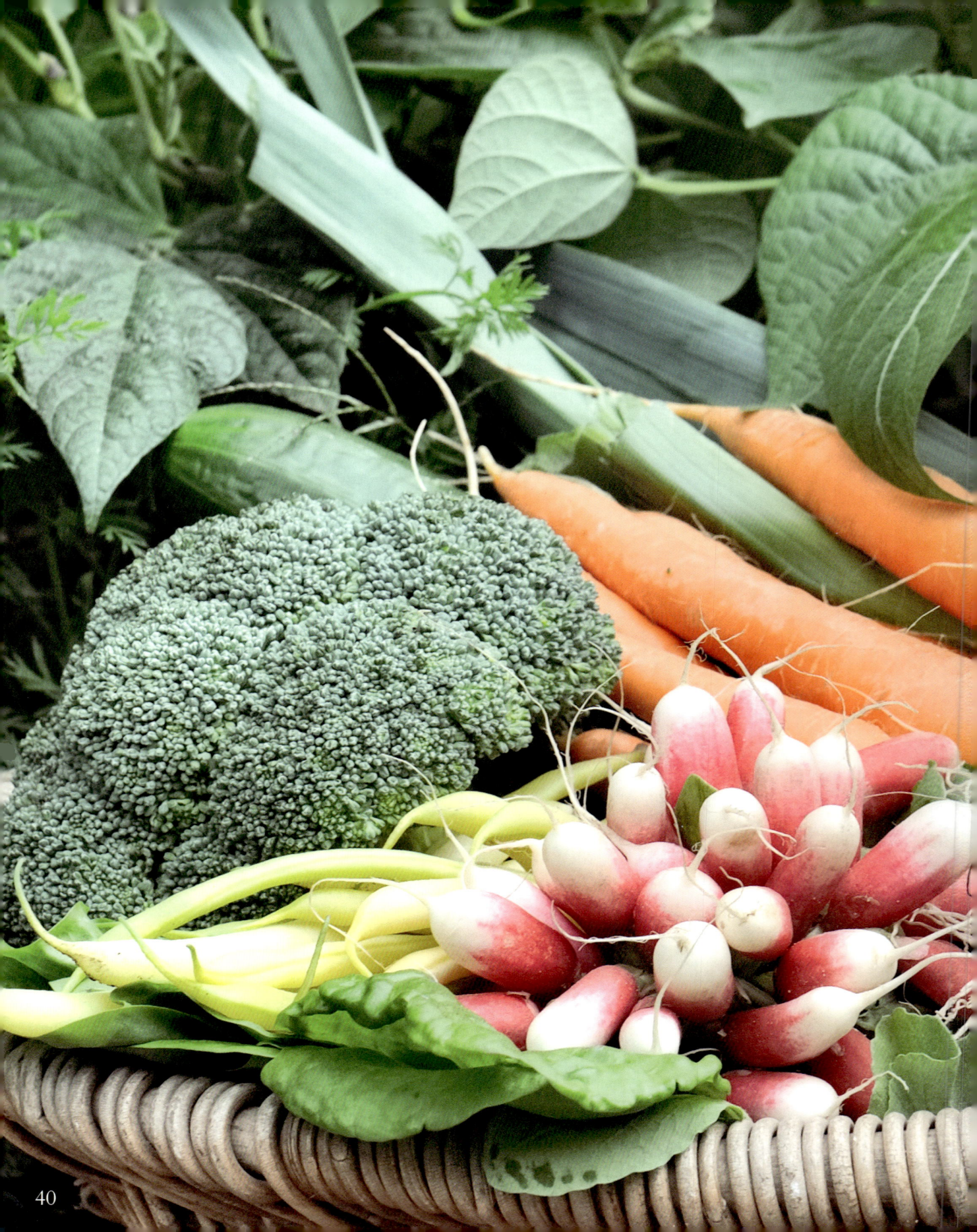

How to get the most value out of your 5-star dining experience!

For beginner to intermediate home chefs, grocery shopping can feel overwhelming—especially after a long day at work with only a little time to spare! Each recipe in this book is designed to stand alone, so you can enjoy it on its own or as part of a complete menu.

When you're ready to try a full menu, I've created a master shopping list for each week's 5-Star menu, guiding you to find each ingredient effortlessly. Follow these simple steps to make your time in the kitchen joyful and fulfilling!

1. **Plan ahead by shopping the day before.**
2. **Invite family or friends to cook together.**
3. **Consider hosting a Cooking Party! Each person brings a few ingredients. It's so fun and easy on the budget!**

When I lived in Europe, I learned the joy of lingering over fresh, vibrant ingredients. Savoring the process of choosing quality foods is part of the art of living. I hope you'll find the same pleasure as you make these recipes your own!

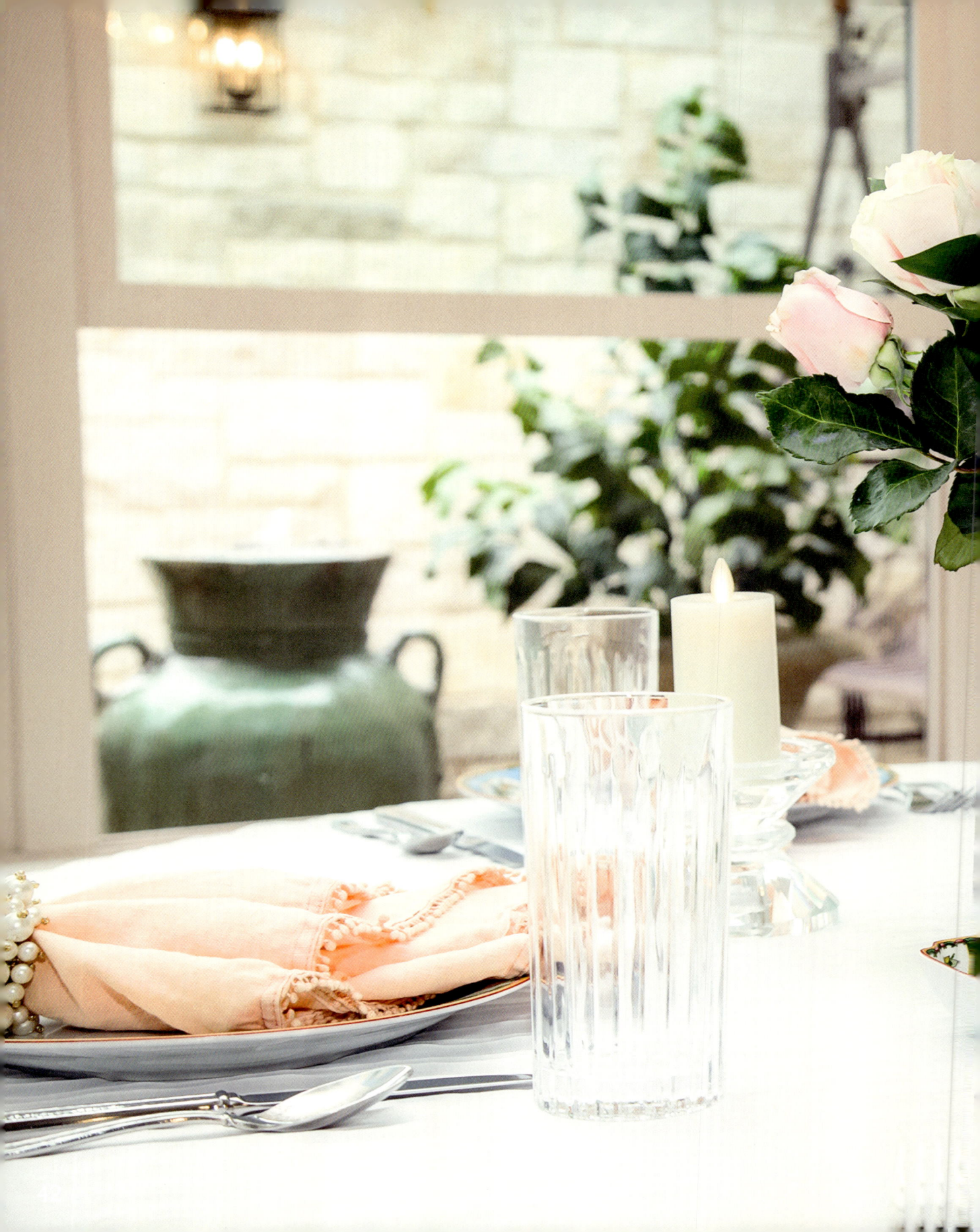

Eating For *Life* Teri Secrest

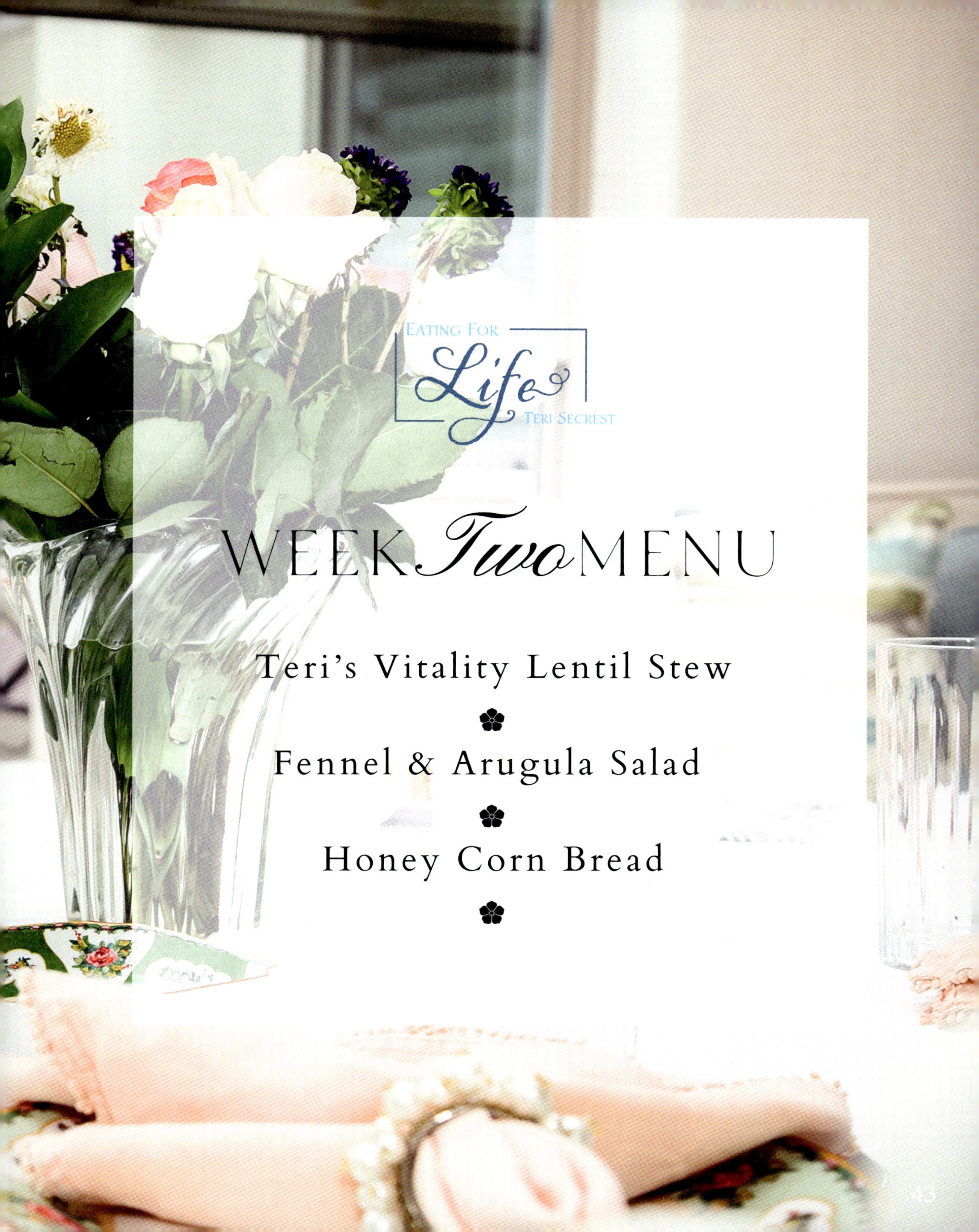

Week *Two* Menu

Teri's Vitality Lentil Stew

Fennel & Arugula Salad

Honey Corn Bread

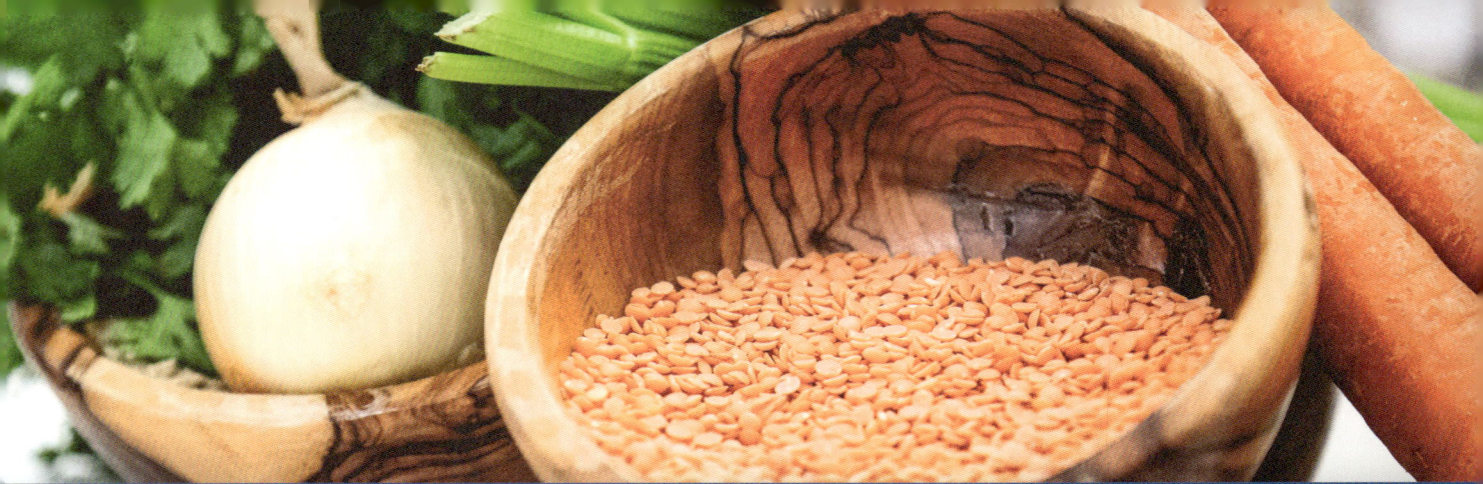

TERI'S VITALITY STEW

Ingredients

1 Tbsp coconut oil

1 medium onion, minced

2 large carrots, sliced

3 stalks celery, chopped

1 cup millet or brown rice
(rinse and drain)

8-10 cups organic chicken stock

1 cup of fresh cilantro chopped
and divided

1 cup green or red lentils
(rinsed and drained)

3 cloves garlic

2 tsp red curry paste

1 Tbsp curry powder

2 tsp cumin

Salt and pepper to taste

1 can full-fat coconut milk

*5 drops YL Vitality Celery
Seed oil

*1 drop YL Vitality Black
Pepper oil

*1 drop YL Vitality Thyme oil

*1 drop YL Vitality oregano oil
*(Order YL Vitality Essential Oils
on page 39)*

1/2 cup Parmesan cheese, shaved

Dash Bragg Liquid Aminos®
(optional)

> "If you want a real treat, combine my Vitality Stew with the Honey Cornbread and a simple salad... it will put a smile on your face and warm your heart!"

Preparation

1. In large soup pot, heat coconut oil over medium heat. Sauté minced onion, carrots and celery, until soft, about 5 minutes. Stir in millet or brown rice.

2. Add chicken stock, red curry paste, dry seasonings, salt and pepper to taste. (YL Vitality oils will be added later) Bring to a boil and then lower the heat, cover and simmer gently for 25 minutes. Be sure it is not boiling!

3. Add green lentils, the coconut milk and 1/2 cup of the cilantro. Simmer gently for another 20 minutes until lentils are tender. If using red lentils simmer for only 10 minutes. If the soup feels too thick you can add more chicken broth.

4. Remove from heat. Stir in the YL Vitality celery seed oil, YL Vitality Black Pepper oil, YL Vitality Thyme oil, and YL Vitality Oregano oil. Adjust the seasonings to taste.

5. Serve in bowls, sprinkled with Parmesan cheese, a little cilantro and a dash of Bragg Liquid Aminos (optional.)

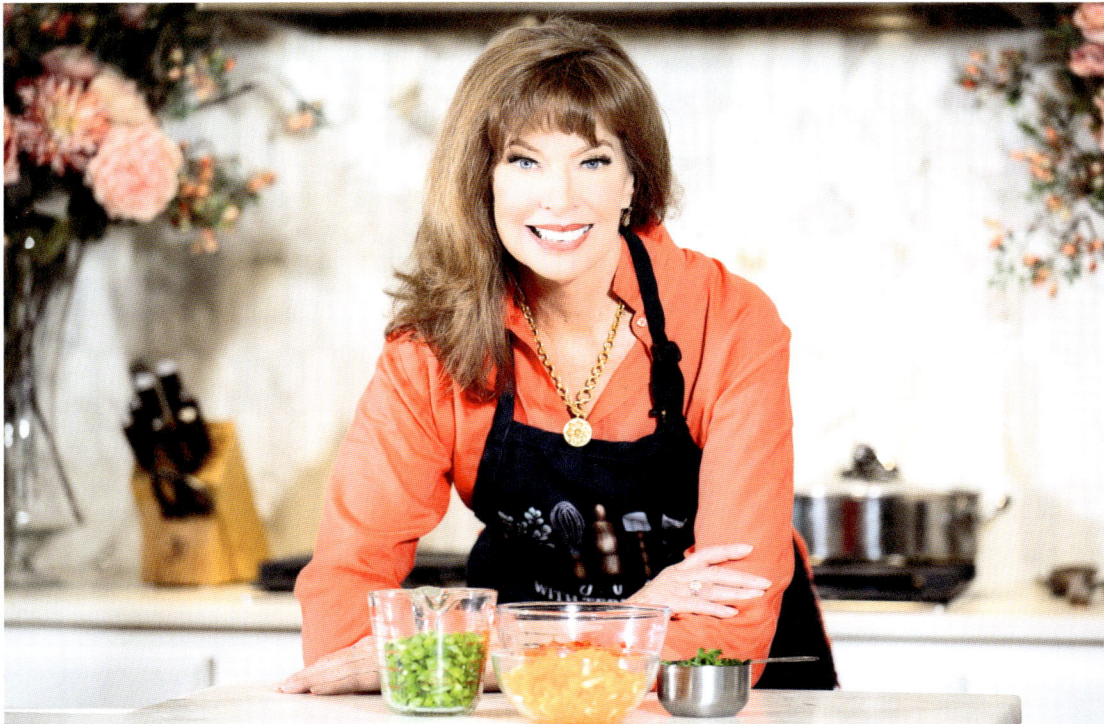

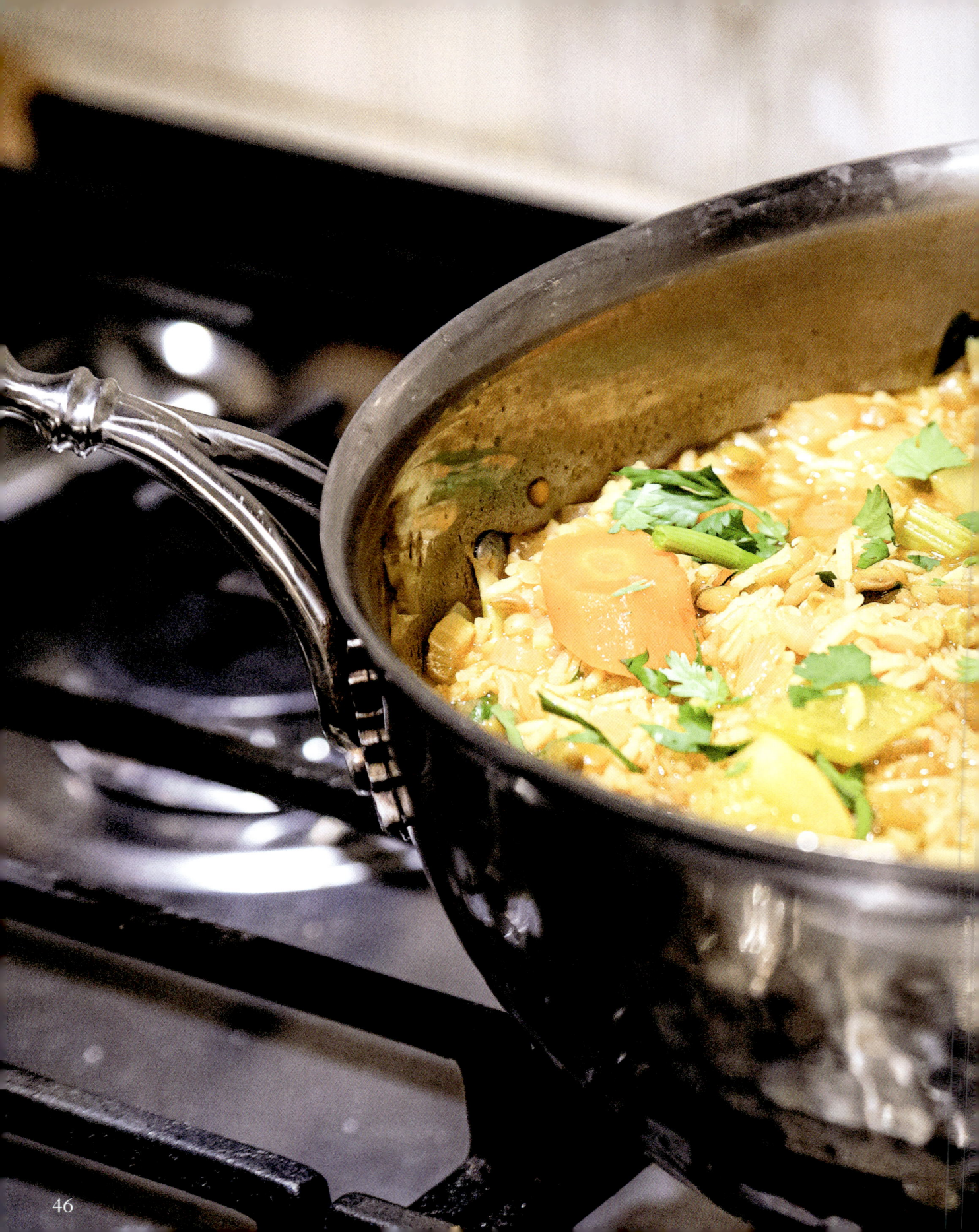

Friend, may I let you in on a little secret?
When your neighborhood children come for a visit
hyper on sugar, try feeding them this delicious stew and
notice how they suddenly calm down!

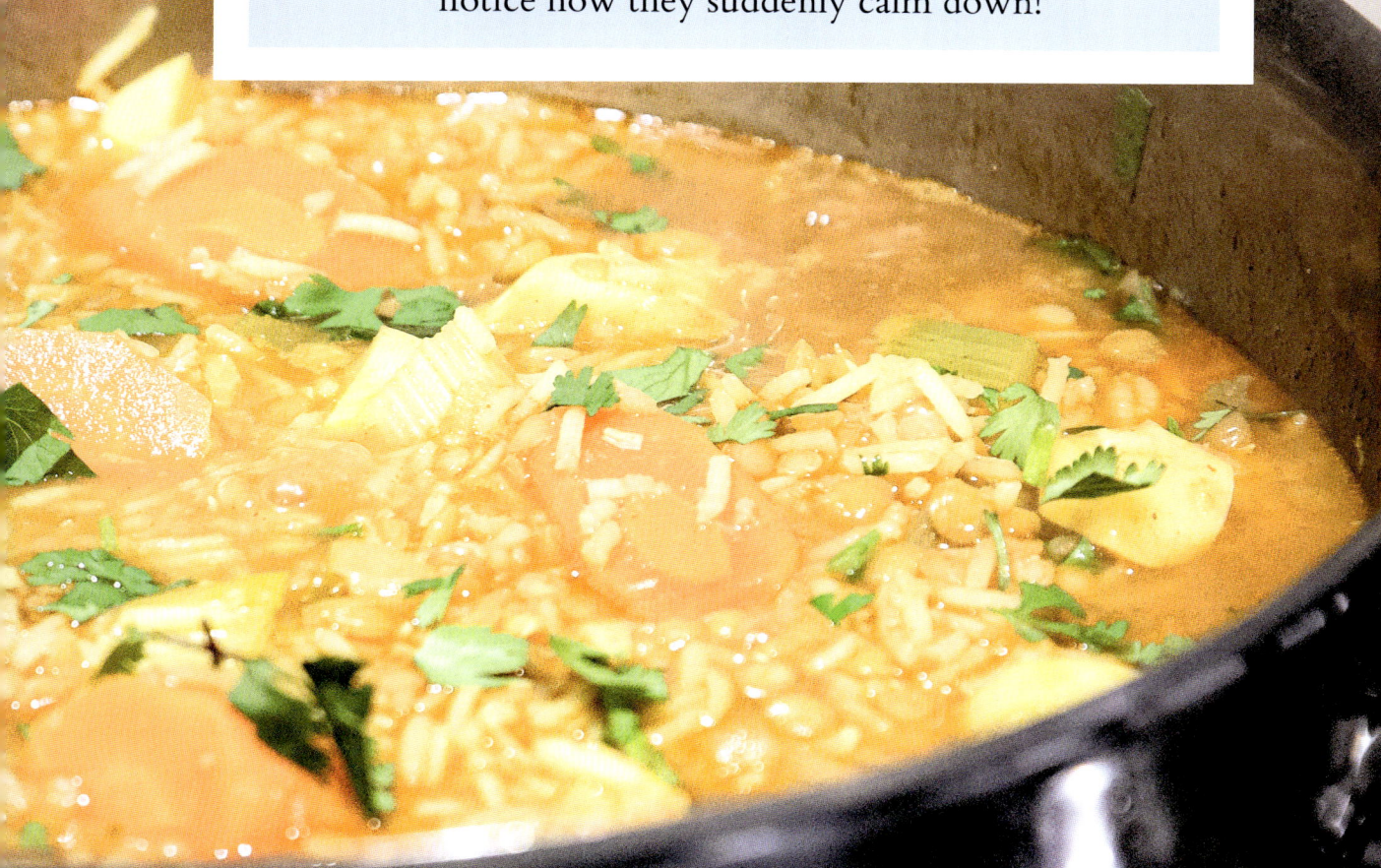

Let's celebrate these life giving ingredients!

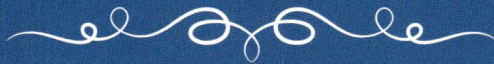

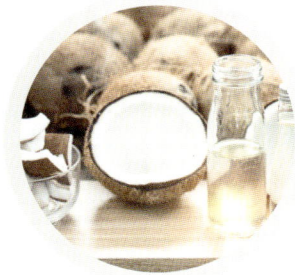

Coconut Oil

- Rich in medium-chain fatty acids, especially auric acid
- Supports heart health
- Boosts metabolism
- Great addition to a hormone supporting diet
- Reduces inflammation
- Suitable for cooking at high temperatures

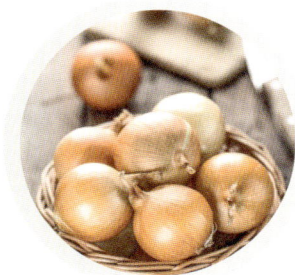

Onions

- Rich in antioxidants, including flavonoids and sulphur compounds
- Anti-inflammatory
- Immune-boosting properties
- Reduces the risk of heart disease and cancer
- High in vitamin C, vitamin B6, and dietary fiber
- Supports brain health

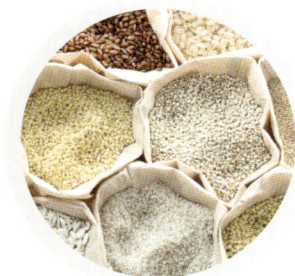

Millet

- Packed with protein
- Rich in magnesium, phosphorus, and manganese
- Promotes bone health
- Boosts energy production
- Gluten-free
- High fiber
- Helps regulate blood sugar levels

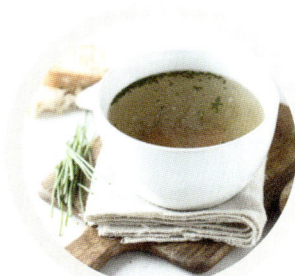

Organic Chicken Stock

- Rich in collagen, gelatin, and amino acids
- Supports joint health, digestion, and immune function
- Provides essential vitamins and minerals like calcium, magnesium, phosphorus, and potassium

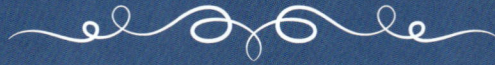

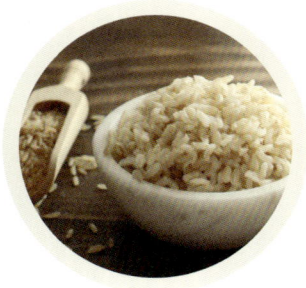

Organic Brown Rice

- Contains vitamin B1 (thiamine) which plays a crucial role in energy metabolism and nerve function
- Contains niacin (B3), which is important for energy production, DNA repair, and skin health
- Provides vitamin B6, which is great for metabolism and immune function
- A natural source of folate
- Has small amounts of vitamin E, a powerful antioxidant
- It has vitamin K which plays a key role in blood clotting
- Phytochemicals in brown rice help lower cholesterol levels, reduce blood pressure, and decrease the risk of heart disease
- Has a lower glycemic index then white rice
- Full of beneficial gut bacteria

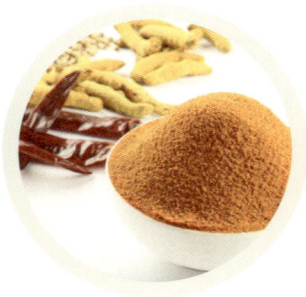

Curry Powder

- Potent antioxidant
- Reduces inflammation
- Support joint health
- Digestive benefits
- Alleviates nausea
- Reduces muscle pain
- Supports immune function

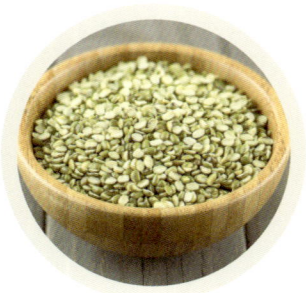

Lentils

- Packed with protein
- Full of fiber
- Rich in plant-based protein
- Good source of iron, folate, potassium, and magnesium
- Supports energy production
- Supports heart health
- Helps regulate blood sugar levels
- Supports weight management

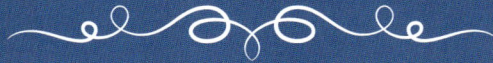

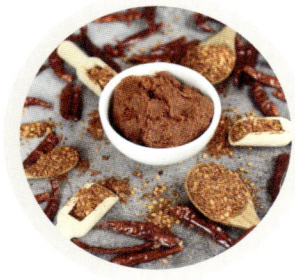

Red Curry Paste

- Bursting with antioxidants
- Helps protect cells from damage
- Anti-inflammatory properties
- May boost metabolism
- Aids in weight management
- Ginger and turmeric in the red curry paste support digestive health

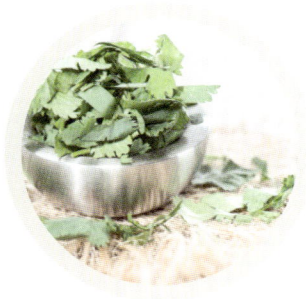

Fresh Cilantro

- Excellent source of vitamin K, which is essential for blood clotting and bone health
- Contains vitamin A, which supports eye health and immune function
- Provides small amounts of vitamin C, an antioxidant that helps protect cells from damage caused by free radicals
- Contains minerals like potassium, manganese, and iron, which play important roles in various bodily functions, including muscle function, metabolism, and oxygen transport

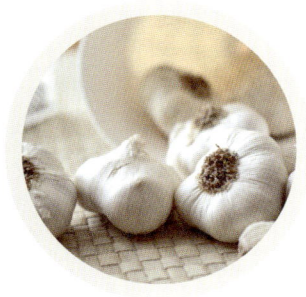

Garlic

- Renowned for natural antibiotic and antimicrobial properties
- Helps combat infections and boost the immune system
- Rich in antioxidants, including allicin
- Reduces oxidative stress
- Can help lower blood pressure and improve cholesterol levels
- Reduces the risk of cardiovascular diseases
- Anti-inflammatory properties

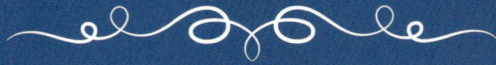

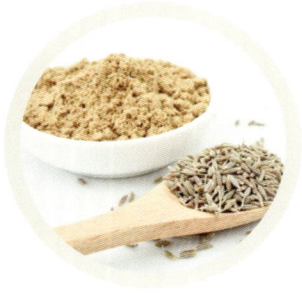

Cumin

- Contains iron, manganese, and magnesium
- Supports healthy blood cells
- Supports bone strength
- Maintains nerve function
- Contains flavonoids and phenolic compounds
- Helps protect cells from damage caused by free radicals
- Aids in digestion
- Promotes weight loss
- Improves cholesterol levels

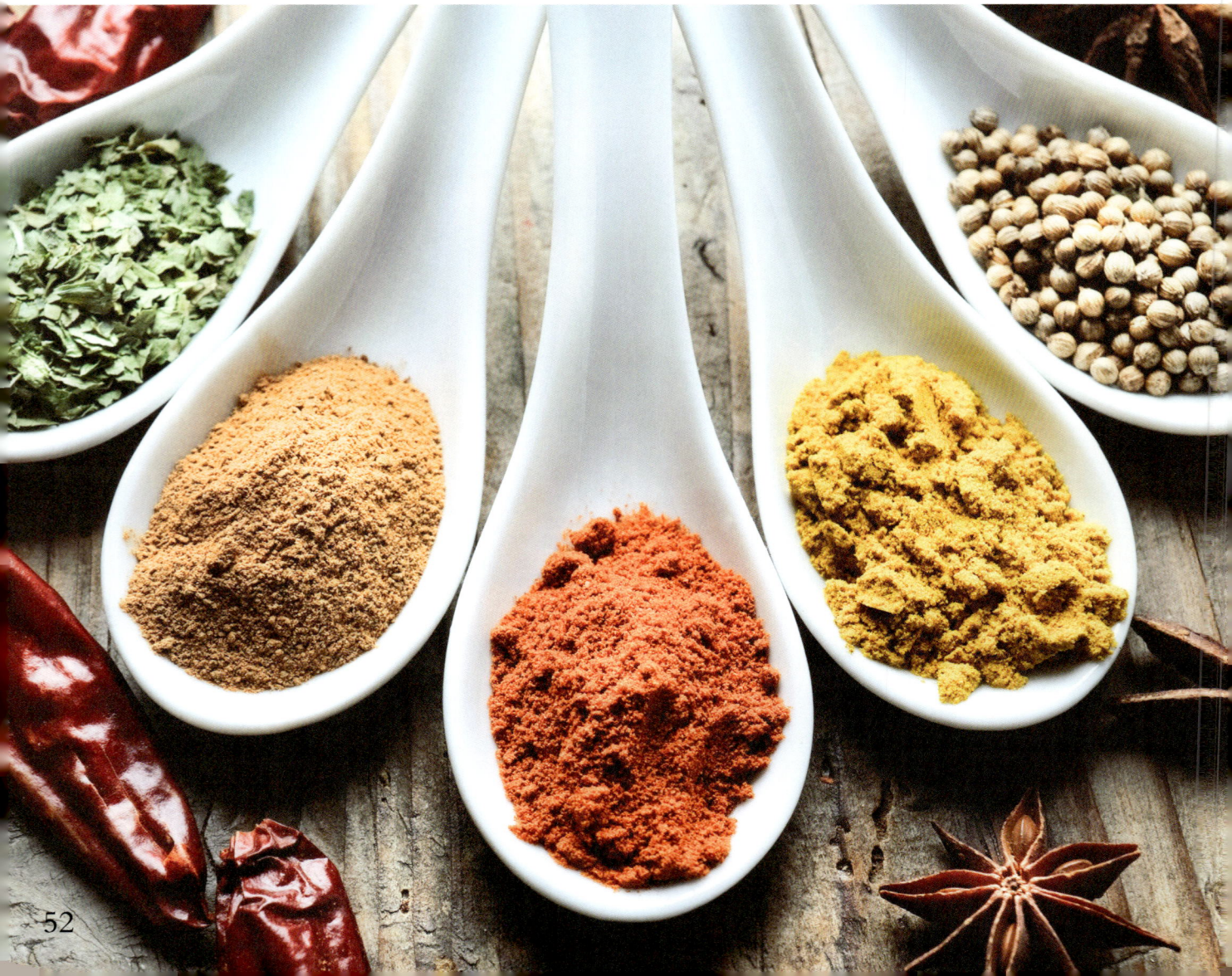

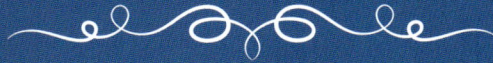

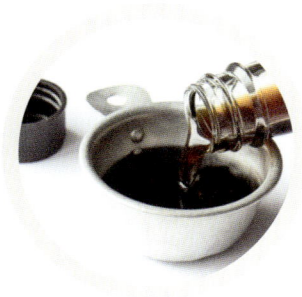

Braggs Liquid Aminos

- Bragg Liquid Aminos is a popular alternative to soy sauce
- Rich in essential amino acids, which are the building blocks of protein and essential for muscle repair and growth
- Low in sodium compared to traditional soy sauce, making it a suitable option for those watching their salt intake

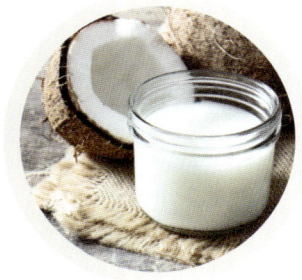

Coconut Milk

- Rich in healthy fats known as medium-chain triglycerides (MCTs)
- Boosts metabolism
- Supports brain function
- Provides quick energy
- Antimicrobial
- Antiviral fatty acid
- Strengthens the immune system
- Provides potassium, magnesium, and iron

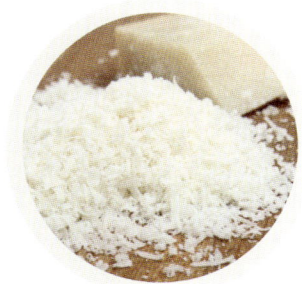

Parmesan Cheese

- Packed with protein and calcium
- Supports muscle health
- Supports bone strength, and overall growth and development
- Contains vitamins and minerals like vitamin A, vitamin B12, and zinc
- Supports immune function
- Supports vision health
- Supports a strong metabolism
- Naturally low in lactose

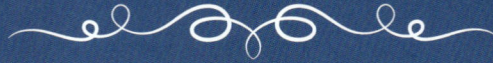

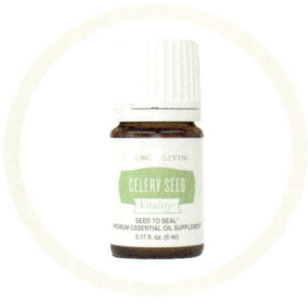

YL Vitality Celery Seed Essential Oil

- Rich in antioxidants
- Anti-inflammatory compounds
- Lowers oxidative stress
- Known for diuretic properties
- Promotes urine production
- Supports kidney health
- Alleviates bloating, gas, and indigestion
- Helps lower blood pressure
- Lowers cholesterol levels

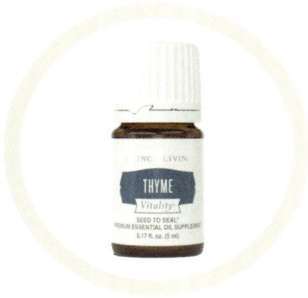

YL Vitality Thyme Essential Oil

- Contains thymol, which possesses strong antimicrobial properties
- Packed with antioxidants that help combat oxidative stress and inflammation
- May aid in respiratory health

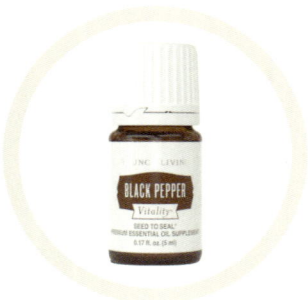

YL Vitality Black Pepper Essential Oil

- Aids in digestive health
- Promotes enzyme activity, helping to alleviate digestive discomfort
- The scent invigorates the mind and boosts alertness, making it a refreshing addition to your daily routine

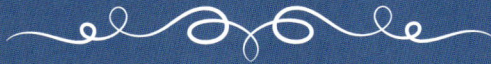

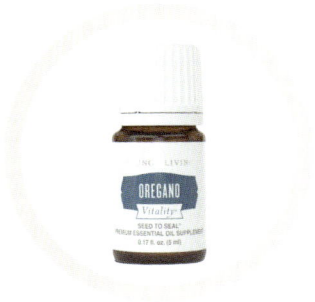

- Contains compounds like carvacrol and thymol, which have strong antimicrobial properties and can help combat harmful bacteria and viruses
- Rich in antioxidants
- May support digestion and alleviate digestive discomfort

YL Vitality Oregano Essential Oil

"Essential oils are the life force of the plant and they are very compatible with the human body."

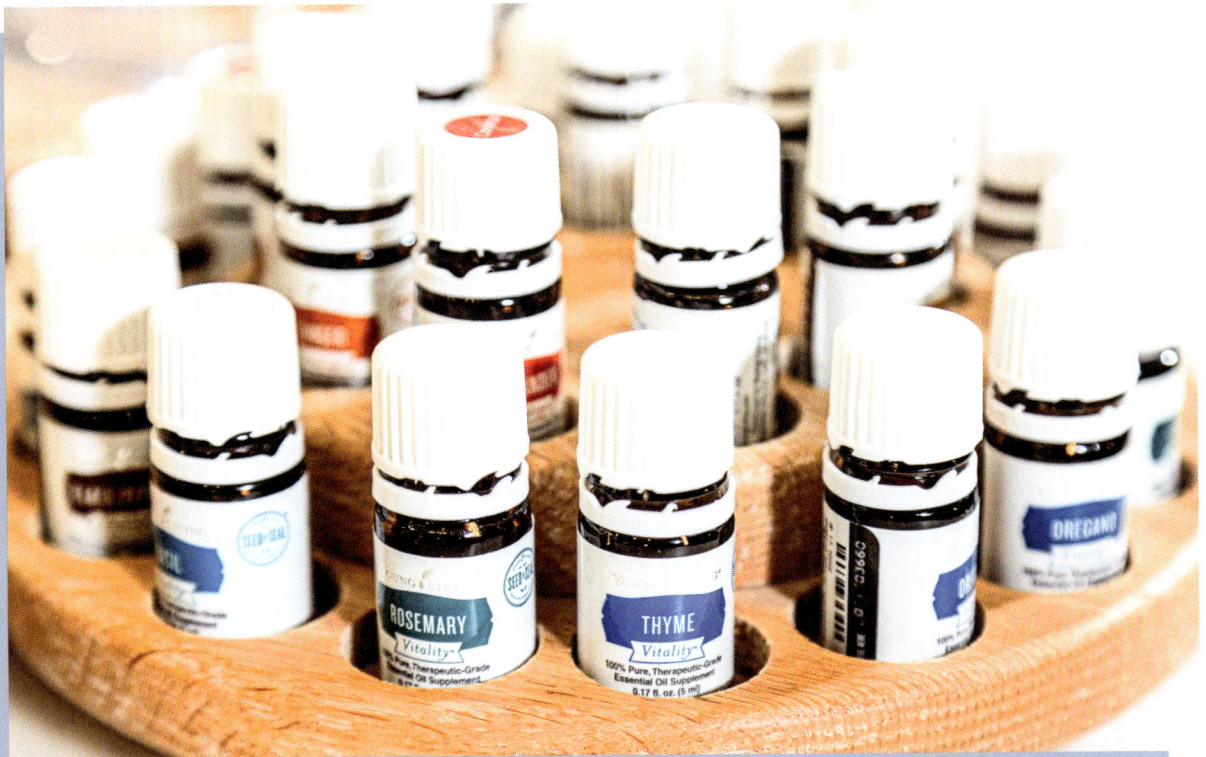

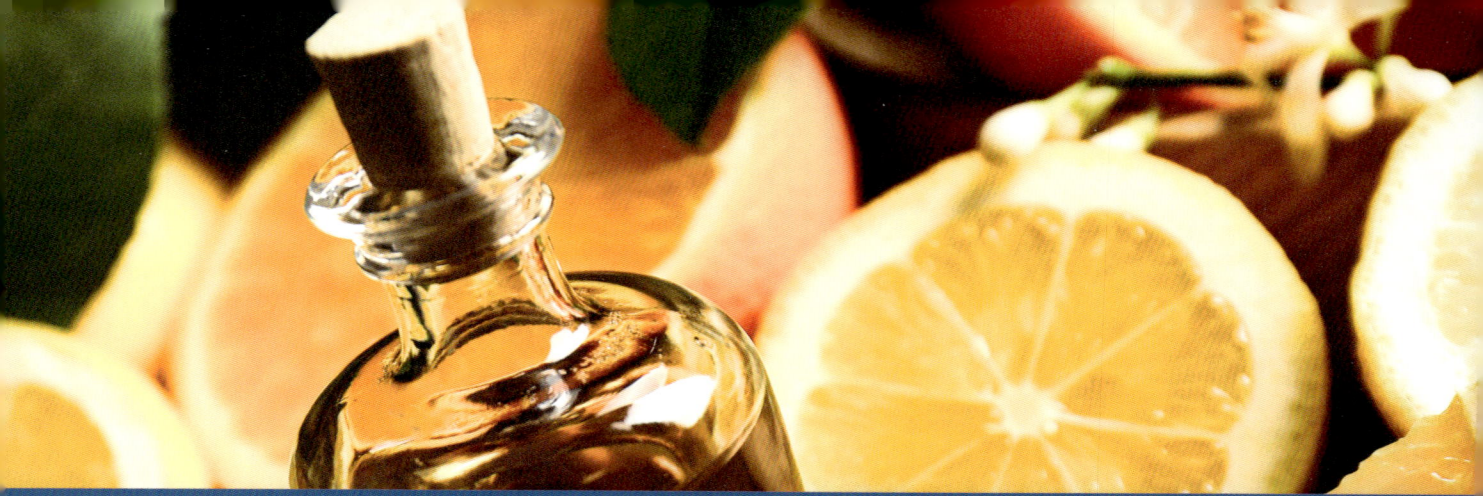

FENNEL & ARUGULA SALAD

Ingredients
Serves 4 - 6

2 oranges

1 large bulb fennel

Extra virgin olive oil

Splash of champagne vinegar

2 cups baby arugula

Kosher salt

Black pepper

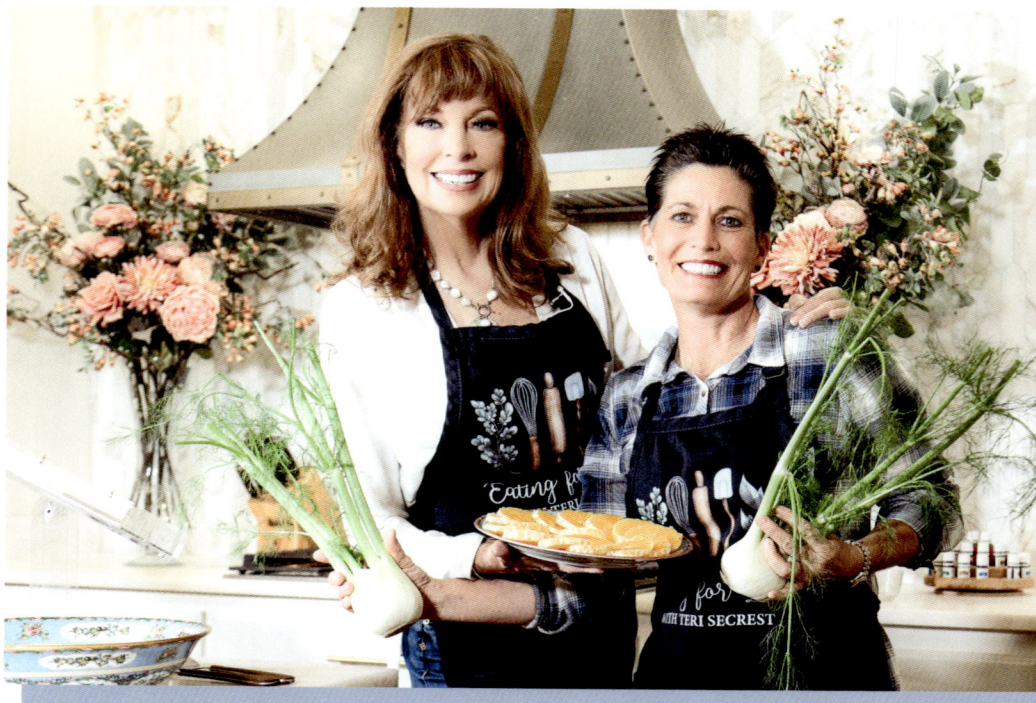

Preparation

1. Peel the oranges. Slice the orange in half vertically. Then slice thinly. Set aside.

2. Remove leaves and stems from the fennel--everything but the bulb. Slice the fennel bulb horizontally into paper-thin slices. The best tool for this is a mandoline. Place in a large bowl.

3. Drizzle the sliced fennel with olive oil and a splash of champagne vinegar.

4. Add the arugula and toss gently with two forks. Season to taste with kosher salt and pepper.

5. To serve, arrange the salad decoratively on a plate and finish with the orange slices.

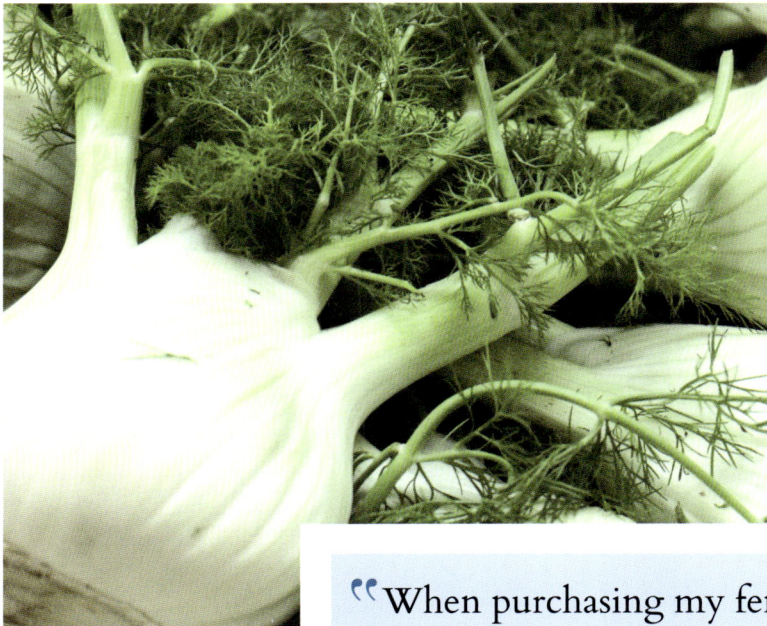

"When purchasing my fennel in the grocery store, the young cashier asked, 'What are these?' As I began explaining what a fantastic vegetable fennel is, his eyes got bigger and bigger until finally he exclaimed, 'I'm going to go buy some right now and try it!'"

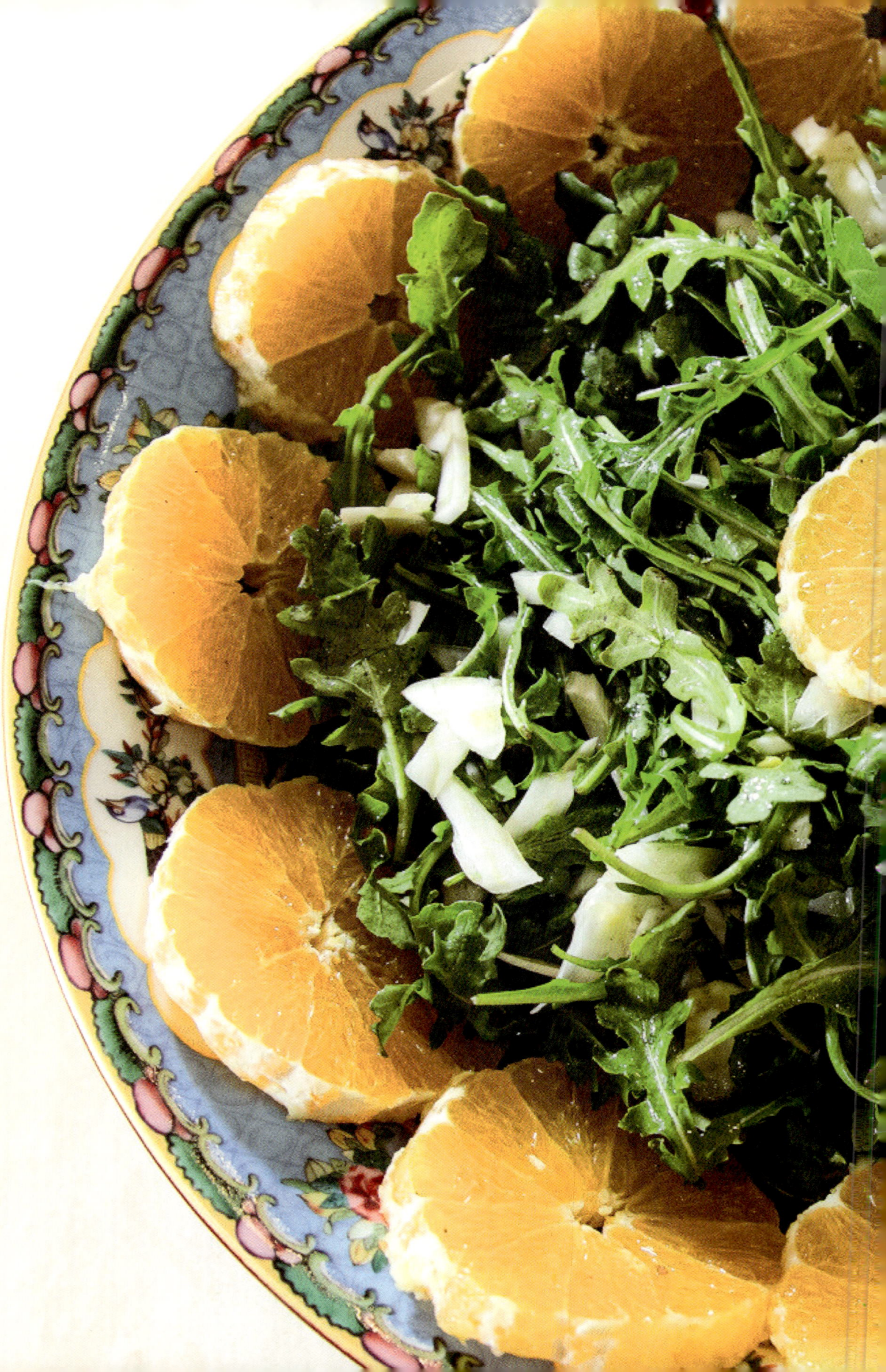

"Did you know fennel supports healthy blood sugar levels? What a great flavorful food choice for all of us!"

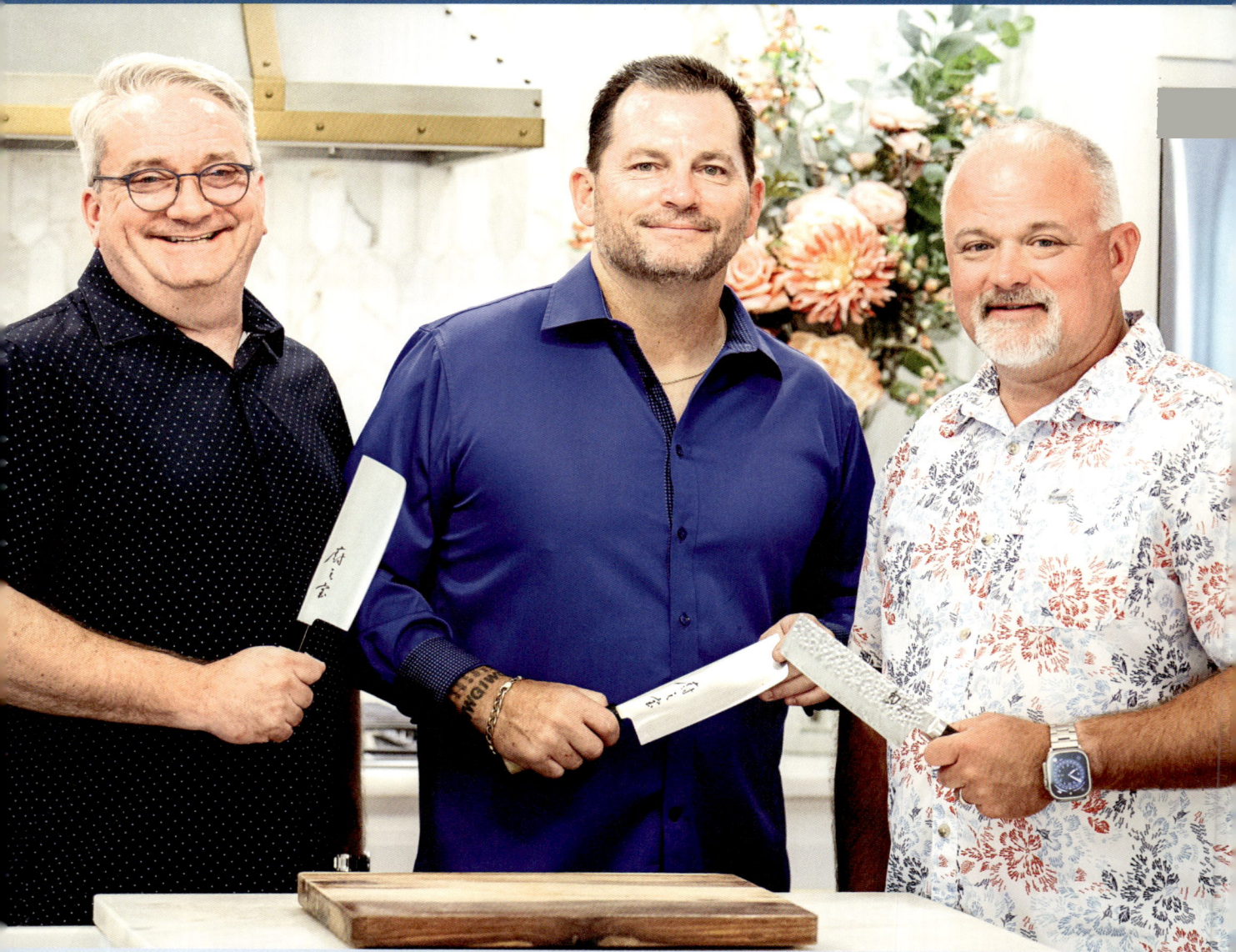

Let's celebrate these life giving ingredients!

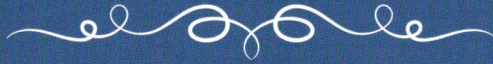

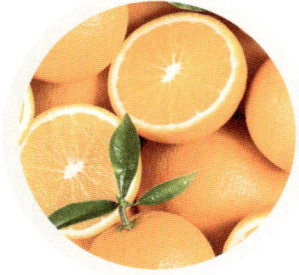

Oranges

- Rich in vitamin C
- Supports immune function
- Skin health
- Collagen production
- Promotes wound healing
- Good source of fiber
- Supports gut health
- Very hydrating
- A quick source of energy
- Contains antioxidants
- Helps reduce inflammation
- Lowers the risk of chronic diseases such as heart disease and cancer

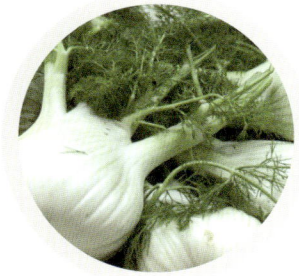

Fennel

- Rich in fiber
- Particularly high in vitamin C
- Helps regulate blood pressure and fluid balance
- Supports immune function
- Supports skin health
- Promotes collagen production
- Contains potassium
- Aids in digestion
- Promotes gut health
- Has antioxidant and anti-inflammatory properties
- Helps reduce gas, bloating, and indigestion

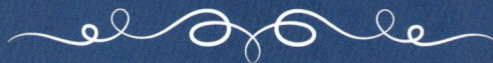

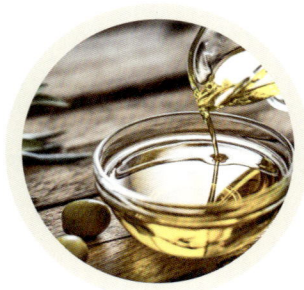

Olive Oil

- Rich in monounsaturated fats
- Can help lower bad cholesterol levels
- Reduces the risk of heart disease
- Packed with antioxidants
- Protects cells from free radicals and oxidative stress
- Anti-inflammatory properties
- Reduces the risk of chronic diseases like cancer and Alzheimer's

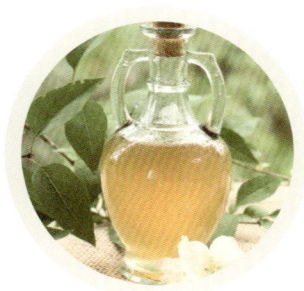

Champagne Vinegar

- Retains antioxidants found in grapes
- Helps reduce inflammation
- Naturally low in calories and fat free
- Improves digestion
- Regulates blood sugar levels
- Supports weight management
- Promotes feelings of fullness and reduces cravings

"This recipe was shared with me by my good friend and Chef Lisa Dahl. Lisa is a highly successful restaurateur in Sedona, Arizona. Be sure to visit one of her award winning restaurants in Sedona!"

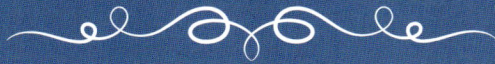

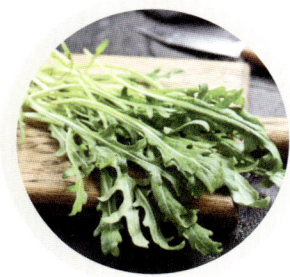

Organic Arugula

- Rich in vitamins, minerals, and antioxidants
- High in vitamins K and C
- Supports bone health
- Supports blood clotting
- Boosts immune function
- Promotes collagen production
- Contains folate, a B vitamin
- Plays a key role in cell growth and metabolism
- Contains potassium
- Helps regulate blood pressure and fluid balance
- High antioxidant content
- Helps reduce inflammation
- High in fiber

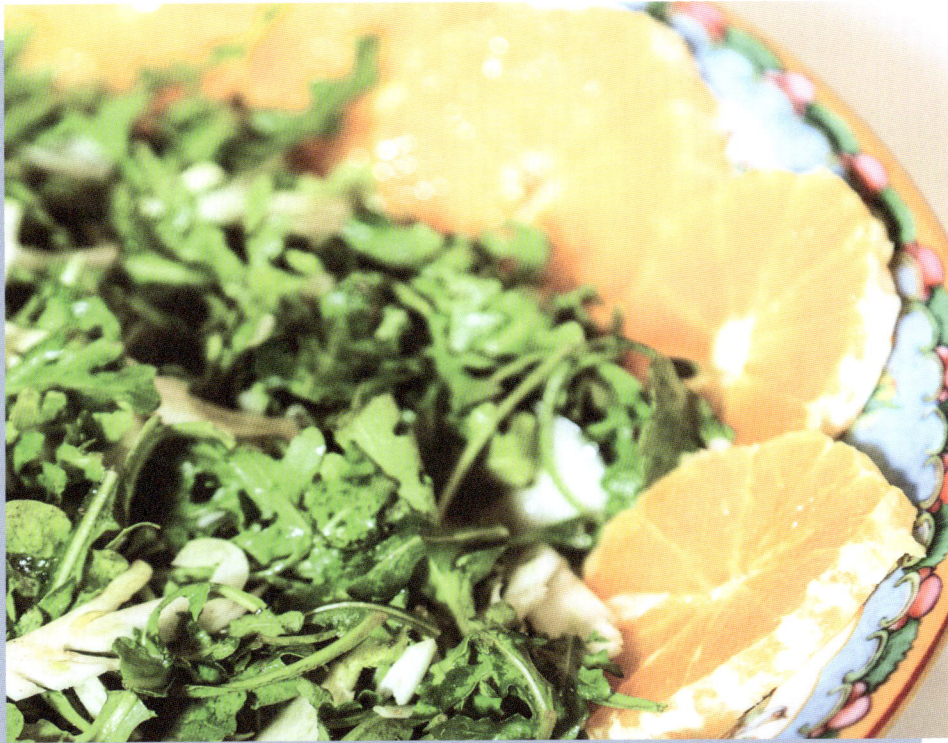

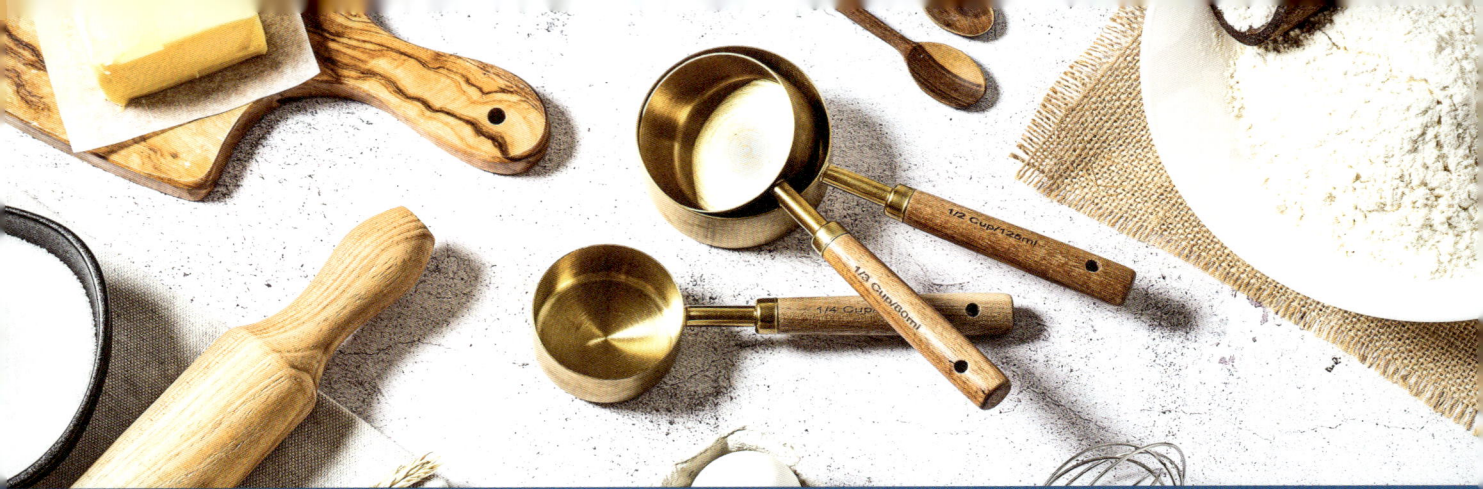

HONEY CORNBREAD

Ingredients

Makes 11 corn muffins or 8″ x 8″ pan

1 cup organic yellow cornmeal

1 cup organic, all-purpose flour

1/2 tsp sea salt

1 tsp baking powder

1 tsp baking soda

1 egg

1-7/8 cups buttermilk (just under 2 cups)

Scant 1/3 cup raw unfiltered honey

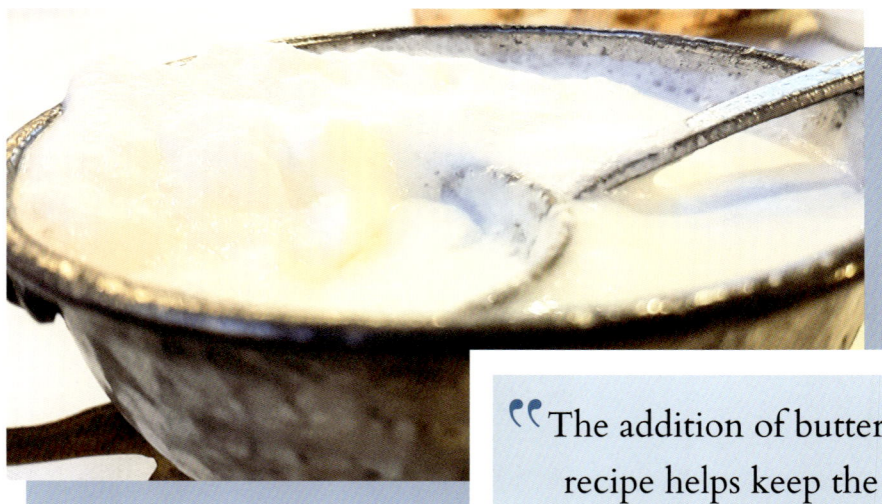

"The addition of buttermilk to this recipe helps keep the cornbread moist and mouth-watering."

Preparation

1. Preheat oven to 425°F. Generously butter or oil a muffin pan or insert cupcake/muffin liners. You can also use an 8"x 8" baking pan.
2. Combine dry ingredients in a large bowl.
3. Mix wet ingredients together in separate bowl.
4. Add wet ingredients to dry ingredients. Mix lightly by hand as cornbread batter must be a little lumpy.
5. Pour batter into the prepared pan. Bake until golden brown, about 20-25 minutes (15 minutes if using muffin tin.) Before you remove from the oven, test for doneness by inserting a toothpick in the center of the bread. It should come out clean.

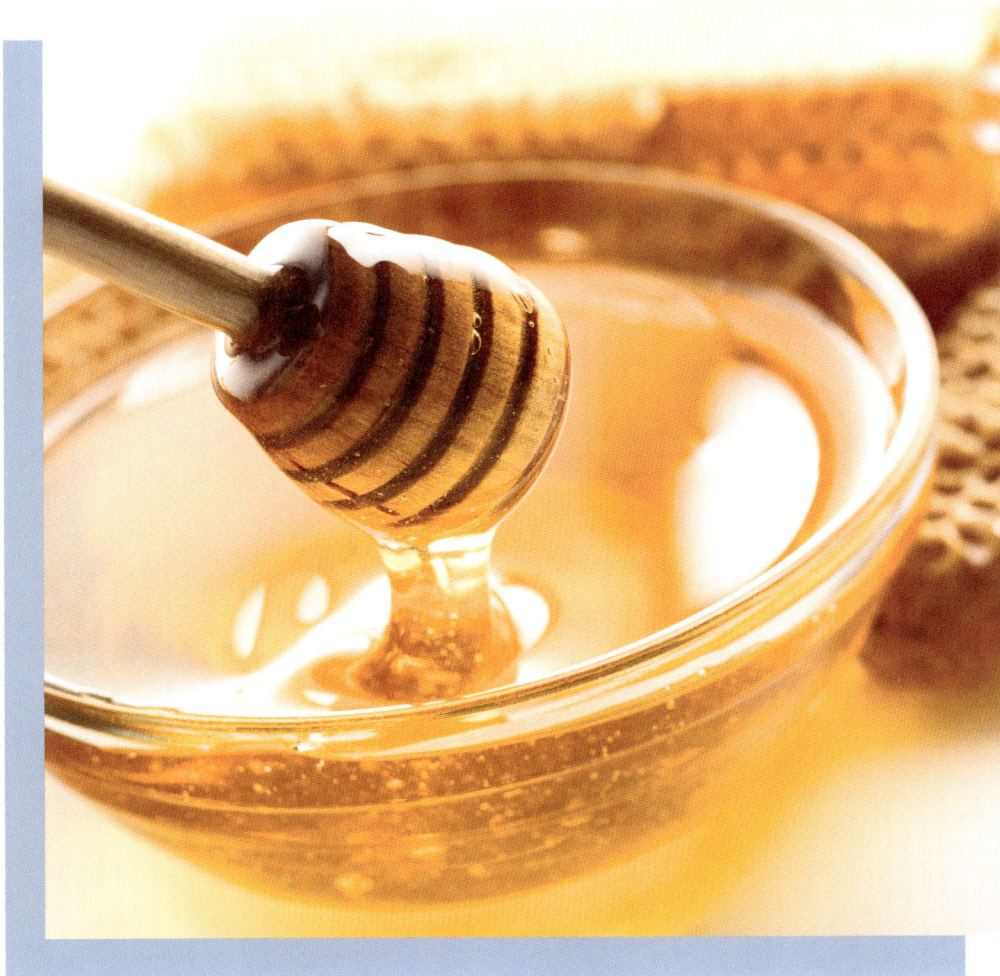

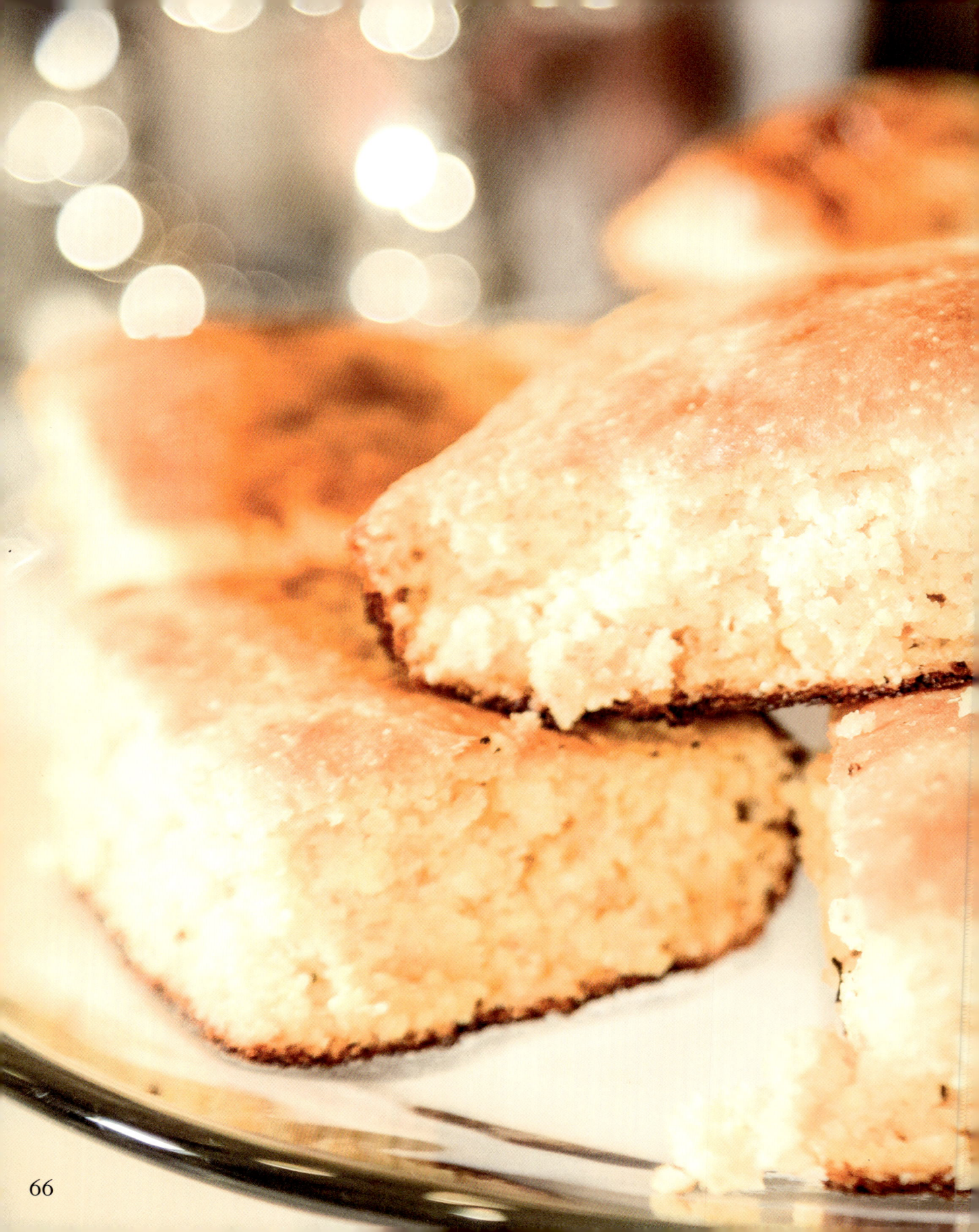

"Not your Momma's cornbread! By investing in organic, non GMO cornmeal, you will experience a difference in flavor and your body will love you for it!"

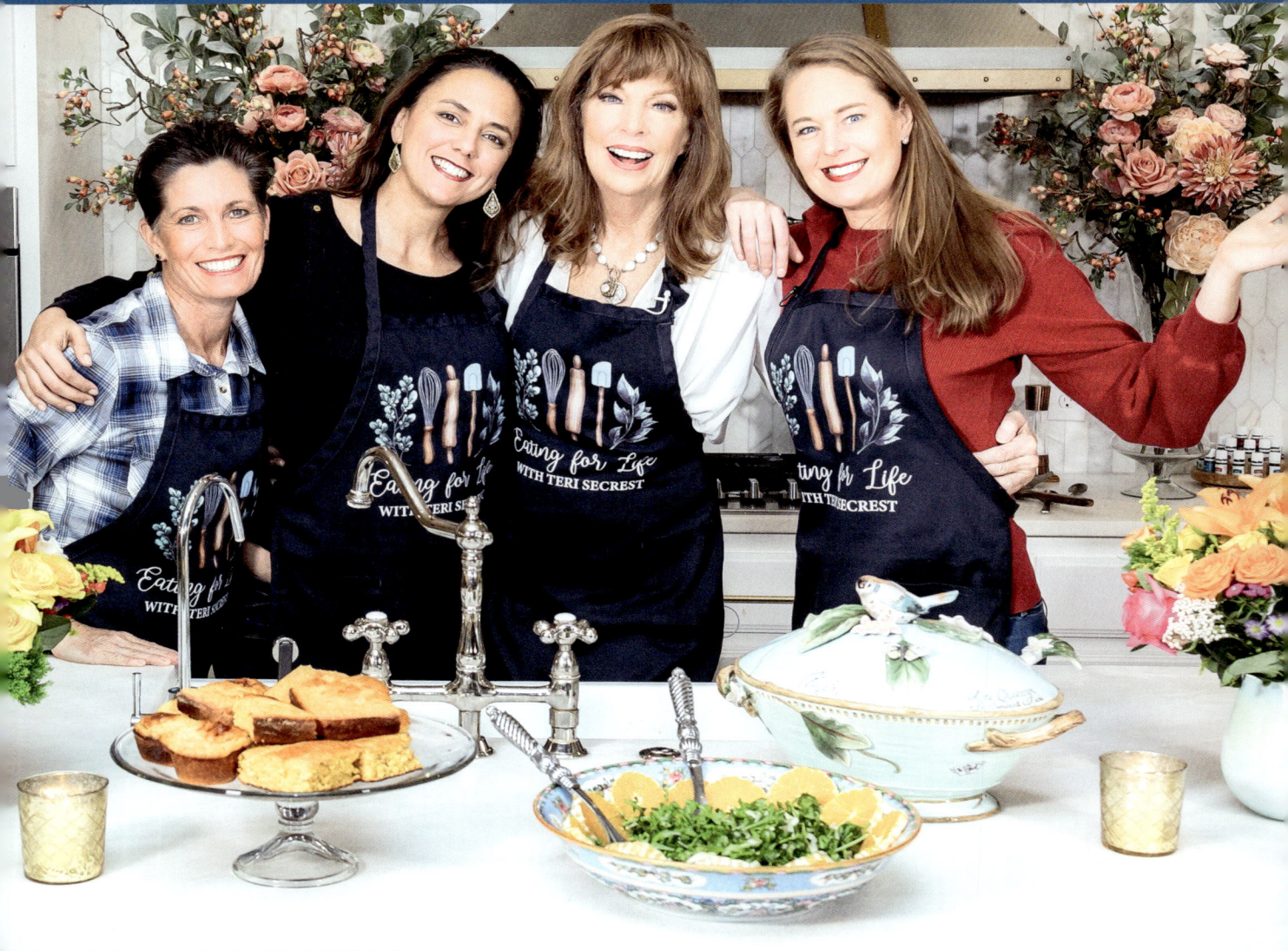

> # Let's celebrate these life giving ingredients!

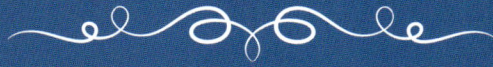

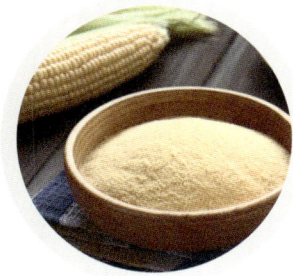

- Provides steady energy
- Contains fiber for digestive health and regular bowel movements
- Contains iron, magnesium, and phosphorus
- Naturally low in fat and cholesterol

Non GMO Cornmeal

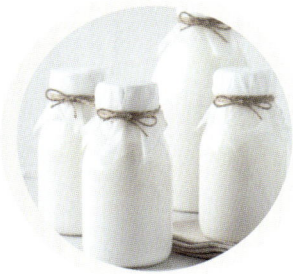

- Source of calcium and vitamin D
- Supports bone health
- Aids in mineral absorption
- Probiotic-rich beverage
- Contains beneficial bacteria for digestive health and improved gut flora
- Aids in nutrient absorption

Buttermilk

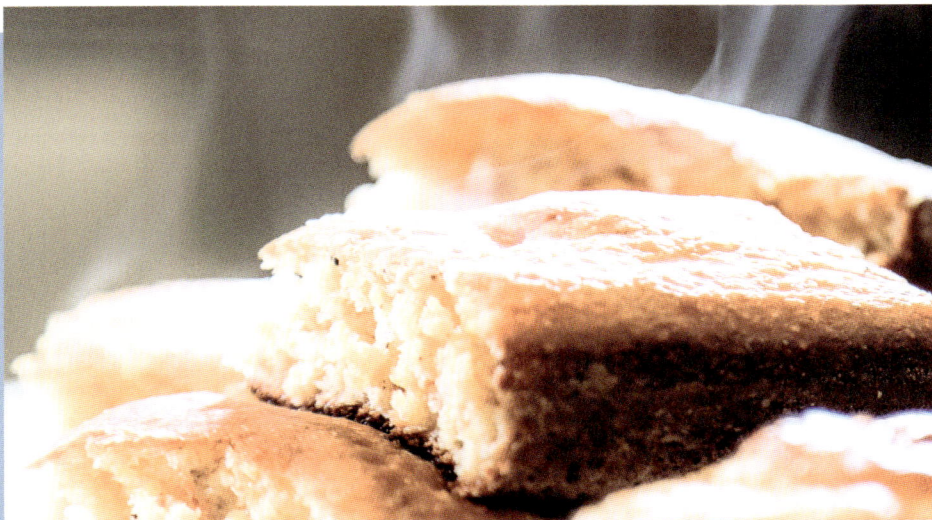

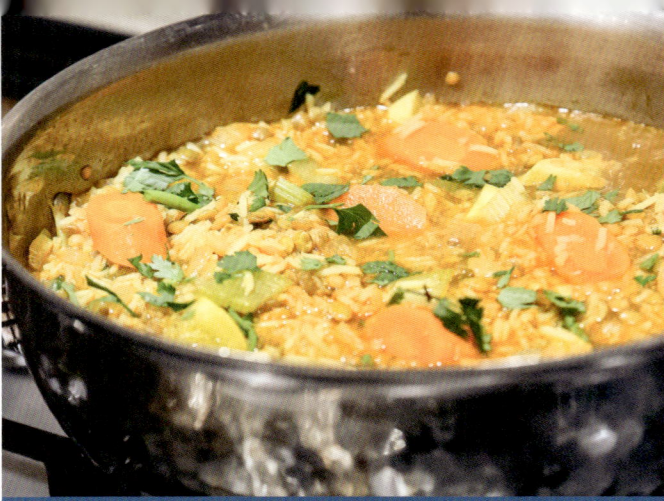

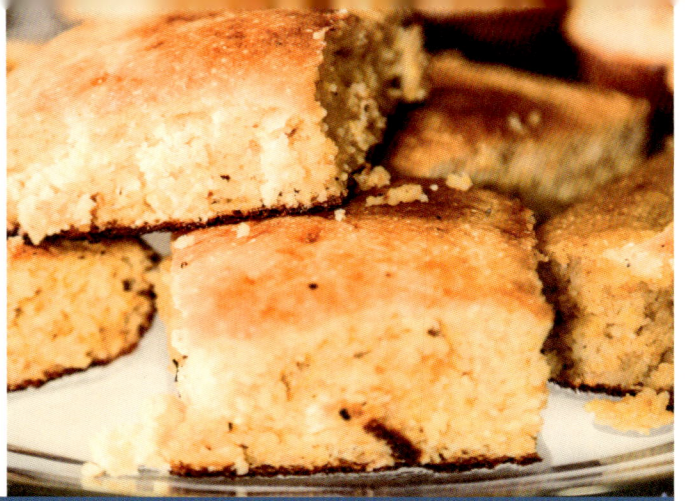

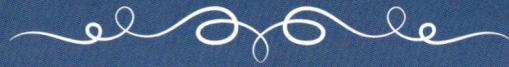

Week 2
Full Menu Shopping List

Produce

1 medium onion

2 large carrots

3 stalks celery

2 oranges

1 large bulb fennel

1 cup fresh cilantro

2 cups baby arugula

3 cloves garlic

Canned Goods

8 cups organic chicken stock
(usually 2 standard cartons)

Baking & Spices

Coconut oil

Cumin

Curry powder

Splash of champagne vinegar

Extra virgin olive oil

Kosher salt

Sea salt

Black pepper

Scant 1/3 cup raw, unfiltered honey

Cupcake wrappers (optional)

Baking powder

Baking soda

Organic, unbleached all-purpose flour

Organic yellow cornmeal

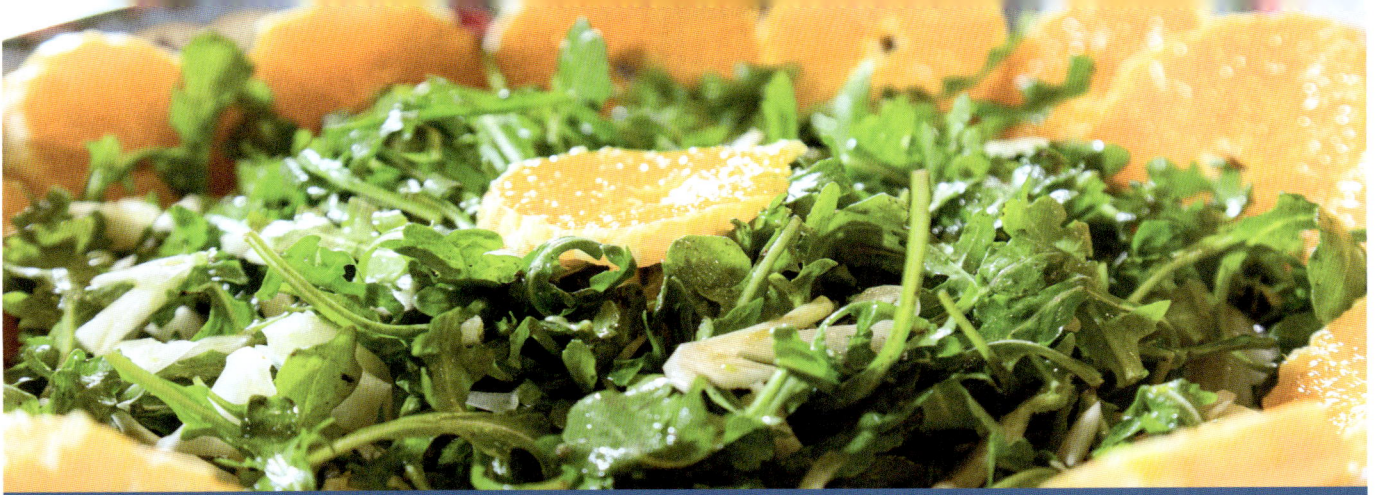

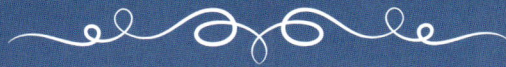

Full Menu Shopping List continued

International Section

1 can full fat coconut milk

1 jar red curry paste

Dry Goods

1 cup millet (or brown rice)

1 cup red or green lentils

Dairy

1/2 cup Parmesan cheese, shaved

1 egg

1 7/8 cup buttermilk
(just under 2 cups)

Condiments

Bragg Liquid
Aminos (optional)

From Young Living*

YL Vitality Celery Seed oil

YL Vitality Black Pepper oil

YL Vitality Thyme oil

YL Vitality Oregano oil

SEE PAGE 39 FOR ORDERING DETAILS

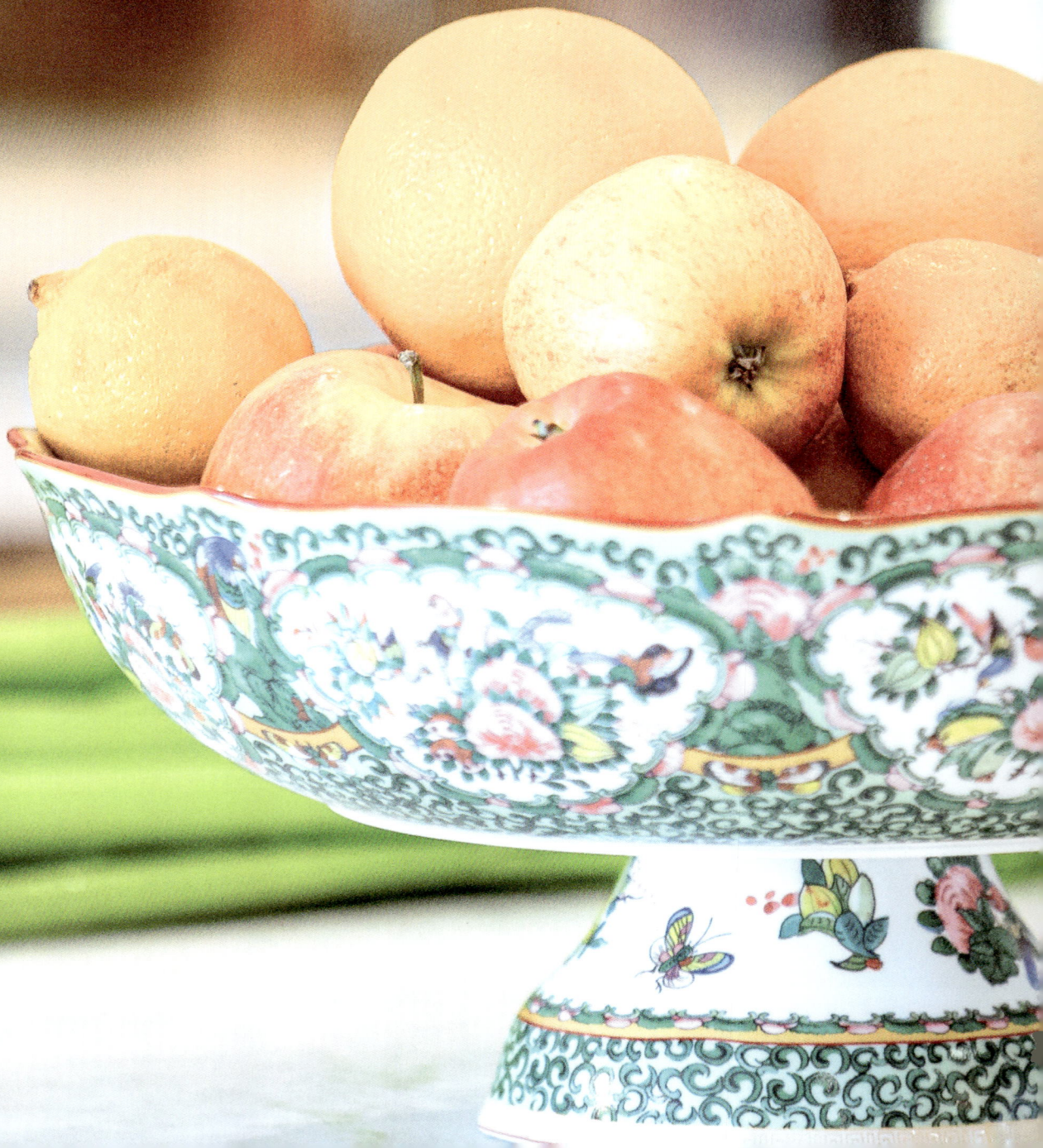

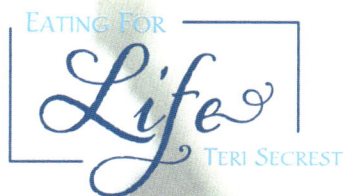

WEEK *Three* MENU

Penne Pesto with Pine Nuts

❀

Teri's Signature Caesar Salad

❀

Lemon Curd

❀

Luscious Lemon Mousse

❀

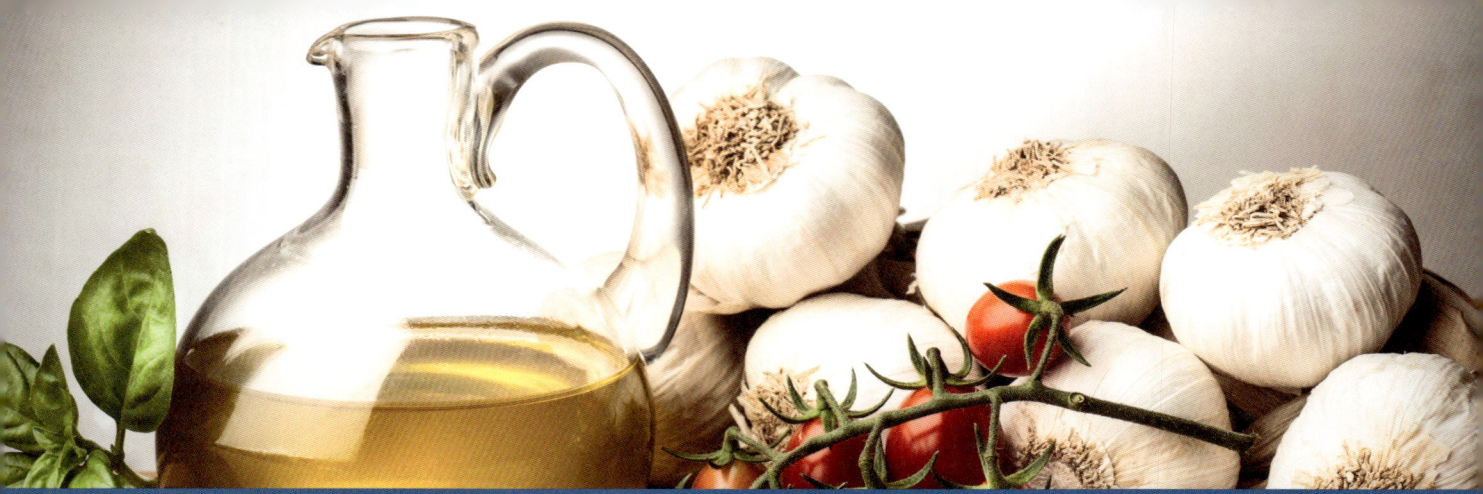

PENNE PESTO WITH PINE NUTS

Ingredients

1 lb organic penne pasta,
(my favorite is made from
Durham wheat)

2 cups fresh sweet basil leaves

1/2 tsp salt for pasta water

3/4 cup olive oil + 1 Tbsp for
cooked pasta

3 cloves fresh garlic, peeled

1/2 cup Parmesan cheese, grated

Finishing Touches

2-3 tomatoes, wedges

1/2 cup Parmesan cheese, shaved

For Roasted Pine Nuts

1/2 cup pine nuts

1 Tbsp butter

Salt to taste

"This is the easiest most flavorful dish ever. We often double the recipe for a large, crowd as people usually eat seconds. Simply heavenly!"

Preparation

Teri's Famous Pesto Sauce (Step 1)

1. In food processor, blend olive oil, basil, garlic, Parmesan cheese and salt together until smooth (about 1 minute.) Set aside.
2. Keeps well up to three days in the refrigerator.

Penne Pasta & Toasted Pine Nuts (Step 2)

1. In a pot, add salt to cold water and bring to a boil.
2. When boiling, add pasta slowly to keep it boiling. Cook pasta until *al dente* (do not overcook.) Drain and immediately toss with 1 Tbsp olive oil to keep from sticking.
3. While pasta cooks, prepare toasted pine nuts.
4. Melt butter in small skillet over medium heat. Add pine nuts and salt. Stir constantly until lightly browned on all sides. Remove and set aside for a finishing touch!
5. Pour pesto sauce over the pasta and toss. Place in warmed serving bowl.
6. Garnish with fresh cut organic tomatoes, sprinkle with shaved Parmesan cheese, and roasted pine nuts.

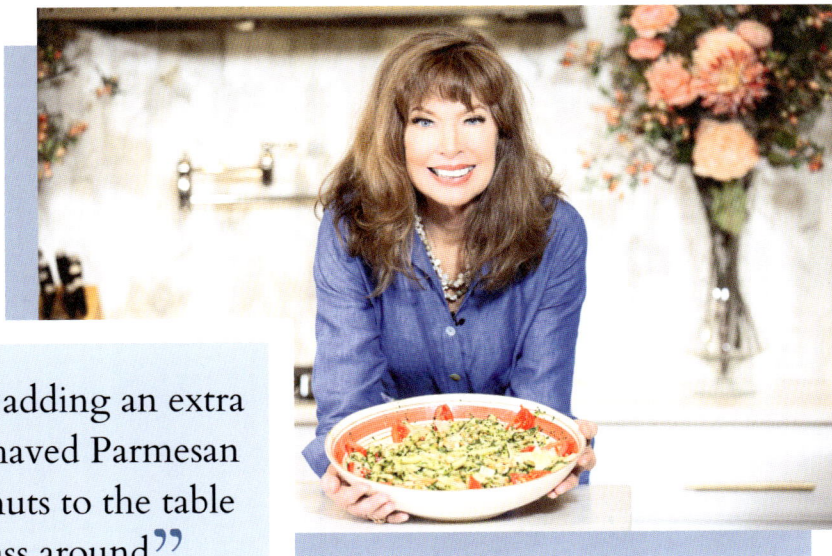

"I just love adding an extra bowl of shaved Parmesan and pine nuts to the table to pass around."

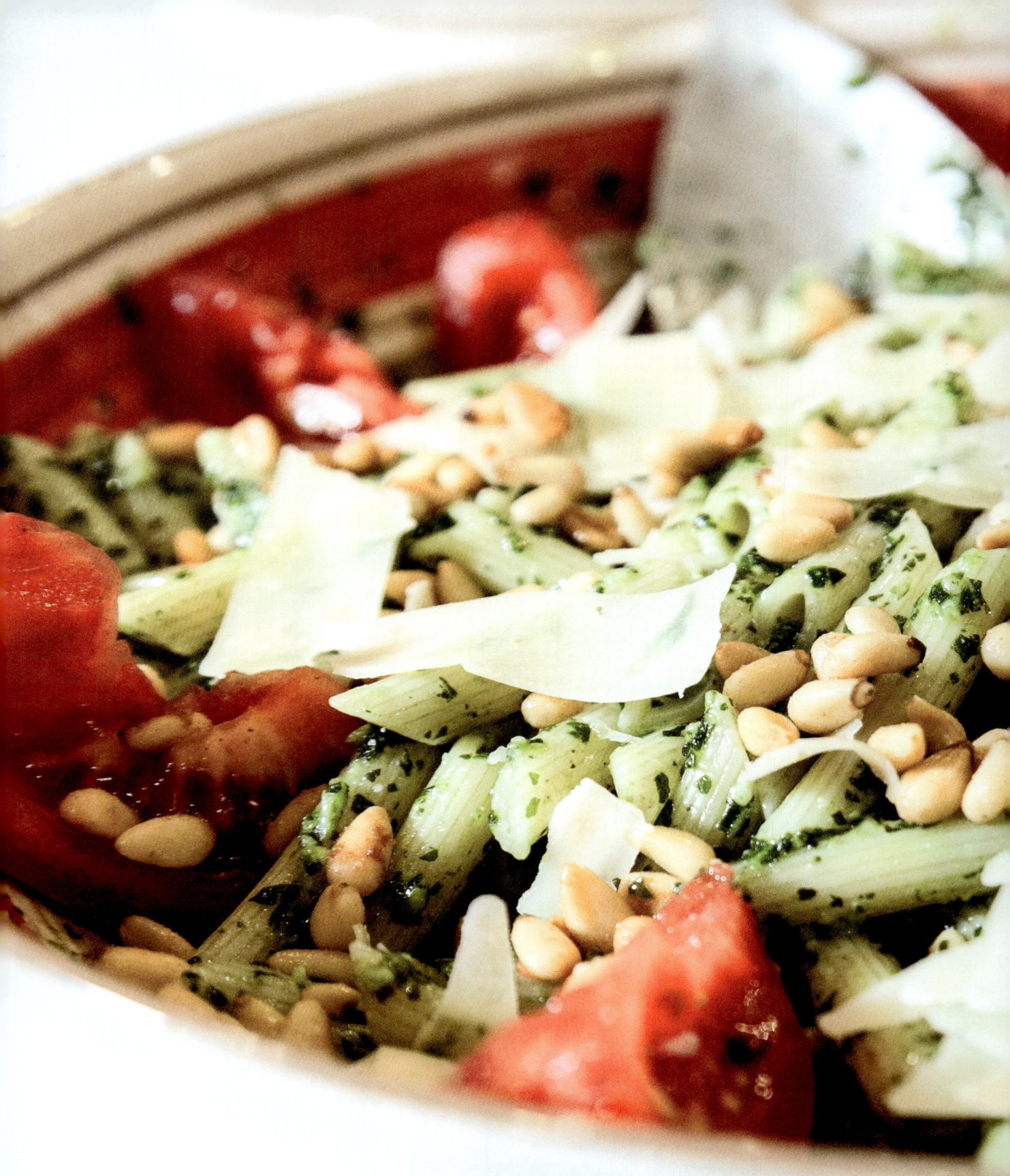

"My kids absolutely love this pesto! It's so quick to make, and the fresh flavors always have everyone asking for seconds. We toss it with pasta, spread it on sandwiches, drizzle it over grilled veggies and so much more! This versatile pesto is a family favorite that never disappoints."

—Beverly Banks

Let's celebrate these life giving ingredients!

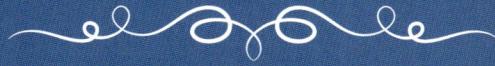

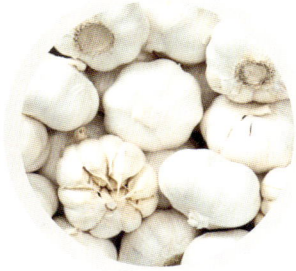

Garlic

- Antibiotic and antimicrobial properties
- Helps combat infections and boost the immune system
- Rich in antioxidants, including allicin
- Lowers blood pressure and improves cholesterol levels
- Reduces the risk of cardiovascular diseases
- Anti-inflammatory properties

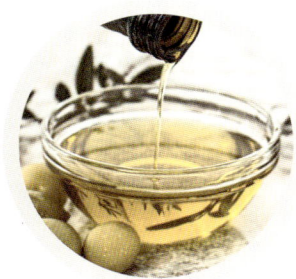

Olive Oil

- Rich in monounsaturated fats
- Helps lower bad cholesterol levels
- Reduces the risk of heart disease
- Protects cells from damage caused by free radicals and oxidative stress
- Has anti-inflammatory properties
- May reduce the risk of Alzheimer's disease

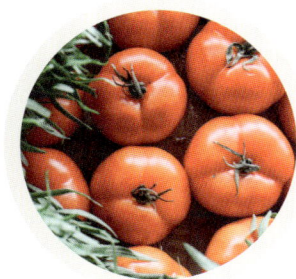

Tomatoes

- Includes vitamin C, potassium, and folate
- Supports the immune system
- Rich in antioxidants like lycopene
- Promotes heart health
- Fiber content aids in digestion

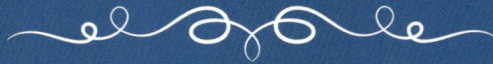

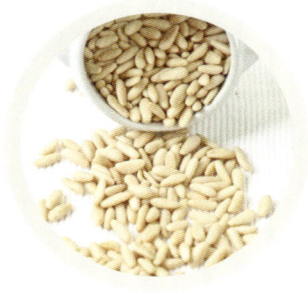

Pine Nuts

- Rich in heart–healthy monounsaturated fats
- Lowers LDL (bad) cholesterol levels
- Reduces the risk of heart disease
- Good source of protein
- Provides essential amino acids for muscle repair and growth
- Contains vitamin E, vitamin K, magnesium, and zinc
- Plays a key role in immune function, bone health, and antioxidant activity

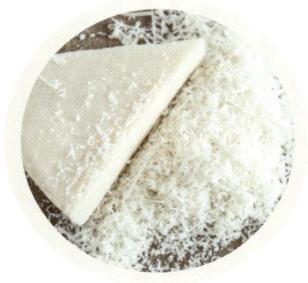

Parmesan Cheese

- Packed with protein and calcium
- Supports muscle health
- Supports bone strength, and overall growth and development
- Has vitamin A, vitamin B12, and zinc
- Supports immune function
- Supports vision health
- Strong metabolism
- Naturally low in lactose

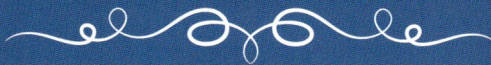

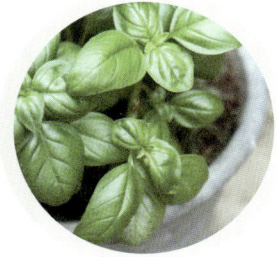

Basil

- Contains vitamins K and C
- Contains vitamin A, which supports eye health and immune function
- Essential for immune function, bone health, and collagen production
- High in antioxidants like flavonoids and polyphenols
- Helps reduce inflammation

"When I walked into Teri's kitchen one day, the aroma of the fresh basil and pine nuts roasting on her cooktop literally stopped me in my tracks. After just one bite the flavors literally burst in my mouth and joy hit my face and heart! I knew I had to have this recipe and look forward to sharing it with others many times over!"

-Lisa Trenary

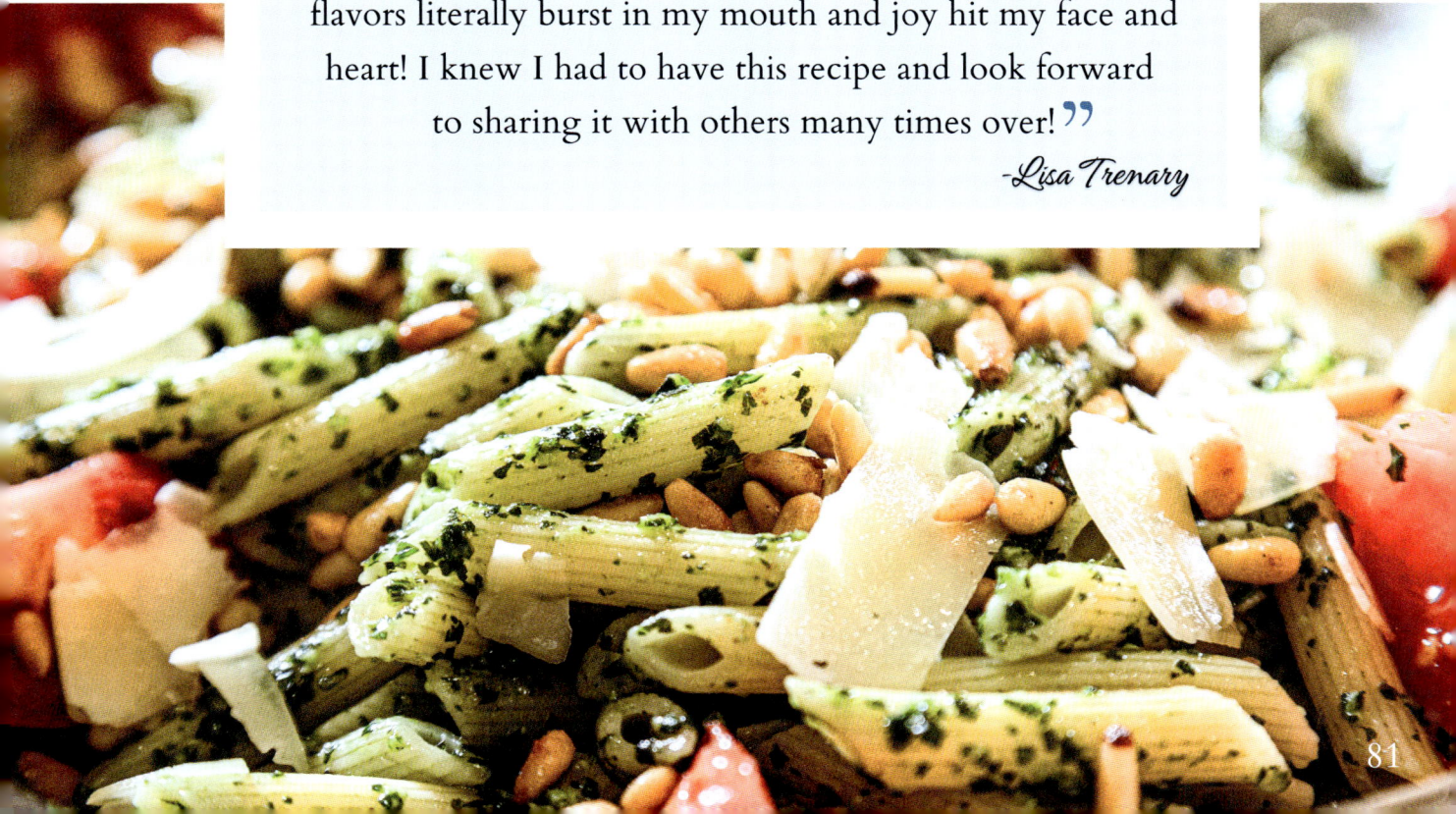

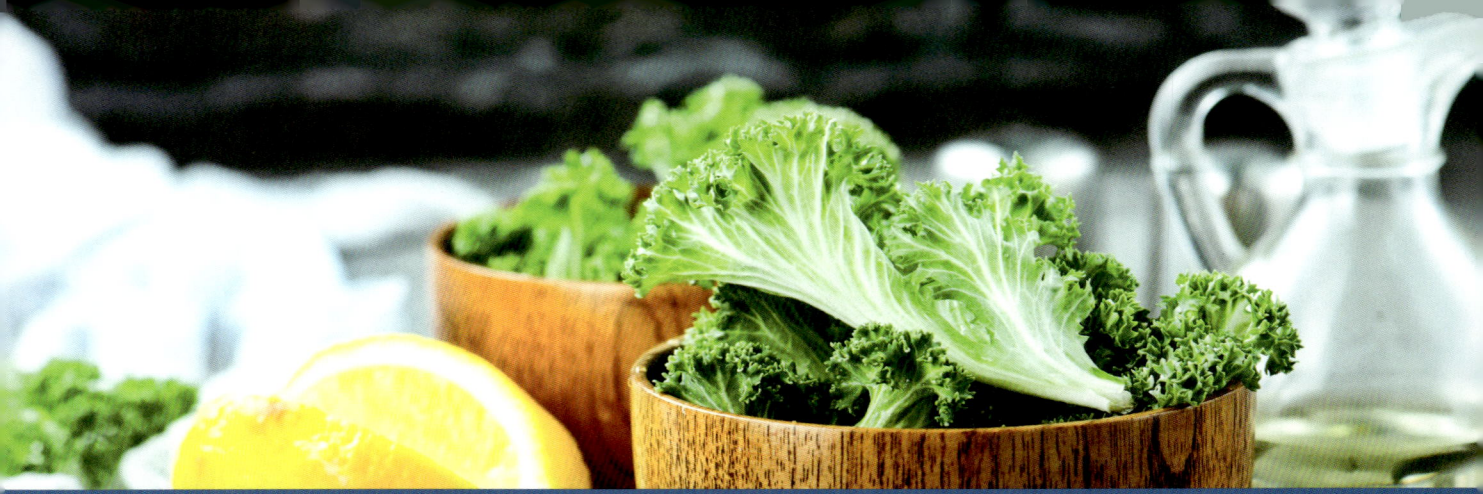

TERI'S SIGNATURE CAESAR SALAD

Ingredients

Teri's Caesar Dressing

2 organic egg yolks

1 Tbsp fresh lemon juice

1 tsp anchovy paste

1 tsp Dijon mustard

2 garlic cloves, minced

2 drops YL Vitality Black Pepper oil

2 drops YL Vitality Lemon oil

(Order YL Vitality Essential Oils on page 39)

1 tsp Worcestershire sauce

1/2 tsp salt

1/2 cup olive oil

2 Tbsp Parmesan cheese, grated

Salad

1 large head of Romaine lettuce

1 cup organic seasoned croutons

1/2 cup Parmesan cheese, shaved

> "My son, Daniel is such a Caesar Salad lover, I created this recipe just for him!"

Preparation

1. In a non-skid heavy bowl, whisk together the egg yolks (you may coddle the eggs if concerned about using the raw egg yokes), lemon juice, anchovy paste, Dijon mustard, garlic, oils, Worcestershire sauce, and salt for about 30 seconds until smooth.

2. Then, whisking constantly, drizzle olive oil slowly in a steady stream, keeping in mind that you don't want to add the oil too fast. It should take about 60-90 seconds to whisk in the olive oil.

3. When the dressing thickens, gently stir in the grated Parmesan cheese.

4. Chill the dressing for at least 15 minutes.

5. Meanwhile, wash, dry, and gently tear the Romain lettuce leaves into bite sized pieces. Place into a beautiful chilled salad bowl.

6. Pour about half of the dressing onto the prepared Romaine leaves and toss well. Add additional dressing if the lettuce feels dry.

7. Top with organic croutons and shaved Parmesan cheese for a beautiful presentation.

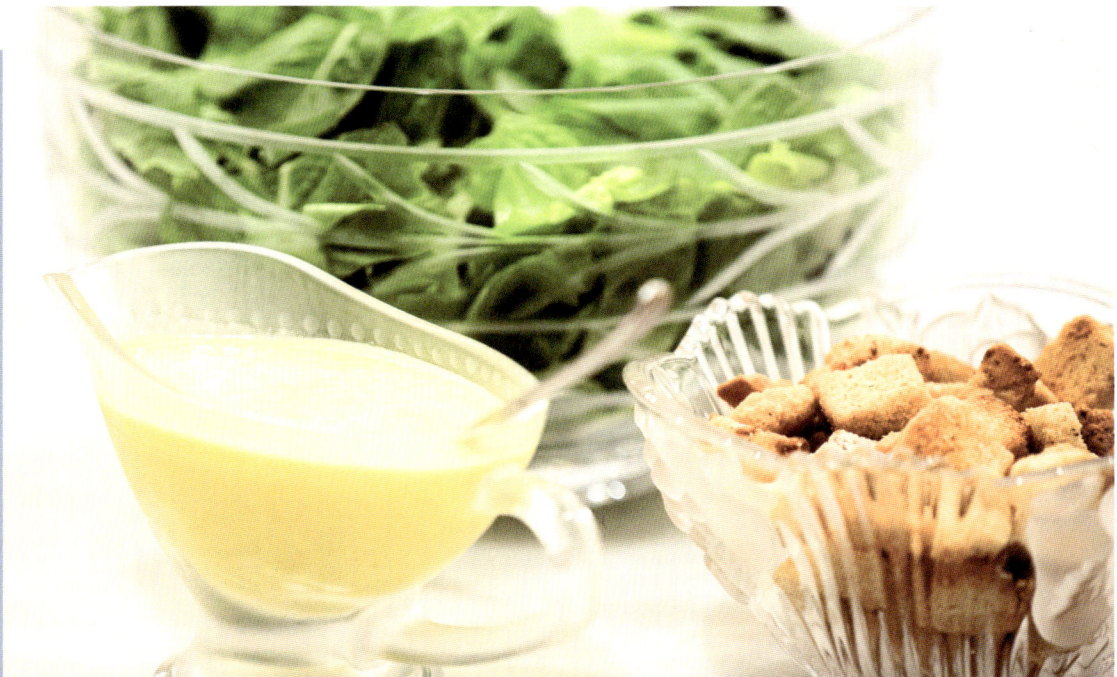

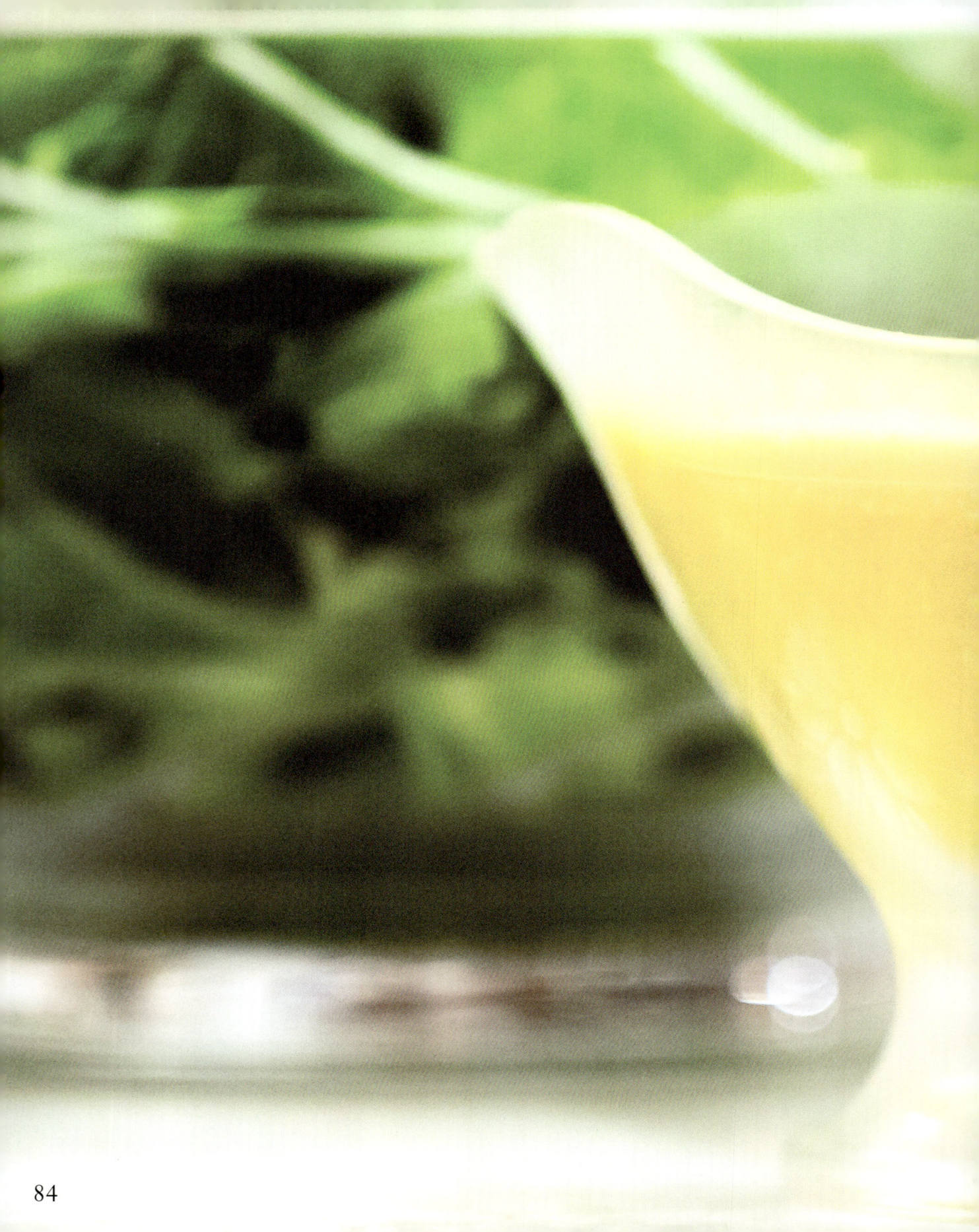

“How would I describe this homemade Caesar Dressing? Just one word, luscious! Store bought dressing simply cannot compare to the flavor and texture!”

Let's celebrate these life giving ingredients!

Eating for Life
WITH TERI SECREST

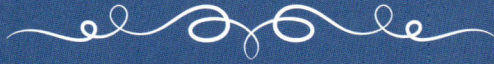

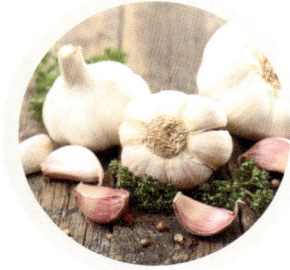

Garlic

- Antibiotic and antimicrobial properties
- Helps combat infections and boost the immune system
- Rich in antioxidants, including allicin
- May reduce oxidative stress and lower the risk of chronic diseases
- Lowers blood pressure and improve cholesterol levels
- Reduces the risk of cardiovascular diseases
- Anti-inflammatory properties may aid in reducing inflammation in the body

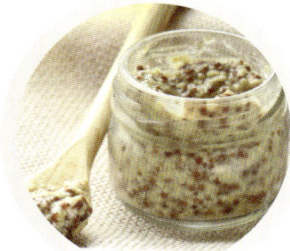

Dijon Mustard

- Contains compounds called isothiocyanates
- Demonstrated antimicrobial properties, aiding in the prevention of foodborne illnesses
- Exhibits anti-inflammatory effects
- Acts as antioxidants, helping neutralize harmful free radicals
- Aids digestion
- Helps alleviate muscle cramps and soreness

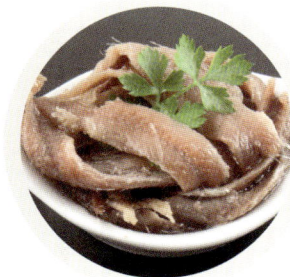

Anchovies

- Rich in omega-3 fatty acids
- Supports heart health and brain function
- Contains protein, vitamins, and minerals

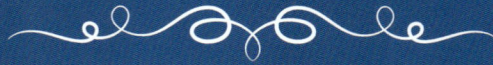

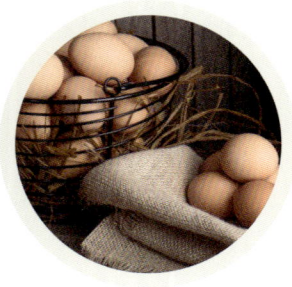

Organic Happy Eggs

- Packed with high-quality protein
- Provides essential amino acids for muscle repair, growth, and overall body function
- Includes vitamin B12, vitamin D, riboflavin, selenium, and choline
- Play crucial roles in metabolism, bone health, brain function, and heart health
- Contains lutein and zeaxanthin, antioxidants that promote eye health
- May reduce the risk of age-related macular degeneration
- Can improve the balance of HDL (good) to LDL (bad) cholesterol

"Making Dressing at home is actually very therapeutic! As you use your wire whisk and begin to see the ingredients come together, you have a silky flavorful creation that is a great edition to every salad."

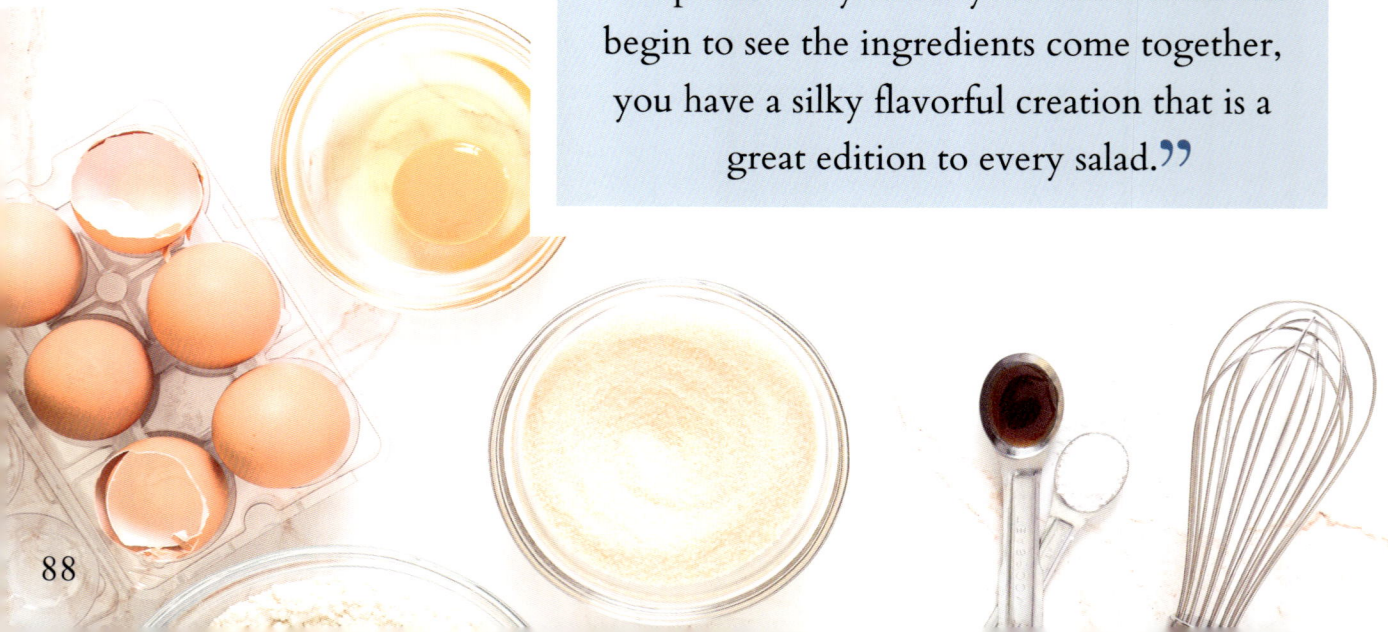

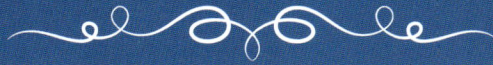

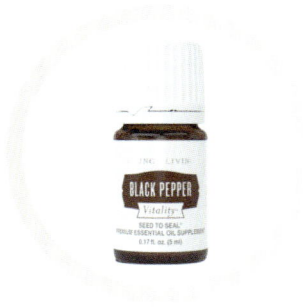

YL Vitality Black Pepper Essential Oil

- Aids in digestive health
- Promotes enzyme activity, helping to alleviate digestive discomfort
- The scent invigorates the mind and boosts alertness, making it a refreshing addition to your daily routine

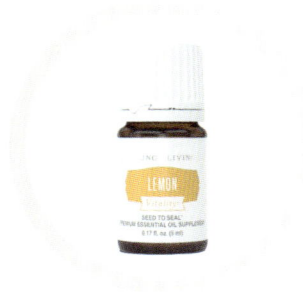

YL Vitality Lemon Oil

- Antioxidant properties
- Helps combat oxidative stress and reduce inflammation
- Supports digestive health
- Alleviates nausea & indigestion
- Immune-boosting properties
- Contains d-limonene

"The Young Living Vitality essential oils of Black Pepper and Lemon take this already great dressing to the next level!"

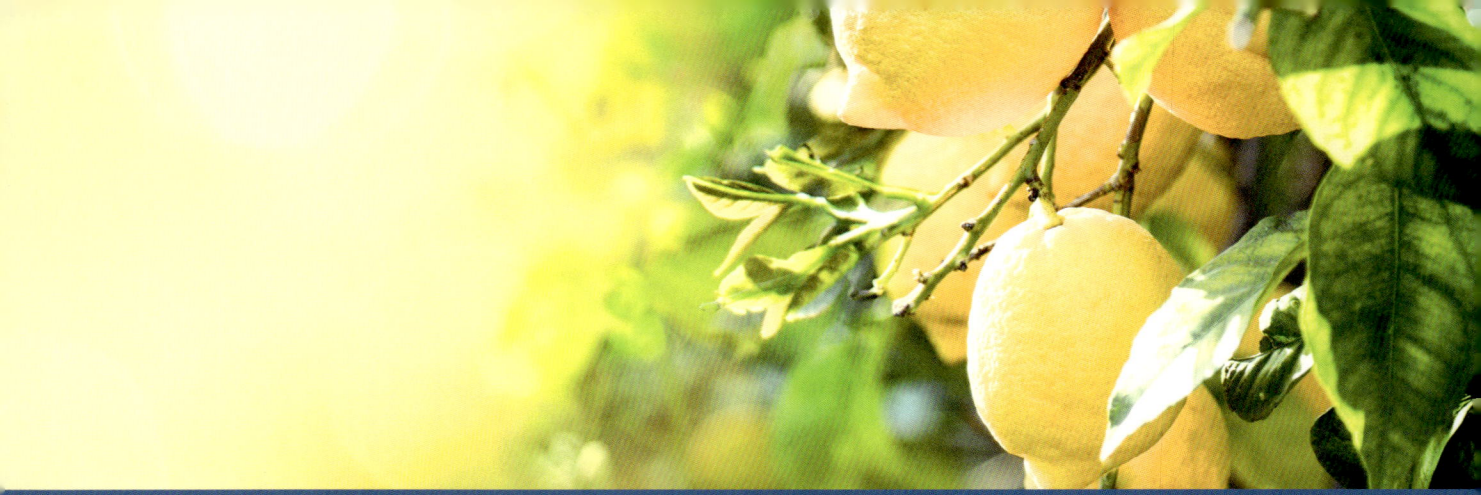

LUSCIOUS LEMON MOUSSE

Ingredients

Makes 4 mouth watering parfait cups

Lemon Curd
(Step 1)

Makes 2 cups of curd
4 large eggs at room temperature

1/2 cup coconut oil

Zest of 2 lemons

1/3 cup raw, unfiltered honey

1/8 tsp fine sea salt

1/2 cup freshly squeezed lemon juice (about 3-4 lemons depending on size)

3 drops YL Vitality Lemon Oil

(Order YL Vitality Essential Oils on page 39)

Luscious Lemon Mousse
(Step 2)

1/2 cup lemon curd from step 1

1 cup cold organic heavy whipping cream or one cup refrigerated coconut cream (for non-dairy option)

1/4 cup powdered sugar

Fresh organic raspberries

Fresh organic blueberries

3 drops YL Lemon Vitality Oil

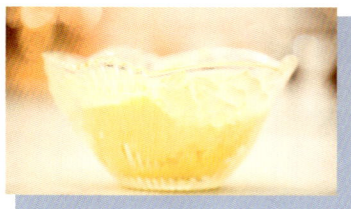

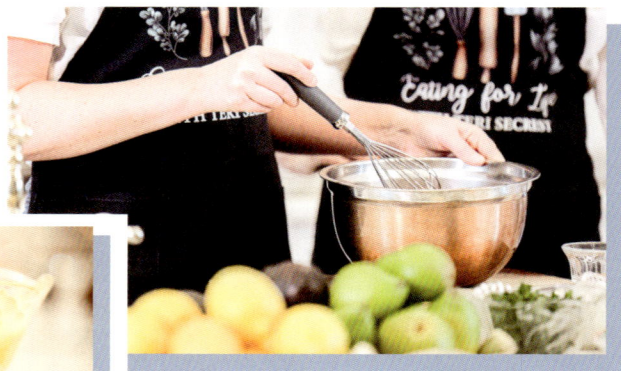

Preparation

Lemon Curd (Step 1)

1. Zest 2 lemons with a zester or hand grater.
2. In a 2-quart, non-stick saucepan, place the eggs, coconut oil, lemon zest, honey, salt and freshly squeezed lemon juice. Whisk together until all ingredients are combined.
3. Heat the mixture over medium-low heat, whisking constantly until thickened to pudding consistency, about 8-10 minutes.
4. Turn off heat and add the YL Vitality Lemon oil.
5. Pour lemon curd into uncovered glass container and allow to come to room temperature.
6. When cooled, cover and refrigerate covered for at least 2 hours, preferably overnight.

Luscious Lemon Mousse (Step 2)

1. In a mixing bowl, combine the chilled Lemon Curd, YL Vitality Lemon oil, chilled heavy whipping cream (or chilled coconut cream), and powdered sugar.
2. Using a hand mixer, begin whipping at a slow speed. Whip for about 3-5 minutes on slow speed. Watch constantly and stop when whipping when silky smooth. Over-whipping will cause the mousse to split!
3. Divide between 4 glasses, cover with plastic wrap, and refrigerate for at least 1 hour.
4. Garnish with raspberries and blueberries for the most exquisite dessert ever!

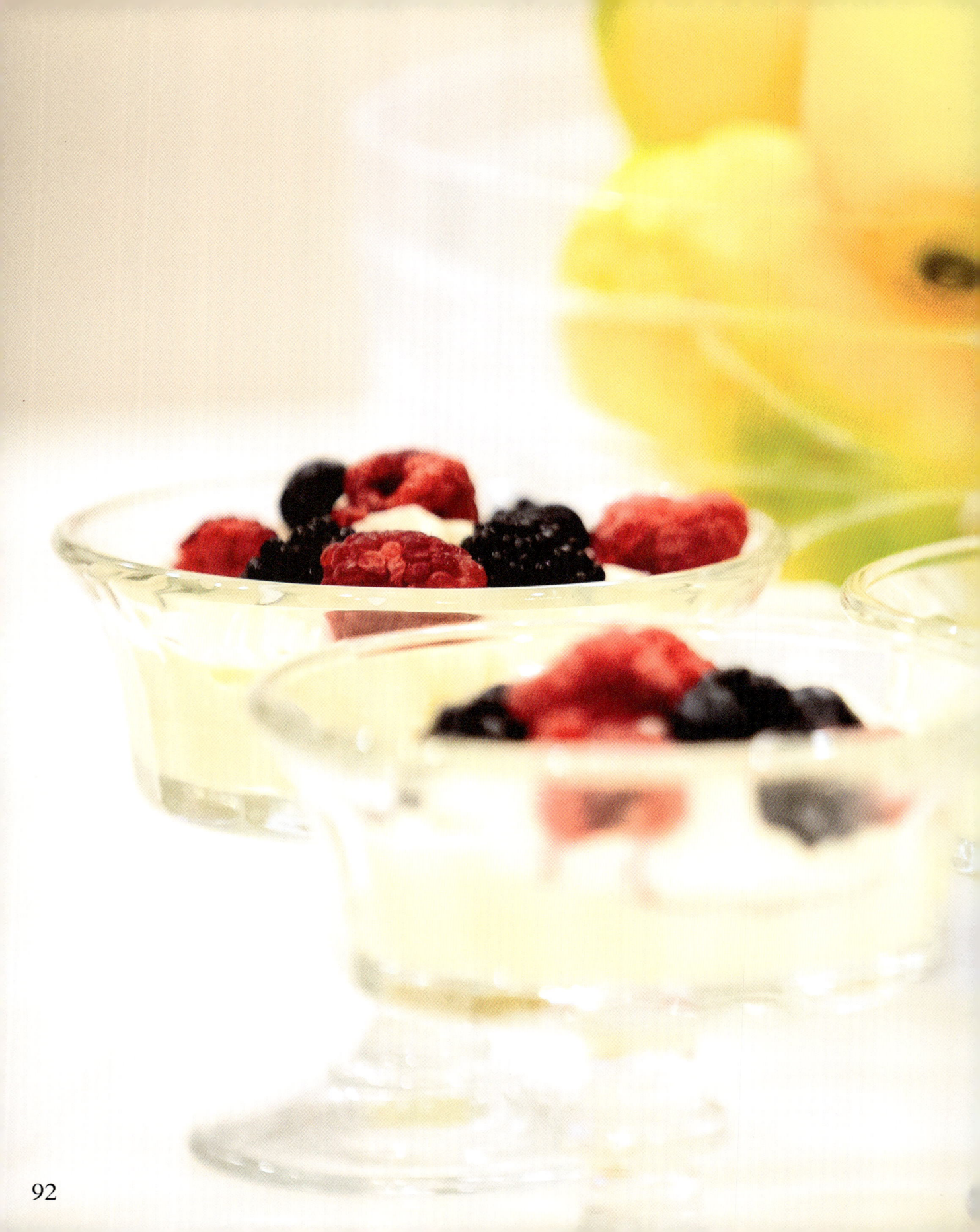

"This Luscious Lemon Mousse has a level of sophistication that deserves a special serving dish. My daughter, Elizabeth and I flipped over these stemmed desserts bowls from France and now we use them several times a week!"

Let's celebrate these life giving ingredients!

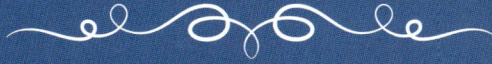

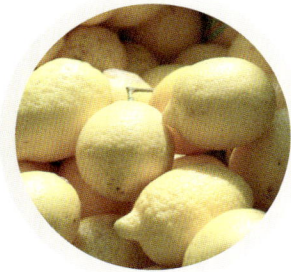

Lemons

- Packed with vitamin C, lemons are a natural immune system booster, helping you fend off colds and infections
- Despite their acidic taste, lemons have an alkalizing effect on the body, promoting PH balance and overall health.
- Start your day with warm lemon water to kickstart digestion, detoxify the body and support liver function.
- The vitamin C in lemons promotes collagen production, keeping skin firm and youthful, while citric acid helps reduce acne and blemishes.

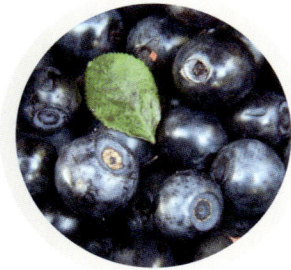

Organic Blueberries

- Packed with antioxidants, particularly anthocyanins
- Protects cells from oxidative damage
- Reduces inflammation
- Great source of vitamins, including vitamin C and vitamin K
- Essential for immune function and bone health

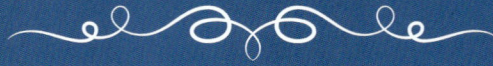

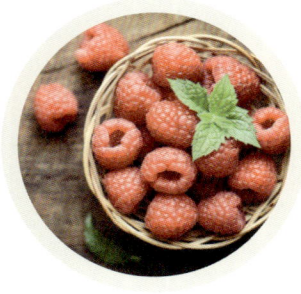

Organic Raspberries

- Rich in antioxidants, particularly vitamin C and quercetin
- Combat free radicals and reduce oxidative stress
- Source of dietary fiber
- Aids digestion
- Beneficial for weight management
- Including vitamin K, manganese, and potassium
- Aids in blood clotting
- Supports healthy heart function

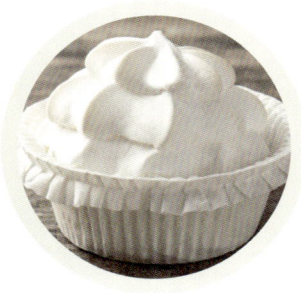

Organic Heavy Whipping Cream

- Natural source of healthy fats
- Maintains stable blood sugar levels
- Source of fat-soluble vitamins like A, D, E, and K.
- Vital for immune health, bone maintenance, and skin integrity

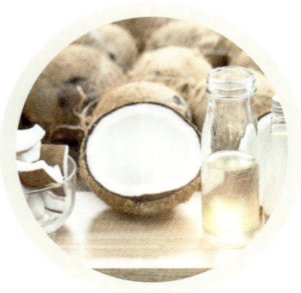

Coconut Oil

- Rich in medium-chain fatty acids, especially lauric acid
- Supports heart health
- Boosts metabolism
- Contains antioxidants
- Reduces inflammation
- Protects against oxidative stress
- Suitable for cooking at high temperatures

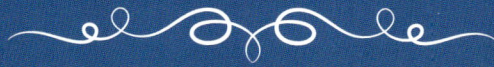

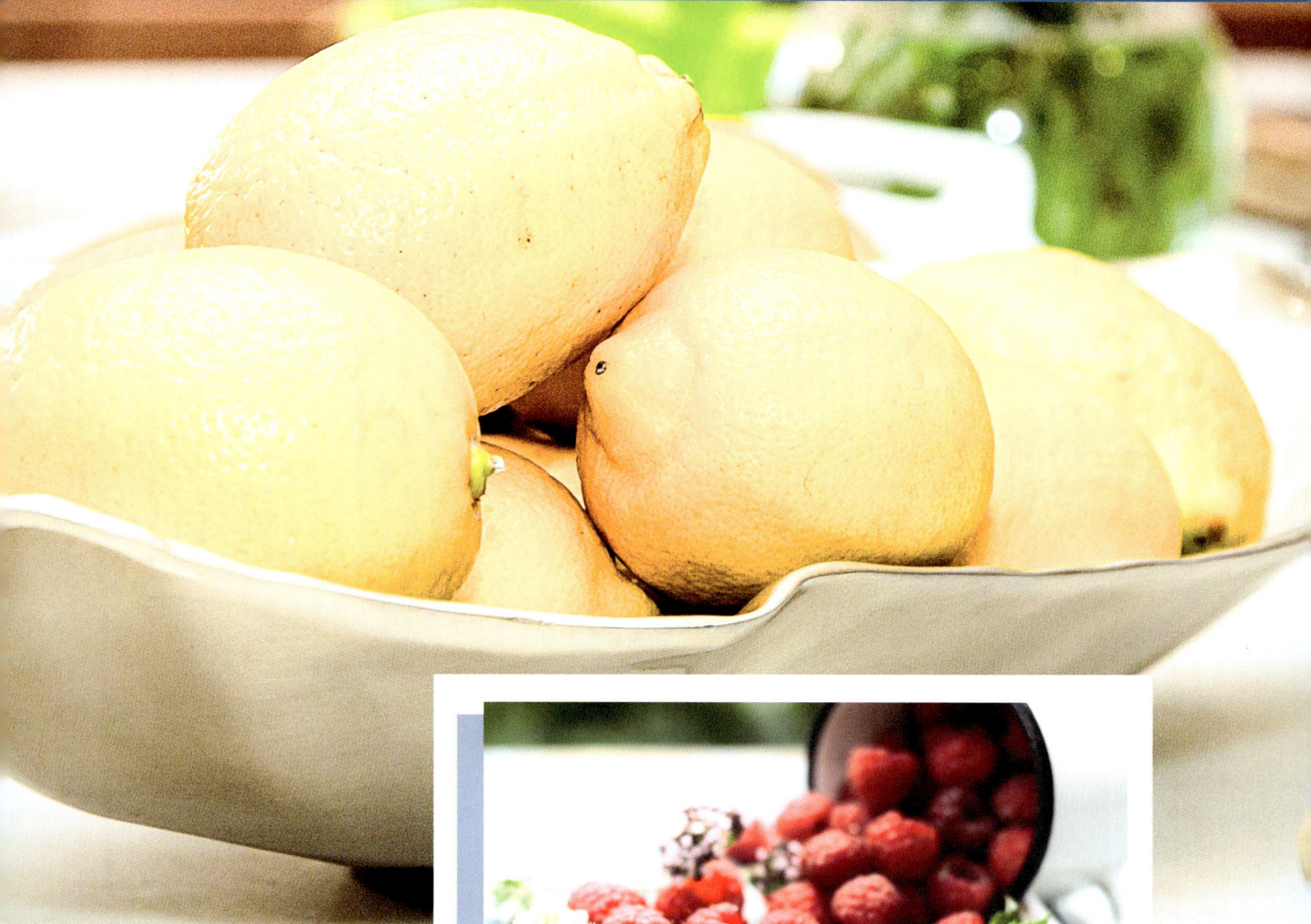

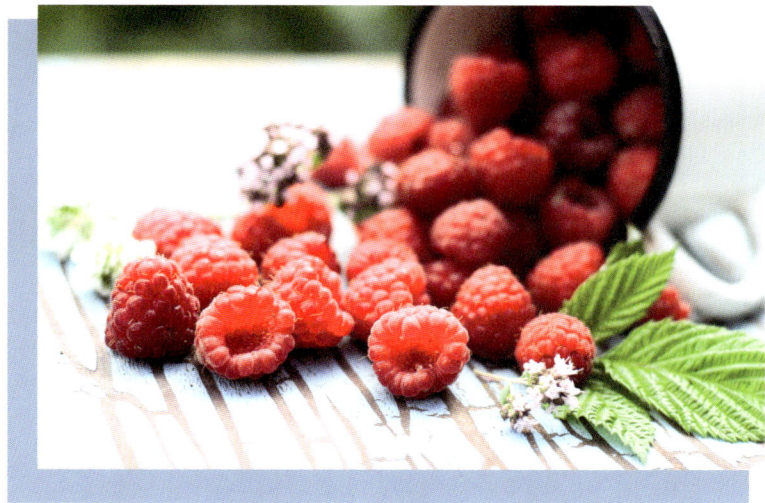

"This Luscious Lemon Mousse literally melts in your mouth! It has been voted the favorite dessert by many of my friends!"

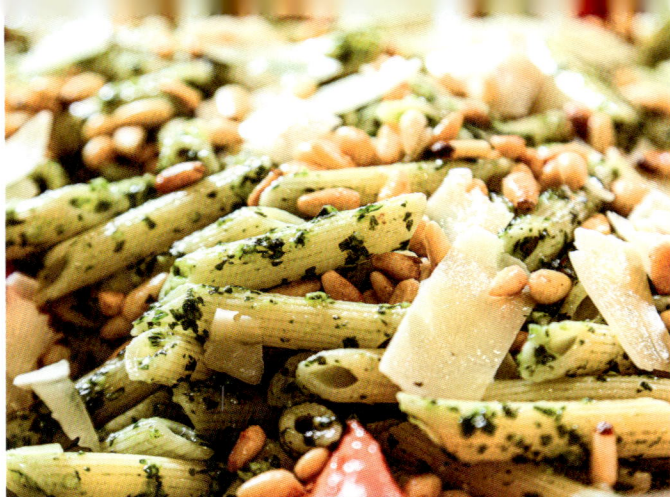

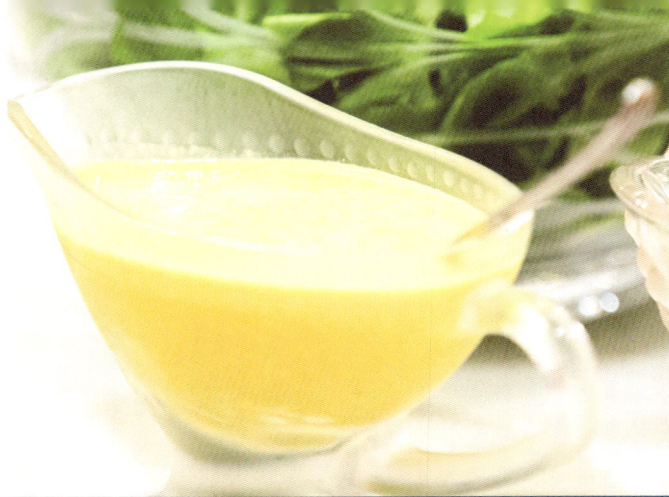

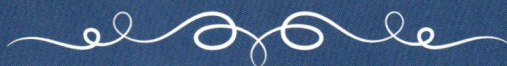

Week 3
Full Menu Shopping List

Produce

2 cups fresh sweet basil leaves

3 cloves fresh garlic

2-3 tomatoes

1 large head of Romaine lettuce

2 garlic cloves

4 lemons

1 container organic raspberries

1 container organic blueberries

Baking & Spices

Olive oil

1/2 cup pine nuts

Coconut oil

Raw, unfiltered honey

Fine sea salt

Powdered sugar

From Young Living*

YL Vitality Lemon Oil

YL Vitality Black Pepper Oil

SEE PAGE 39 FOR ORDERING DETAILS

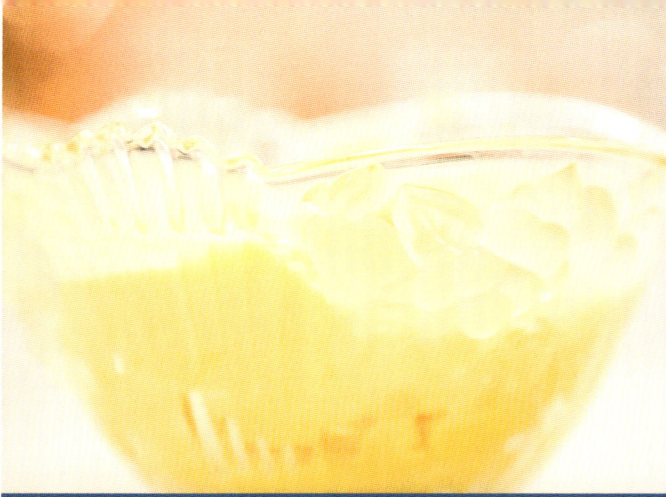

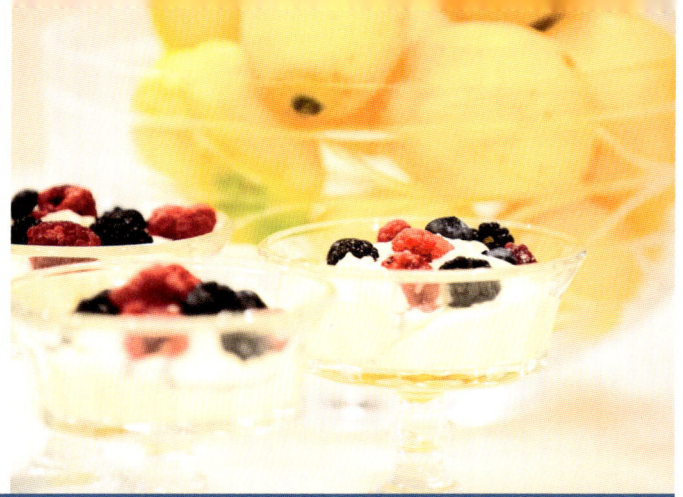

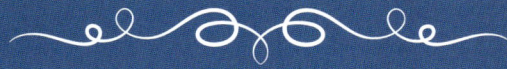

Full Menu Shopping List continued

Condiments

Anchovy paste
Dijon mustard
Worcestershire sauce

Dry Goods

1 lb organic penne pasta,
(my favorite is made from
Durham wheat)
Organic seasoned croutons

Dairy

1/2 cup Parmesan cheese,
grated
1/2 cup Parmesan cheese,
shaved
Butter
6 large organic eggs
1 pt organic heavy whipping
cream
*substitute 1 can of full-fat
coconut cream for a non-dairy
option

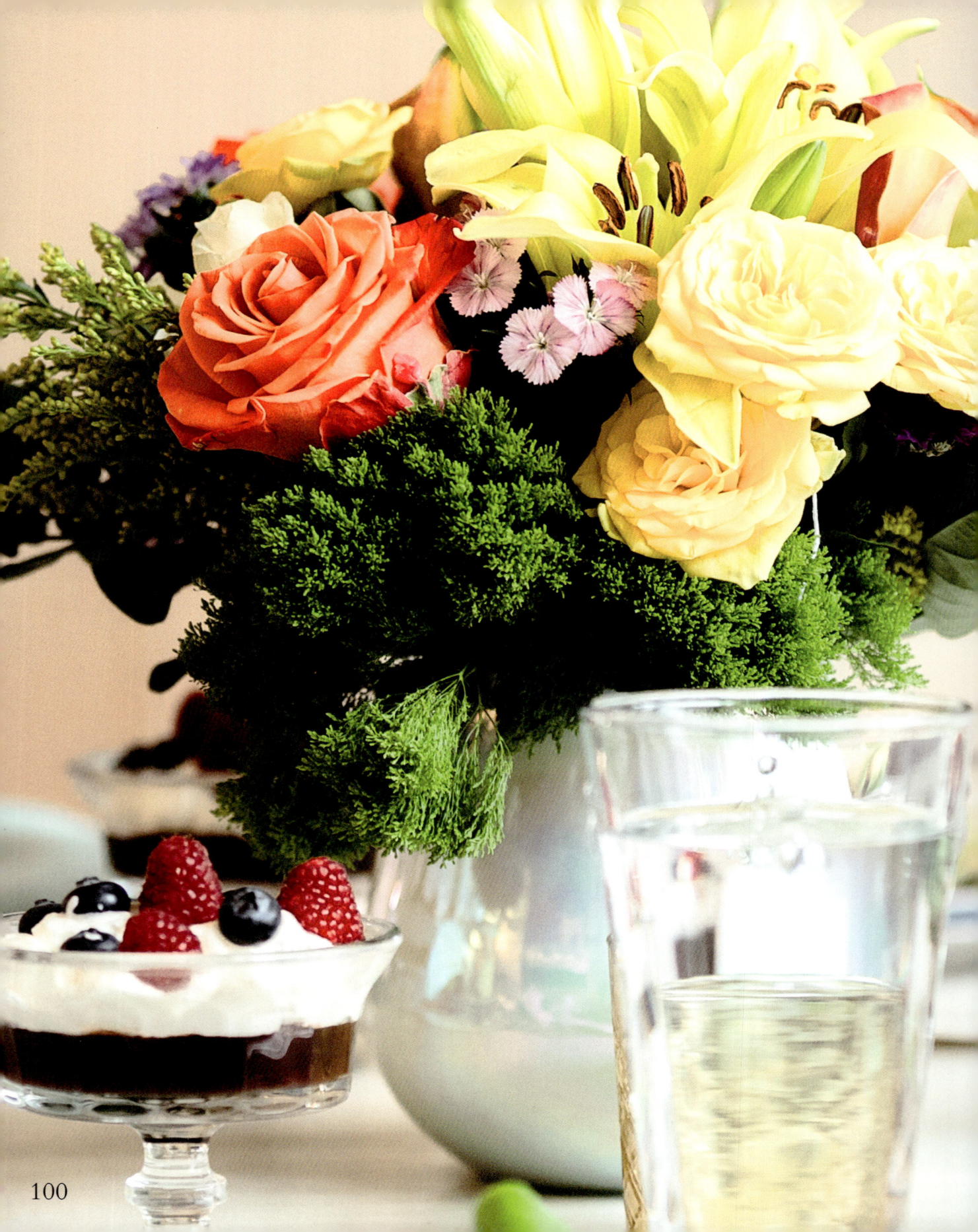

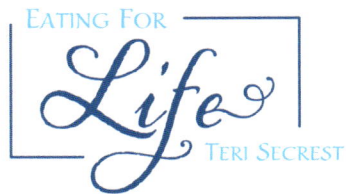

WEEK *Four* MENU

Salmon with Lemon Butter Sauce

❀

Costa Rican Rice

❀

Pear & Avocado Salad

❀

Honey Toasted Pecans

❀

NingXia Red Parfait

❀

Whipped Cream/Coconut Cream

❀

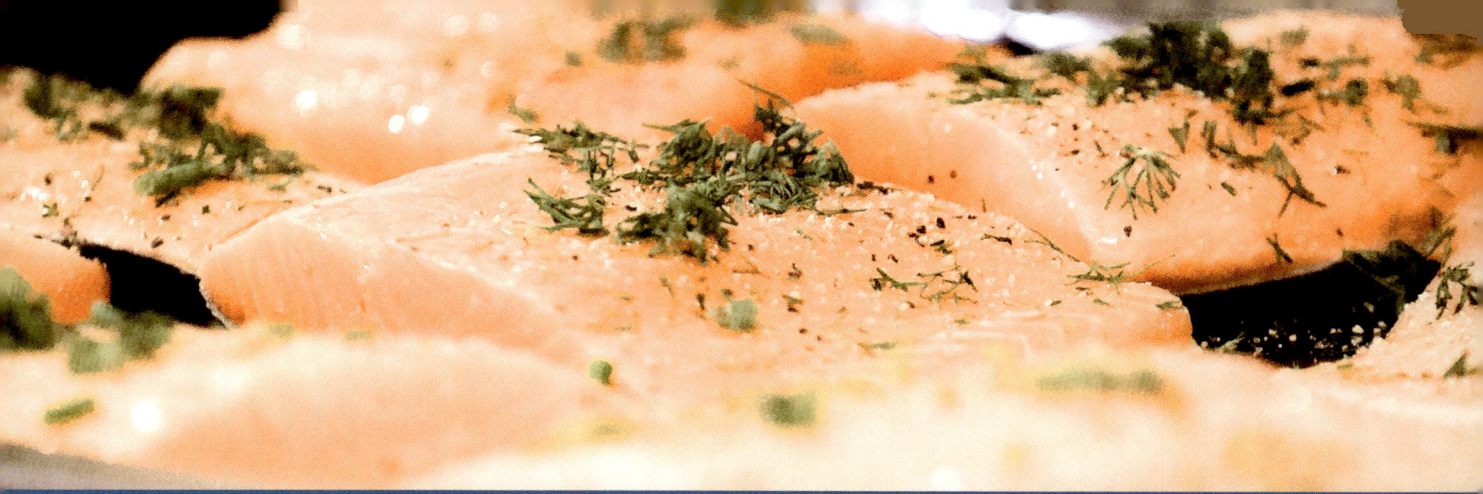

SALMON WITH LEMON BUTTER SAUCE

Ingredients
Create 4 Amazing Portions!

Salmon

Wild-caught salmon, 6 to 8
ounces per person
Olive oil
Lemon pepper seasoning
2 tsp fresh dill, chopped
8 lemon slices, thinly sliced
Butter (optional)

Lemon Butter Sauce

4 Tbsp olive oil
3 tsp capers, smashed with a fork
1/2 tsp fresh Dill, chopped
2-3 Tbsp white wine (optional)
Juice of 2 small lemons
2-3 Tbsp arrowroot powder
1 cup chicken stock
5 Tbsp organic heavy whipping
cream
3 Tbsp butter

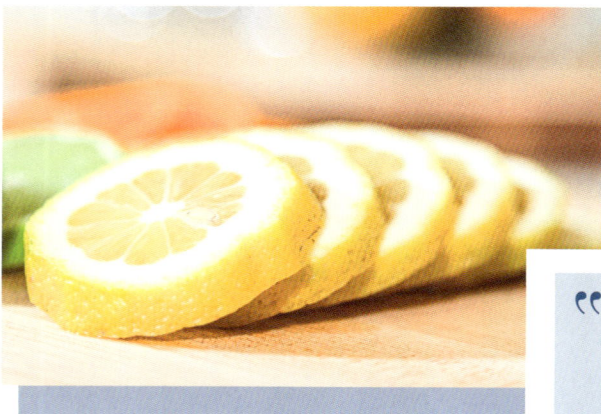

"This spectacular dinner is truly
worthy of candlelight and
thoughtful table settings."

Preparation

Instructions for Salmon

1. Preheat the oven to 350°F and line a baking sheet pan with parchment paper.
2. Rinse the salmon under cold water and pat dry with paper towels.
3. Place the salmon skin side down on the baking pan.
4. Drizzle olive oil over the salmon, ensuring it is evenly coat to prevent it from drying out.
5. Sprinkle lemon pepper seasoning generously over the top of the salmon.
6. Sprinkle freshly chopped dill over the seasoned salmon (about 1/2 tsp per fillet.)
7. Arrange 2 lemon slices on top of each salmon filet.
8. If desired, place small pieces of butter on top of the salmon for added richness.
   Before continuing to step 9, consider pausing here and making the Lemon Butter Sauce.
9. Bake until you see the white come up to the top of each fillet and they flake easily with a fork. Cooking time varies depending on the thickness of the salmon fillet. Thin fillets usually take 10-12 minutes. Thick fillets can take up to 15-19 minutes.

> "Exquisite music adds an unforgetable touch to your evening. Andre Bocceli's Italian music mirrors the high quality of this Alaskan salmon."

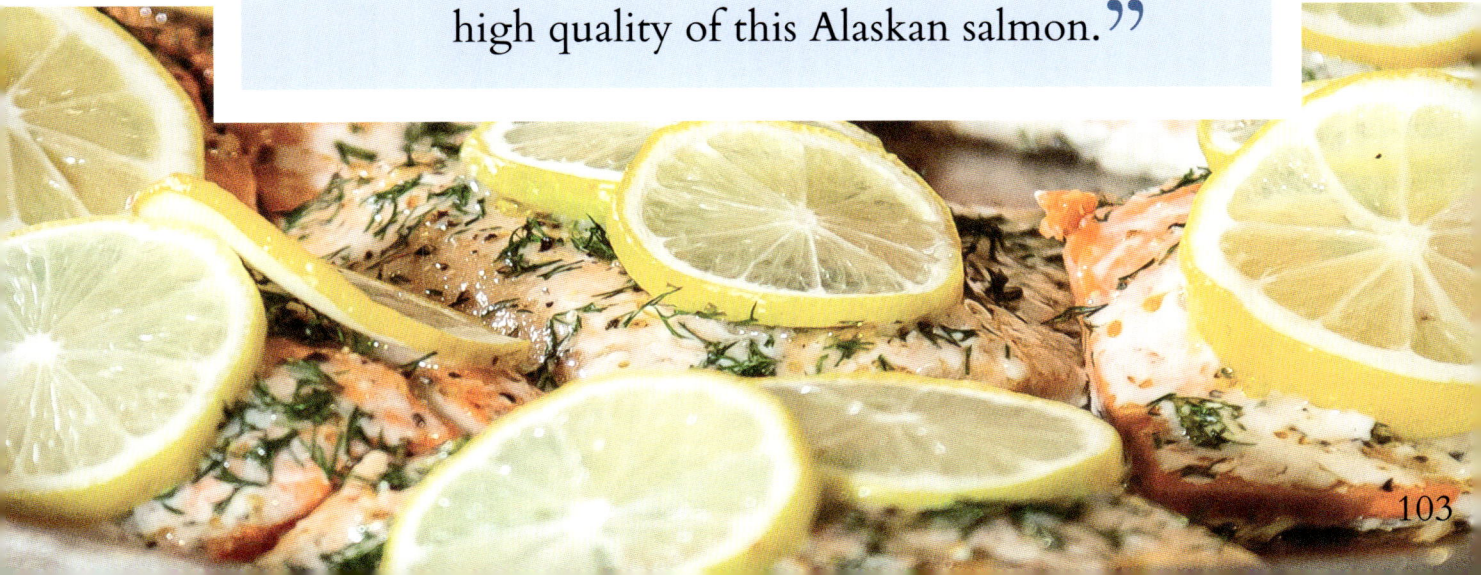

"Once the salmon is cooked, serve it hot with the lemon butter sauce drizzled over the top. Place extra sauce in your favorite sauce dish and set on the dinner table for a delightful topping to your Costa Rican Rice and extra for the salmon."

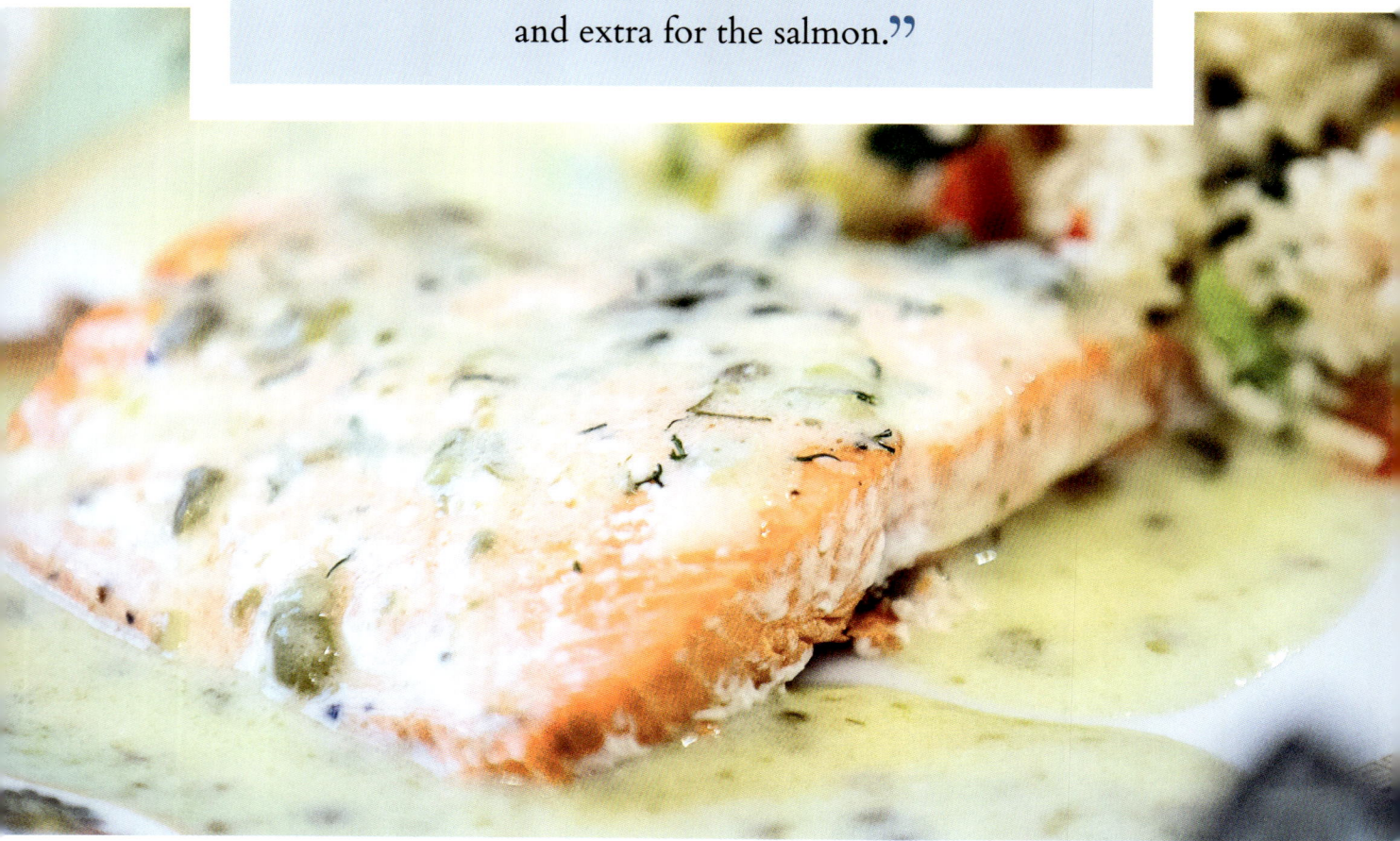

Preparation

Instructions for Lemon Butter Sauce

I recommend making the sauce before putting the salmon in the oven.

1. In a saucepan over low heat, combine olive oil, smashed capers, and fresh dill. Cook for 1-2 minutes until fragrant.

2. Add the lemon juice and white wine (optional) to the saucepan, stirring to combine.

3. In a separate cup, whisk arrowroot with chicken stock until well combined. Pour this mixture into the saucepan, stirring continuously as you pour (For a thinner sauce use 2 Tbs of arrowroot, for thicker sauce use 3 Tbs).

4. Cook the sauce for several minutes on simmer, allowing it to thicken.

5. Stir in the heavy whipping cream and continue to cook for another minute.

6. Finally, add the butter to the sauce, stirring until melted and well incorporated.

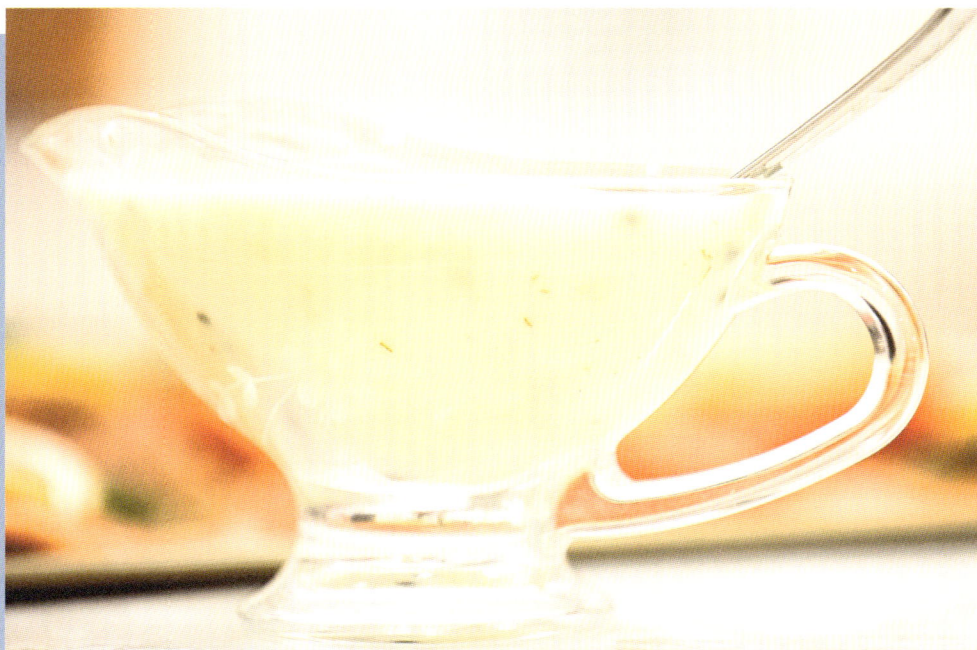

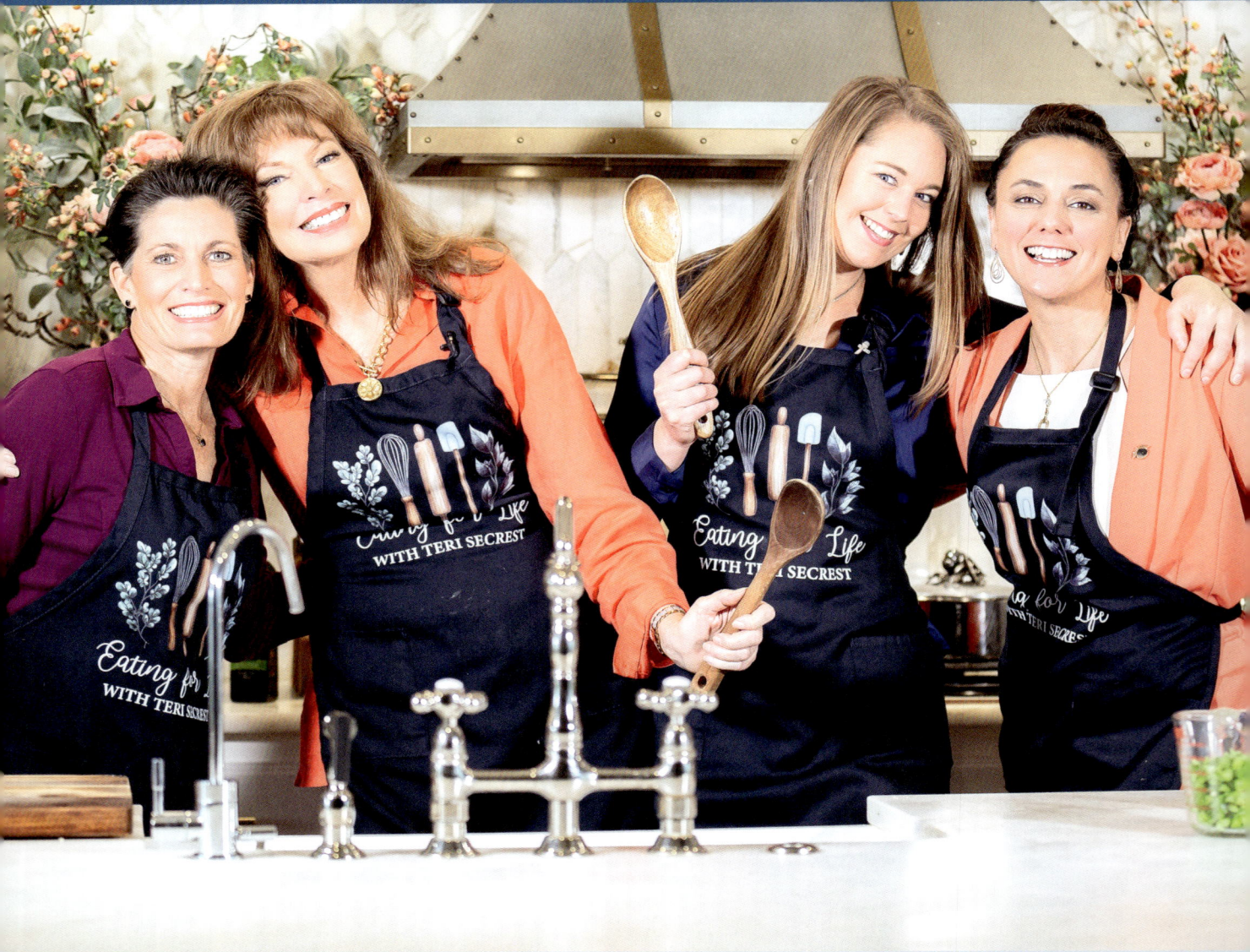

Let's celebrate these life giving ingredients!

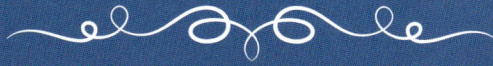

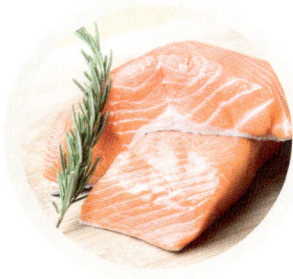

Wild Caught Salmon

- Rich in high-quality protein and omega-3 fatty acids
- Reduces the risk of heart disease
- Supports brain & cognitive function
- Omega-3 fatty acids, particularly EPA and DHA, reduce inflammation
- Has vitamin D for bone health, immune function, and mood regulation
- Minerals like selenium, potassium, and magnesium
- Antioxidant protection
- Supports healthy aging

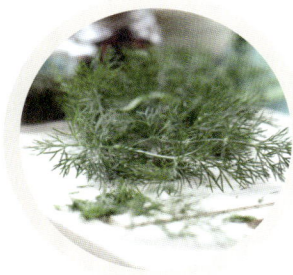

Dill

- Contains flavonoids, and monoterpenes
- Antioxidant and anti-inflammatory properties
- Reduces inflammation
- Rich in vitamin C, vitamin A, manganese, and iron
- Has digestive benefits
- Helps relieve gas, bloating, and indigestion

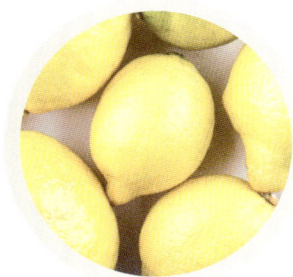

Lemons

- Packed with vitamin C, lemons are a natural immune system booster, helping you fend off colds and infections.
- Despite their acidic taste, lemons have an alkalizing effect on the body, promoting PH balance and overall health.
- Start your day with warm lemon water to kickstart digestion, detoxify the body and support liver function.
- The vitamin C in lemons promotes collagen production, keeping skin firm and youthful, while citric acid helps reduce acne and blemishes.

Organic Heavy Whipping Cream

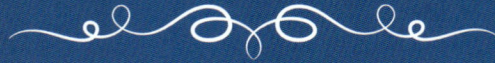

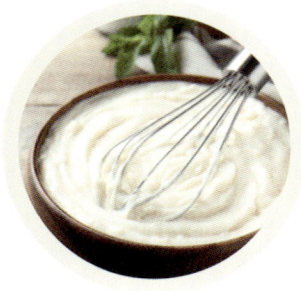

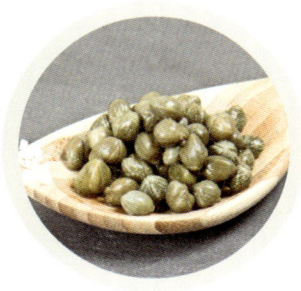

- Good source of healthy fats, including saturated and monounsaturated fats
- Provide essential energy
- Supports hormone production
- Contains vitamins A, D, E, and K
- Good source of calcium

Capers

- Rich source of antioxidants, particularly rutin and quercetin
- Combat free radicals and reduce inflammation
- Antimicrobial properties

"This exquisite dish was shared with me by my late, loving husband Reed. We just loved gourmet cooking and entertaining guests together. This was one of his signature dishes. It is my joy to share this with you."

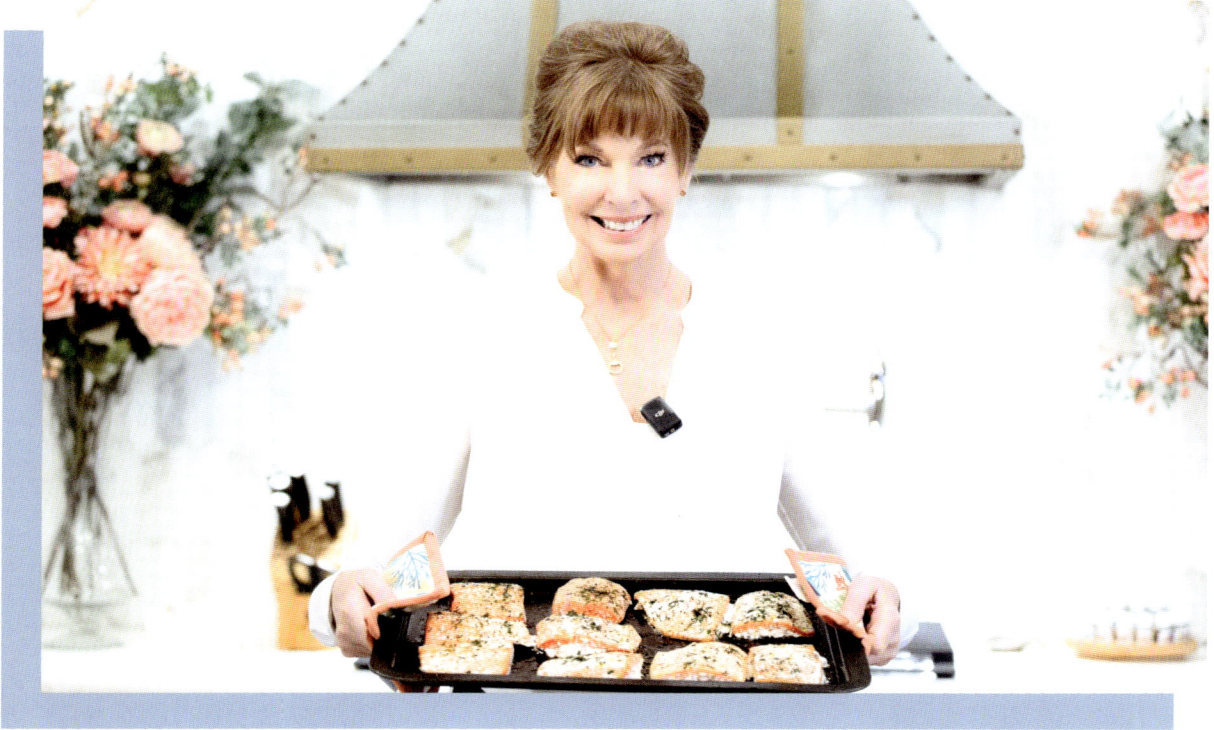

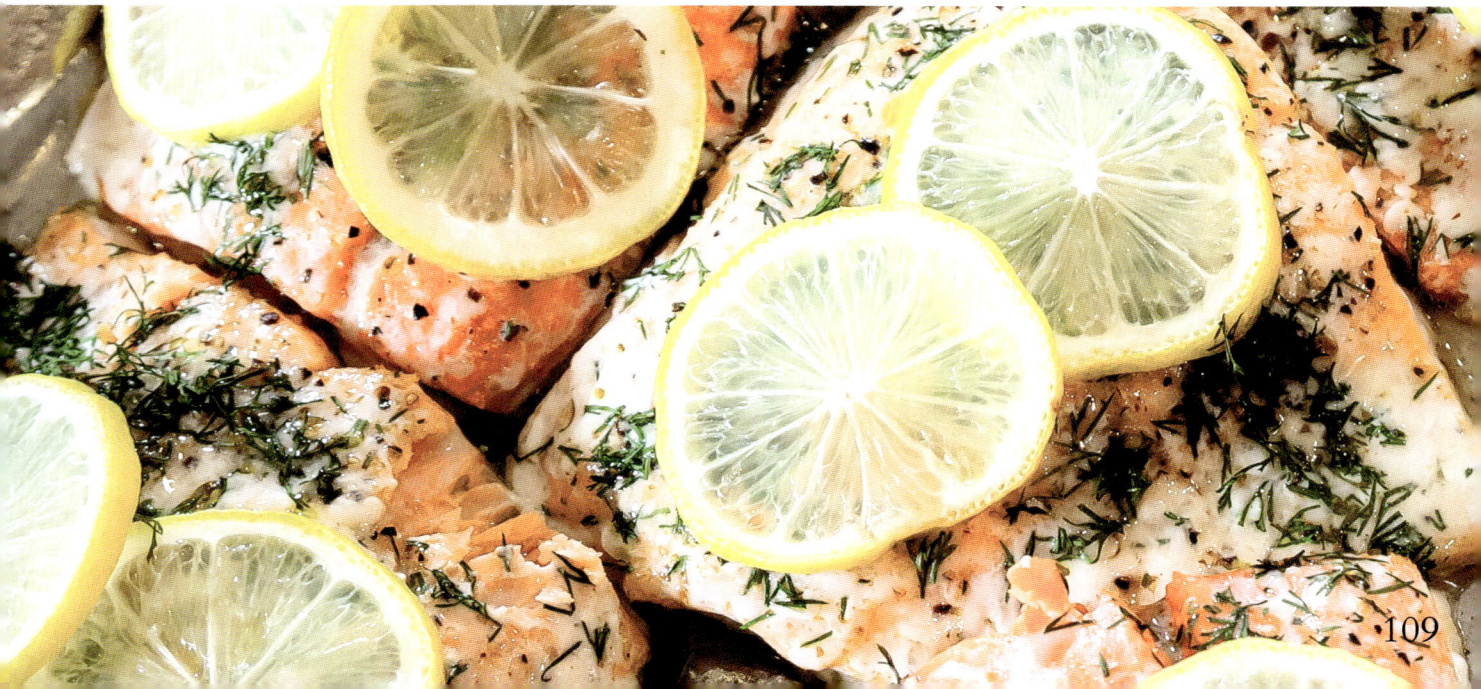

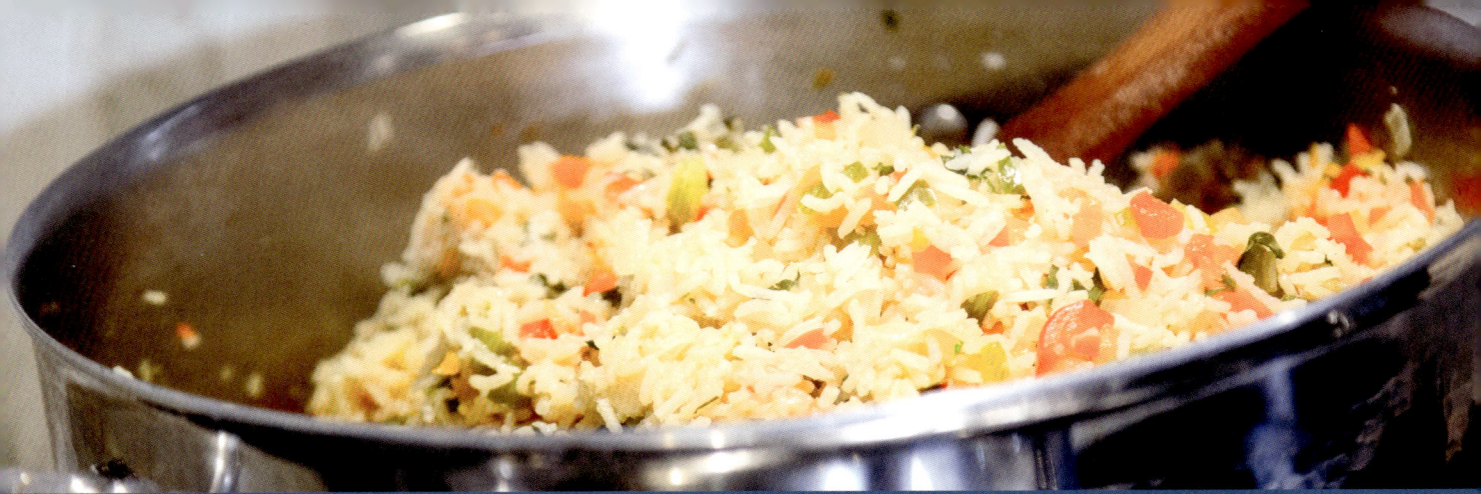

COSTA RICAN RICE

Ingredients
Creates 4 Amazing Portions!

1 cup Basmati rice
2-3 Tbsp olive oil
1/2 each of red, green
and yellow bell
pepper, chopped
1/2 onion, diced
2 garlic cloves, chopped
2 tsp Tony Chachere's
Creole Seasoning
(Blue Label)
2 cups chicken broth
½ cup fresh cilantro

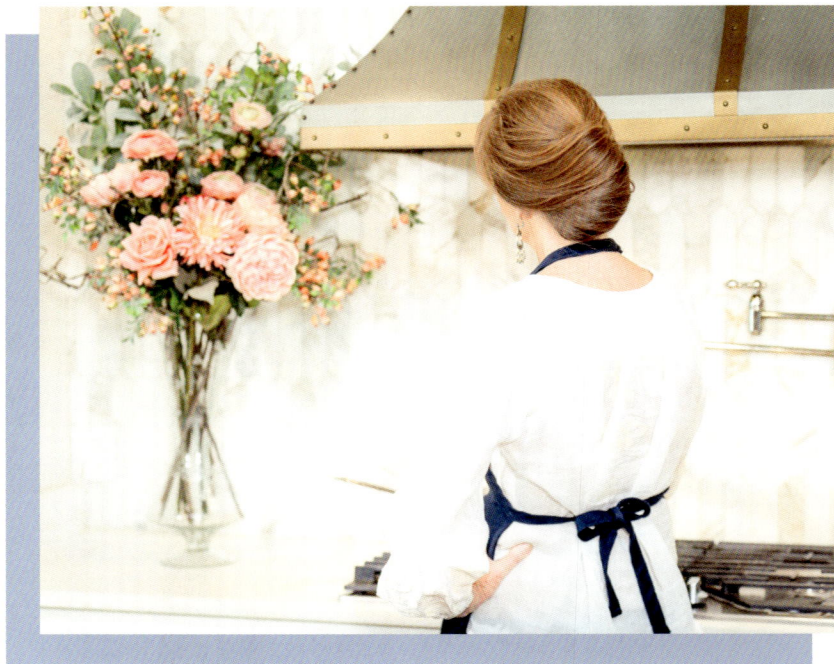

Preparation

> **"**As soon as you bring the rice to the boiling point, simmer is your best friend. I love to simmer my rice and allow the flavors time to come alive!**"**

1. In a skillet, heat the oil over medium heat. Add the chopped onions and garlic, and sauté for a couple of minutes until they become fragrant and translucent.
2. Add the basmati rice to the skillet and stir well. Coat it with the oil, onions, and garlic. Toast the rice for a couple of minutes until it becomes lightly browned.
3. Sprinkle the Tony's Blue Label Seasoning over the rice and stir to incorporate.
4. Pour in the chicken broth and stir well. Bring to a boil and immediately simmer.
5. Cover and let the rice cook for about 15 minutes, or until most of the liquid has been absorbed and the rice is tender.
6. After 15 minutes, add the chopped red, green, and yellow peppers to the skillet. Stir to combine.
7. Cover the skillet again and let the rice cook for an additional 5 minutes or until the peppers are still slightly crisp.
8. Remove the skillet from the heat. Stir in the chopped fresh cilantro, mixing it evenly throughout the rice.
9. Serve the Costa Rican Rice hot as a delicious side dish or as a main course.

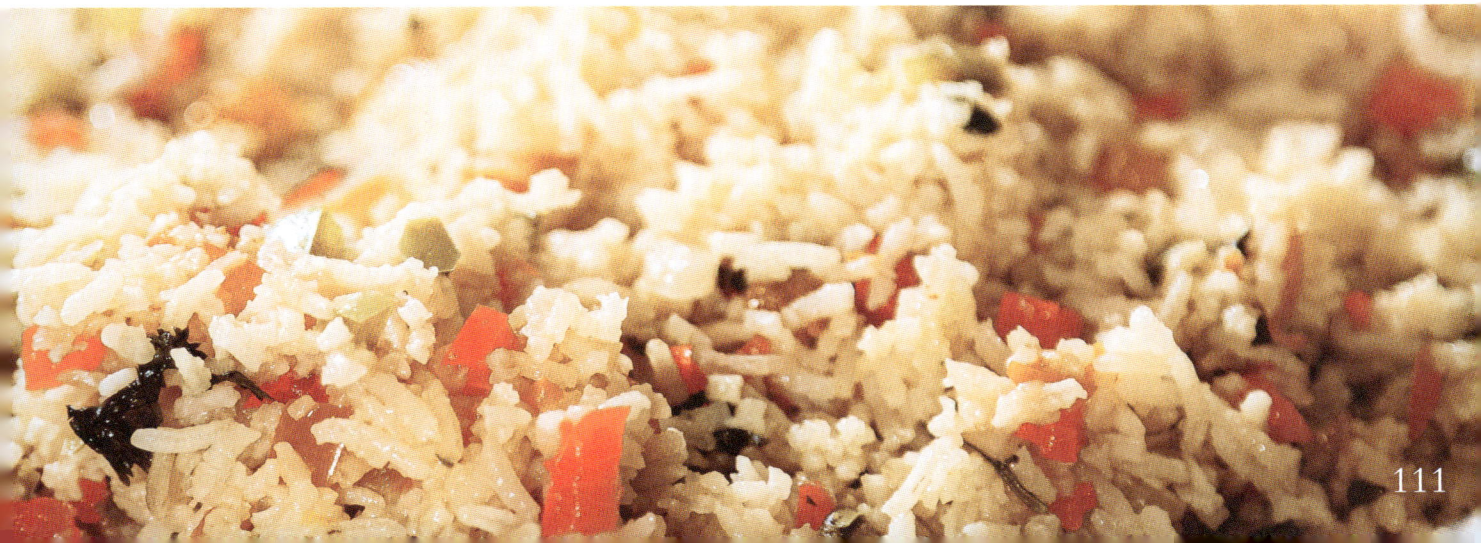

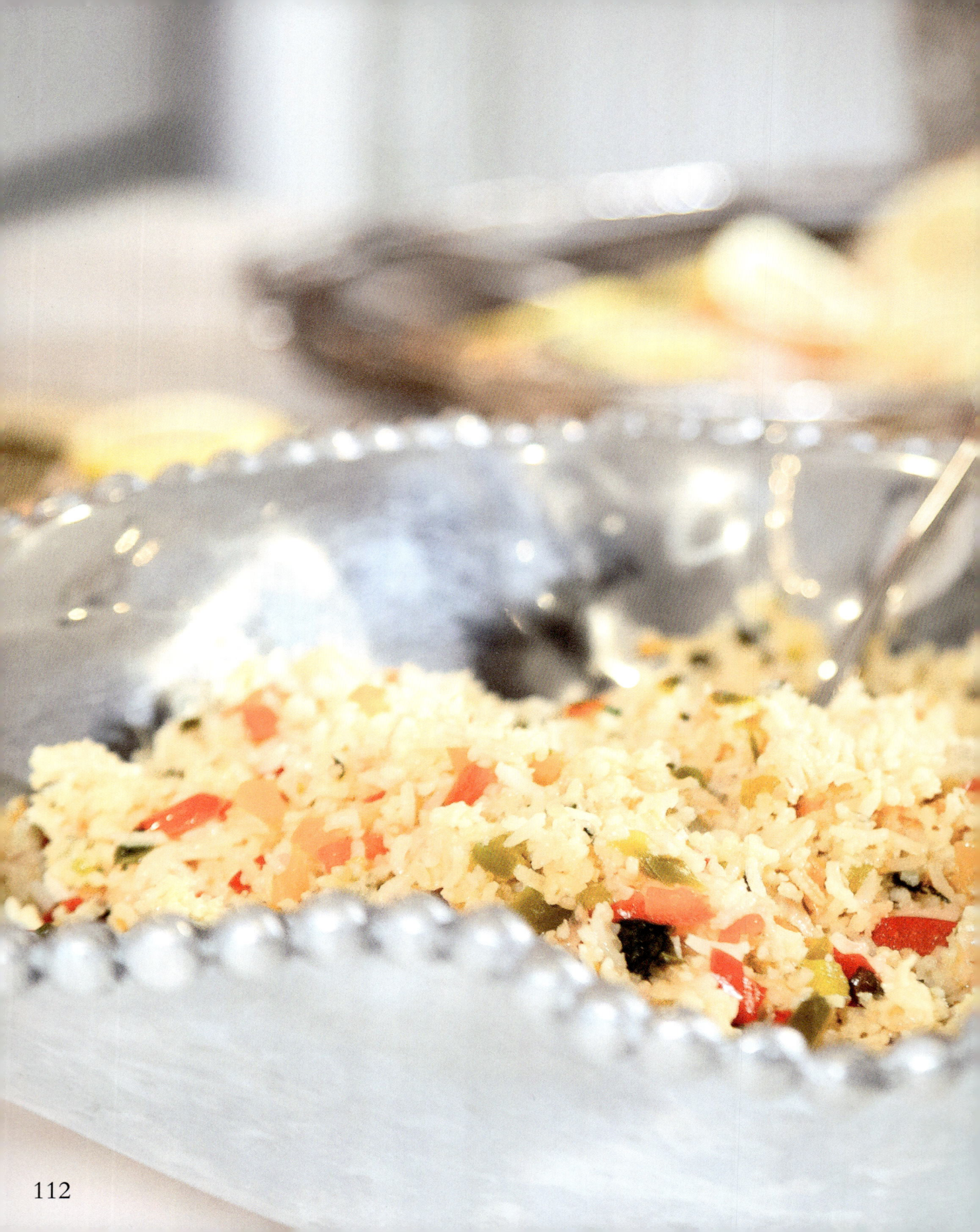

"This is a another spectacular dish that Reed shared with me. I can still hear him saying, "Honey, don't over cook the peppers! Just add them in the last 5 minutes." This dish pairs beautifully with the salmon and it is delicious with the Lemon Butter Sauce on it."

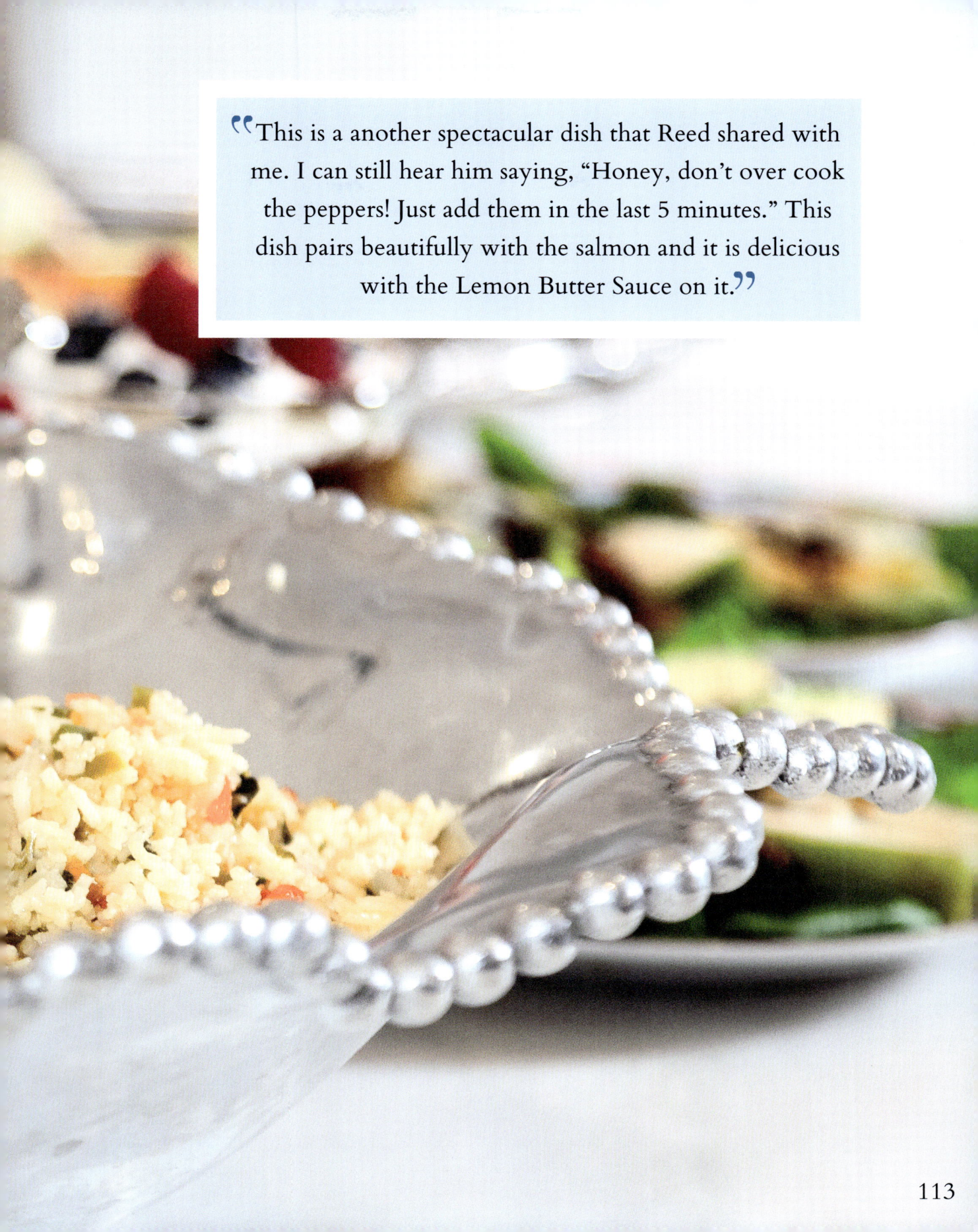

Let's celebrate these life giving ingredients!

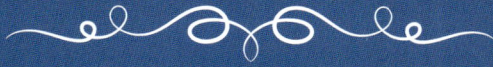

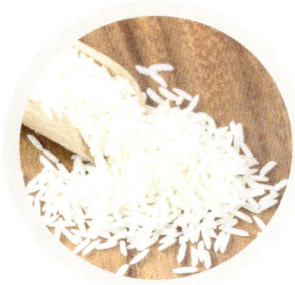

Basmati Rice

- Contains protein
- Source of vitamin B, zinc, and magnesium
- Will not cause rapid spikes in blood sugar levels like white rice
- High fiber content supports digestion

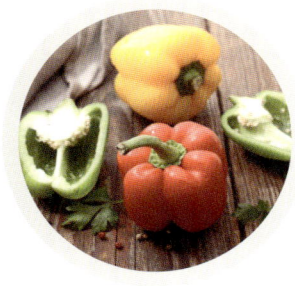

Bell Peppers

- Packed with antioxidants
- Rich in vitamin C, supports immune function and skin health
- High in vitamin A for eye health and vitamin K for bone strength
- Contains a variety of carotenoids like beta-carotene, lutein, and zeaxanthin
- Offers potent anti-inflammatory and antioxidant properties

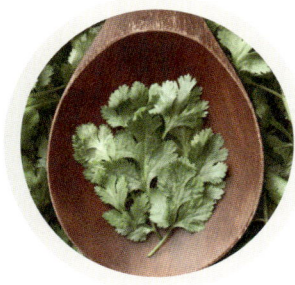

Cilantro

- Contains minerals like potassium, manganese, and iron
- Packed with antioxidants
- Excellent source of vitamin K for blood clotting and bone health
- Provides vitamin A for eye health and immune function
- Immune-boosting properties
- Contains vitamin C, an antioxidant
- Important for muscle function, metabolism, and oxygen transport
- Antimicrobial properties
- Helps lower blood sugar levels and reduce inflammation

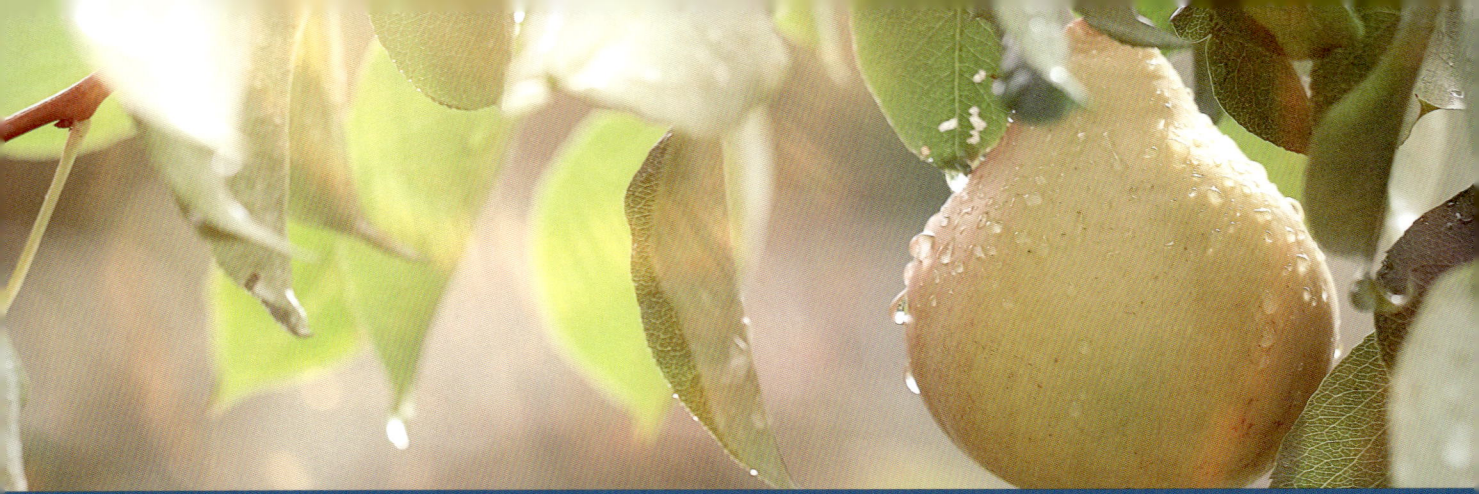

PEAR & AVOCADO SALAD

Ingredients
Creates 4 Individual Portions!

1 head of butter lettuce

2 ripe pears

2 ripe avocados

1/4 cup soft blue cheese
(may substitute Feta)

1/2 cup honey roasted pecans
(see recipe)

2 Tbsp high quality balsamic
vinegar reduction (such as aged
Balsamic Vinegar of Modena)

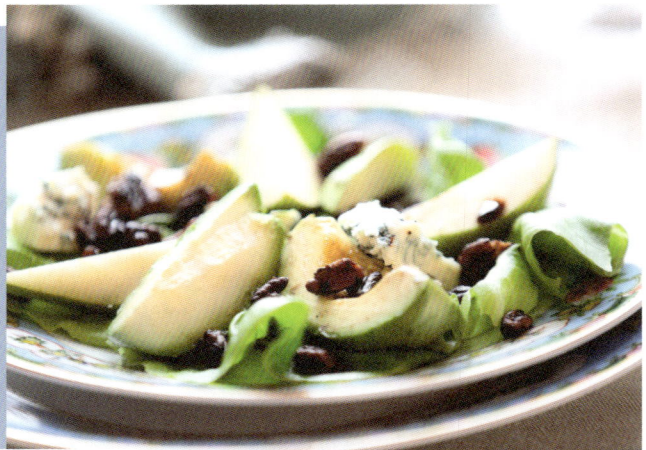

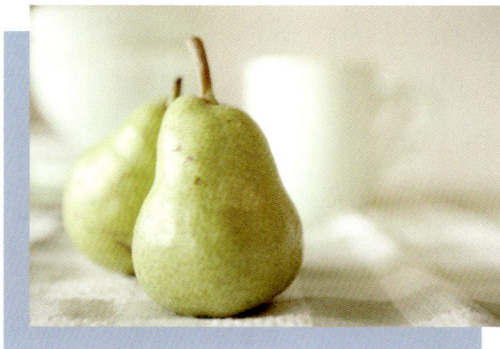

Preparation

1. Wash lettuce and place two whole lettuce leaves on each salad-size plate.
2. Peel and cut avocados in half length-wise. Then cut 3 slices per half and place three slices on each plate.
3. Wash the pears and peel if skin is tough. Cut each pear in half length-wise and core. Then cut 3 slices per half and place three slices on each plate.
4. Cut soft blue cheese into medium-size pieces and place on each plate, about 1 Tbsp per plate.
5. Sprinkle toasted pecans over each salad.
6. Drizzle balsamic all over each salad.

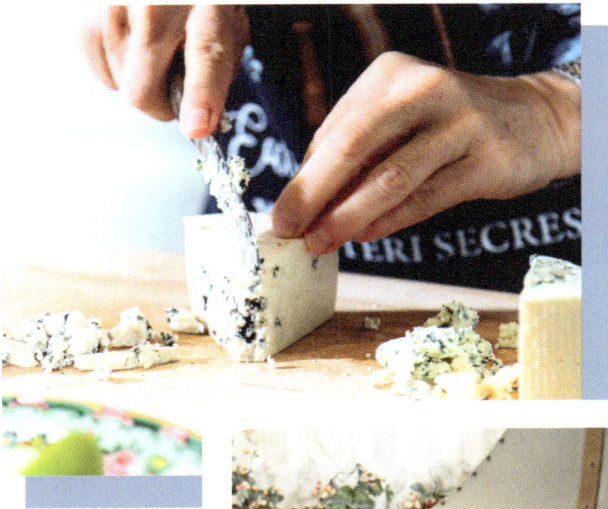

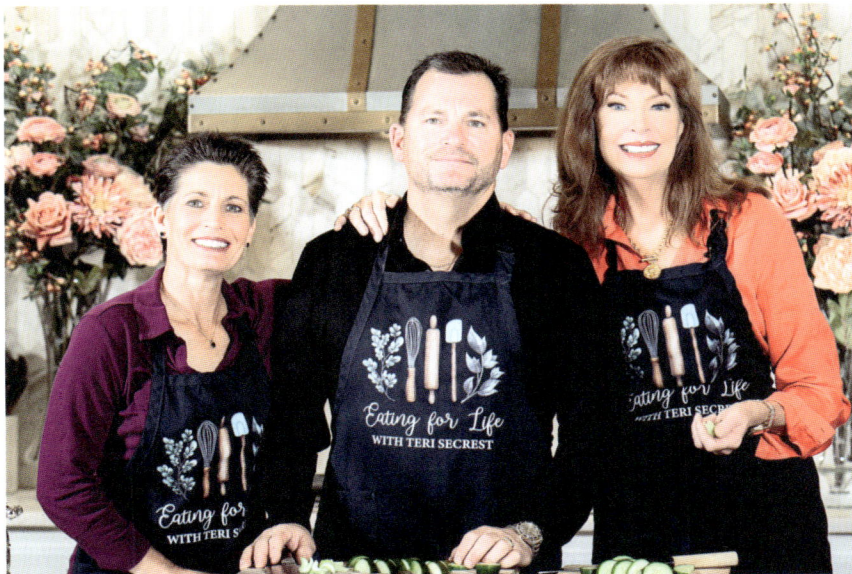

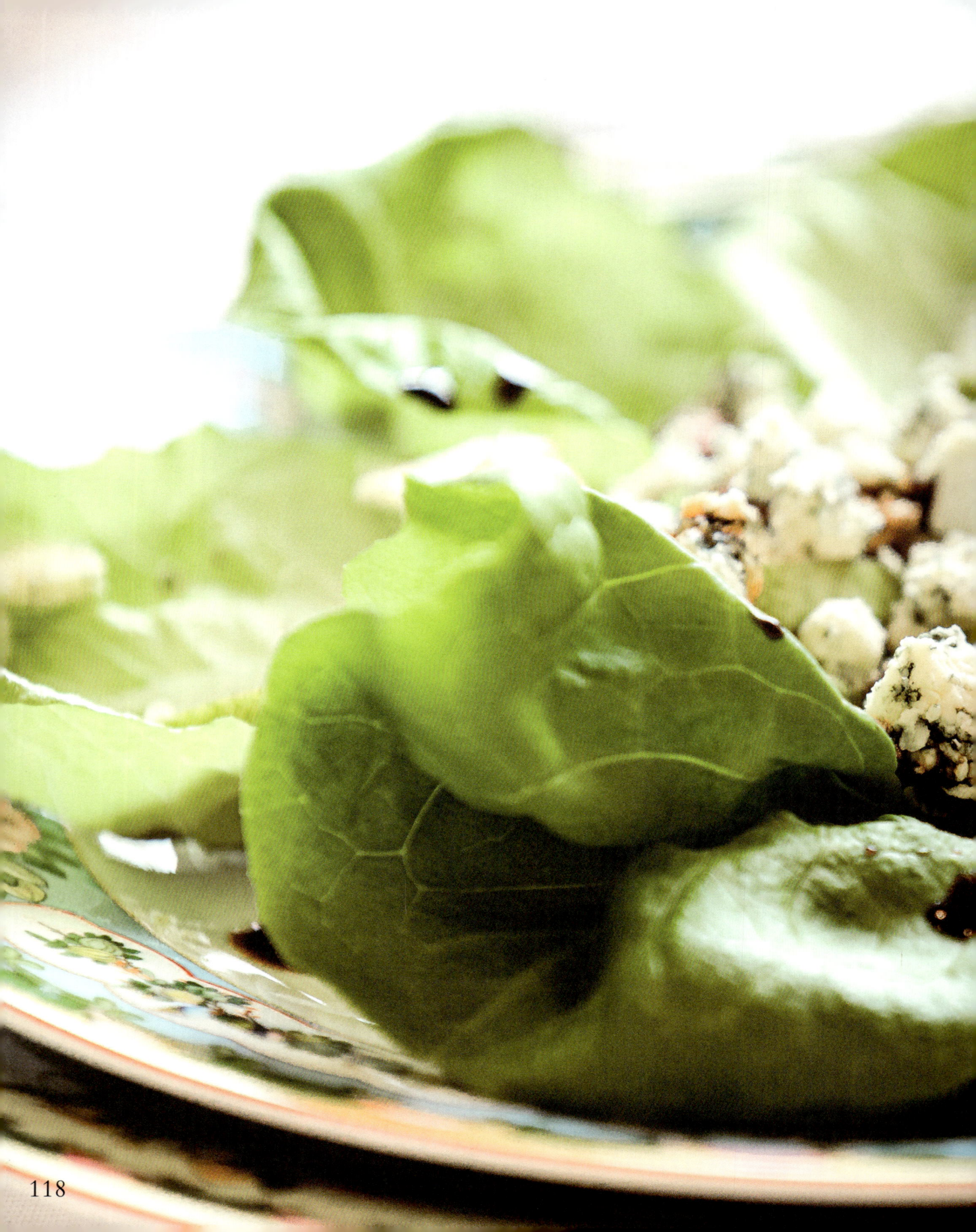

"A balsamic reduction is much thicker than a typical balsamic vinegar. Be sure to use the reduction in this recipe."

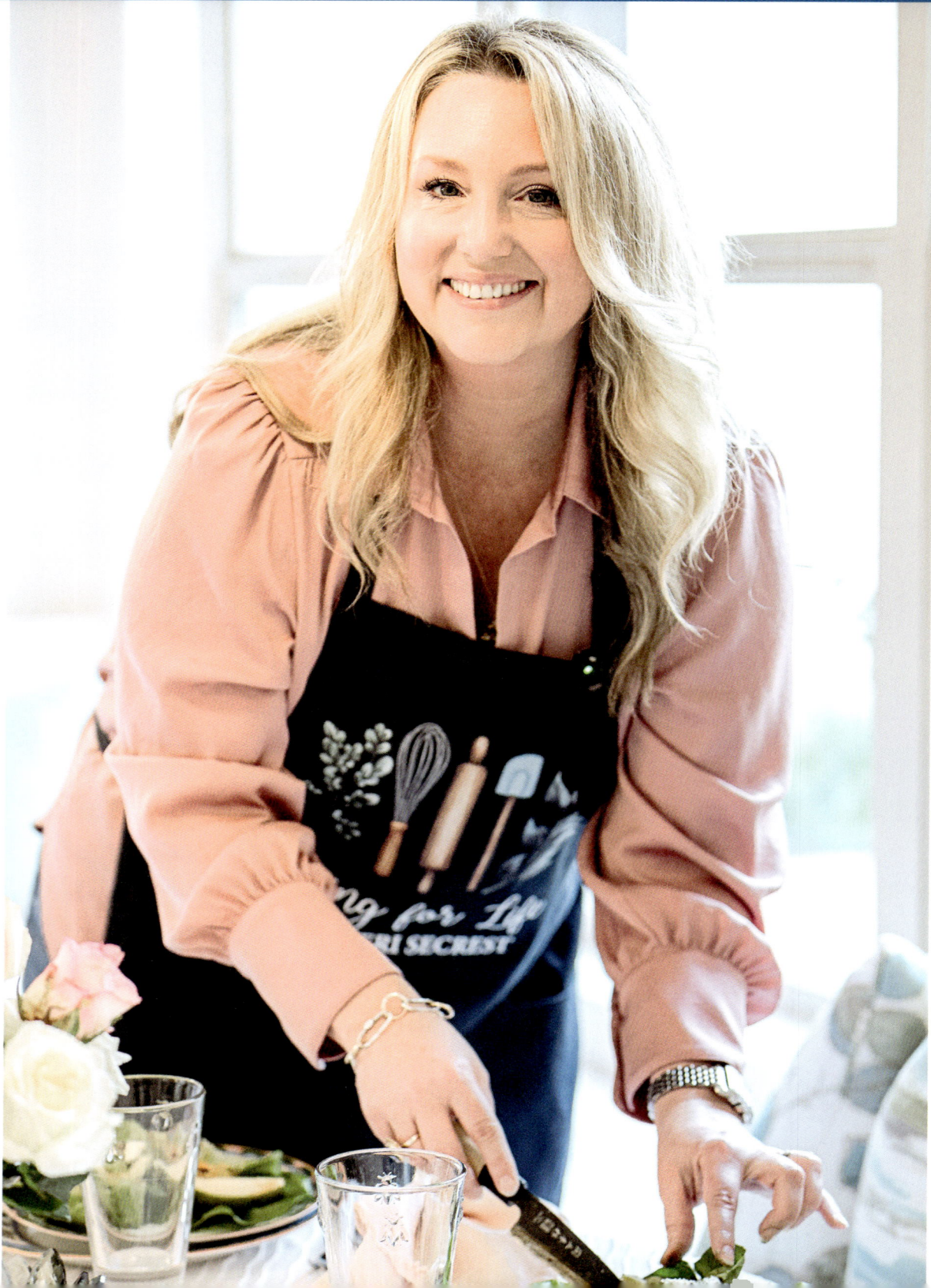

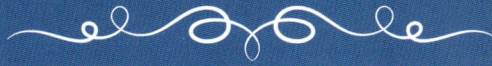

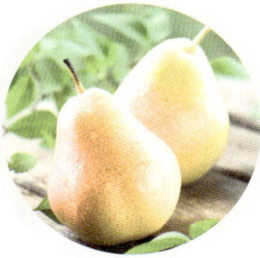

Pears

- Vitamin C supports immune function and skin health
- Potassium helps regulate blood pressure and heart function
- Promotes digestion and gut health
- Contains antioxidants like flavonoids and phytonutrients
- Protects cells from damage caused by free radicals

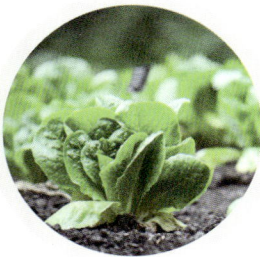

Organic Butter Lettuce

- Source of vitamins A and K for eye health, immune function, and bone strength
- Contains folate, important for cell division and DNA synthesis
- Provides small amounts of vitamin C, potassium, and iron
- Promotes feeling of fullness

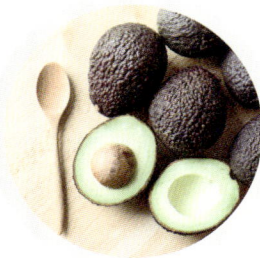

Avocados

- Packed with heart-healthy monounsaturated fats
- Helps lower bad cholesterol and raise good cholesterol levels
- Promotes cardiovascular health
- Fiber for digestion and weight management
- Keeps you feeling full and satisfied
- Contains vitamins E and K for skin health, blood clotting, and bone strength
- Provides potassium, folate, and vitamin C

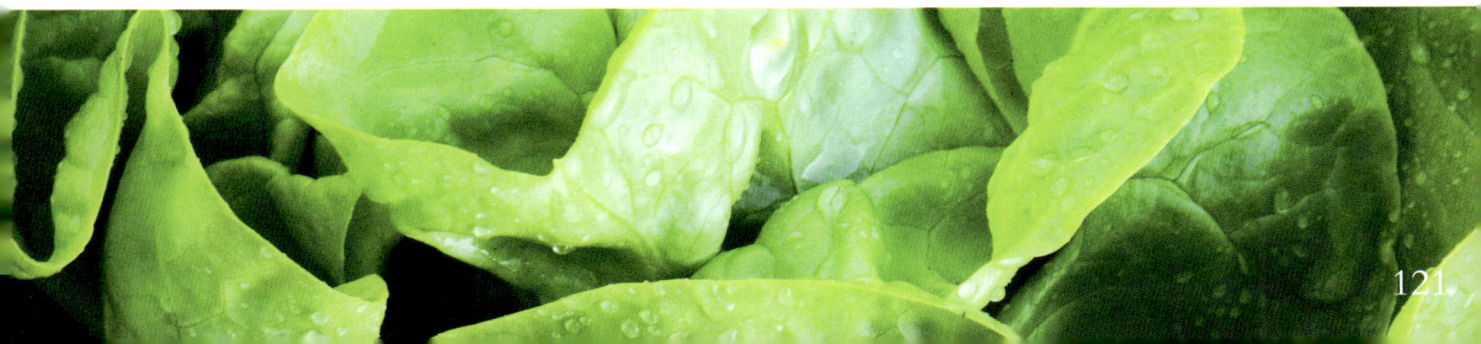

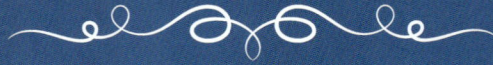

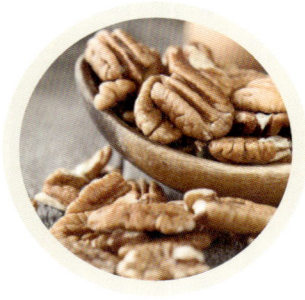

Pecans

- Rich in heart-healthy monounsaturated fats
- Good source of protein and fiber
- Lowers bad cholesterol and reduces heart disease risk
- Aids in weight management and promotes satiety
- Contains vitamin E, a powerful antioxidant
- Protects cells from free radical damage
- Provides manganese for metabolism and bone health

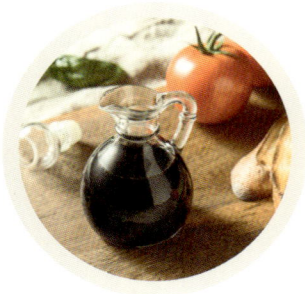

Balsamic Reduction

- Rich in antioxidants
- Contains polyphenols, which protect cells from damage
- Contributes to heart health
- Contains acetic acid linked to improved digestion blood sugar regulation, and appetite control
- Lowers cholesterol
- Promotes weight loss

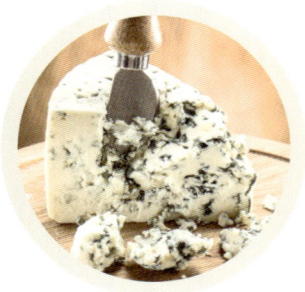

Soft Blue Cheese

- Contains beneficial bacteria and enzymes for gut health
- Promotes digestion
- Provides protein, calcium, and other essential nutrients

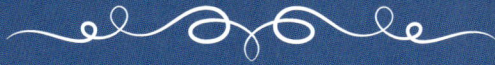

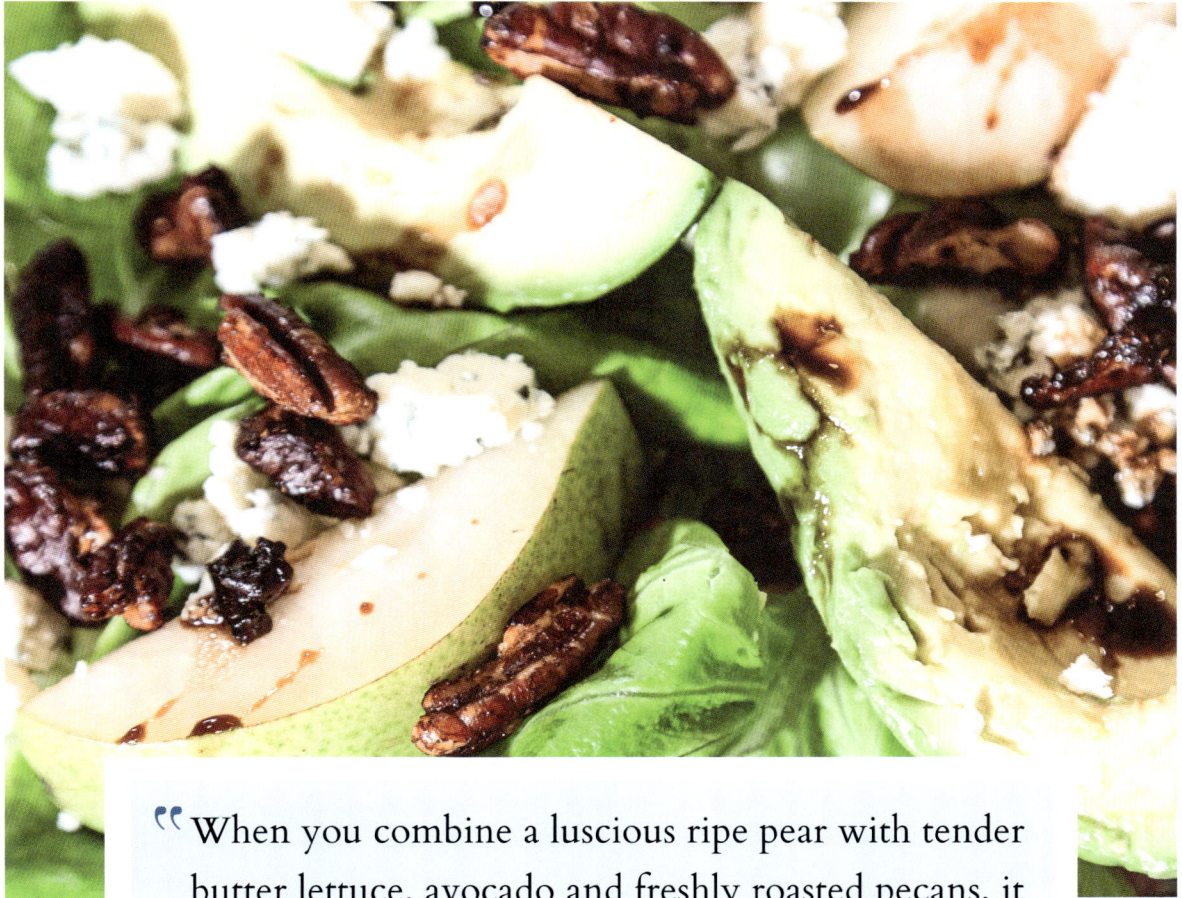

"When you combine a luscious ripe pear with tender butter lettuce, avocado and freshly roasted pecans, it may just 'pucker your palate'...so good!"

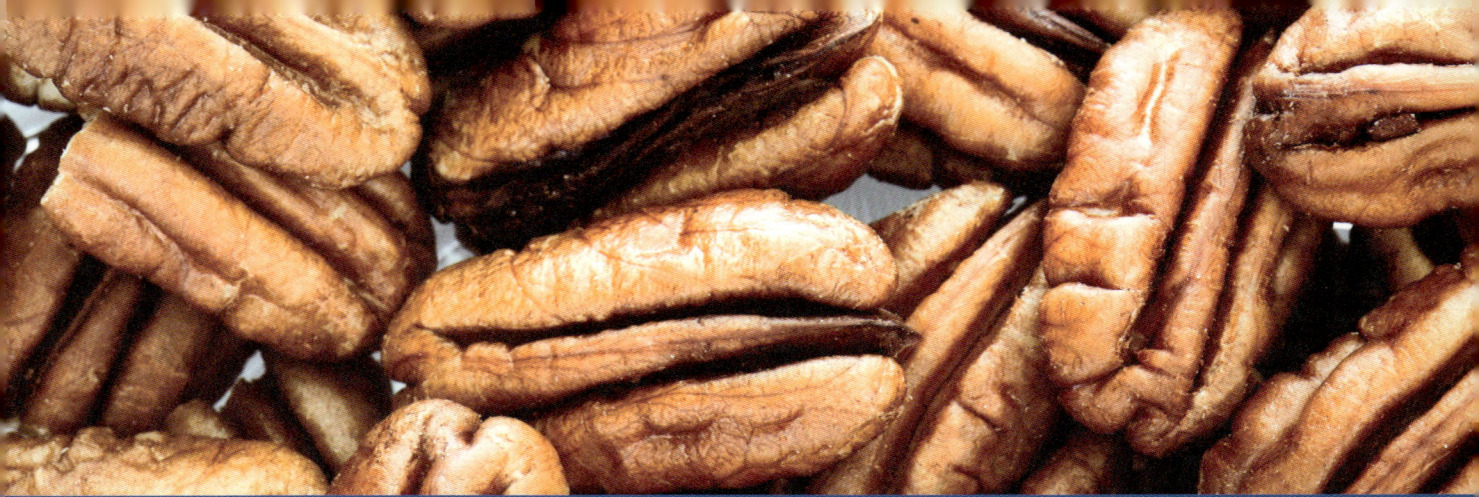

HONEY TOASTED PECANS

Ingredients

2 Tbsp butter

1/2 cup raw pecans

1/4 tsp Tony Chachere's Original Creole seasoning

2 Tbsp raw, unfiltered honey

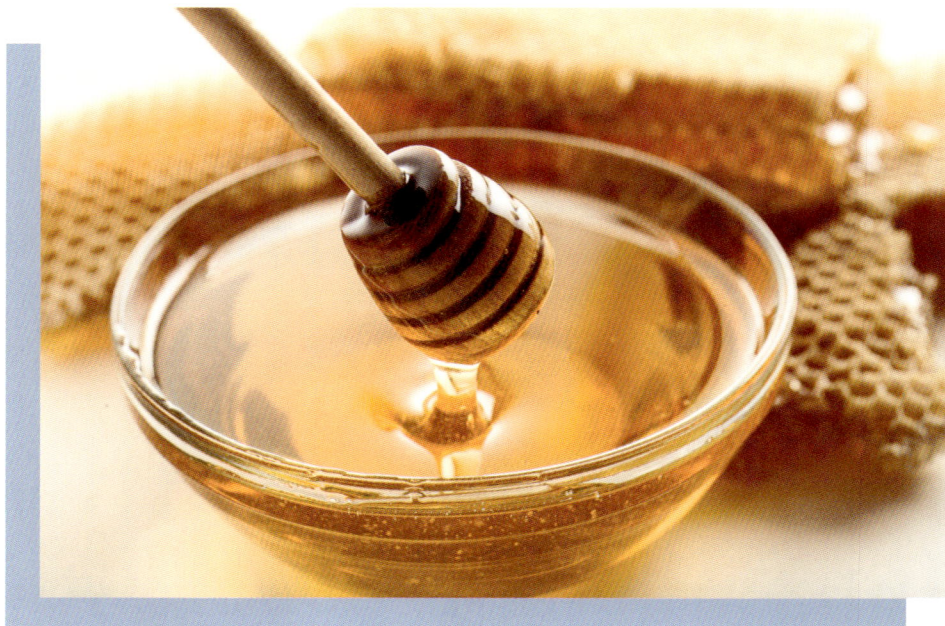

"Enjoy your delicious Honey Toasted Pecans as a snack, topping for salads, or as a tasty addition to your favorite recipes!"

Preparation

1. Heat a skillet or frying pan over medium heat. Add butter.
2. Once the butter is melted, add the pecans to the skillet and stir to coat them evenly.
3. Sprinkle on Tony's seasoning to season the pecans. Start with a little bit and adjust to taste.
4. Drizzle honey over the pecans and stir to coat evenly.
5. Continue to cook the pecans, stirring frequently, for about 5-7 minutes or until they are toasted and fragrant. Check your heat and turn down if needed to avoid burning the pecans.
6. Remove pecans from the heat and let them cool slightly before serving

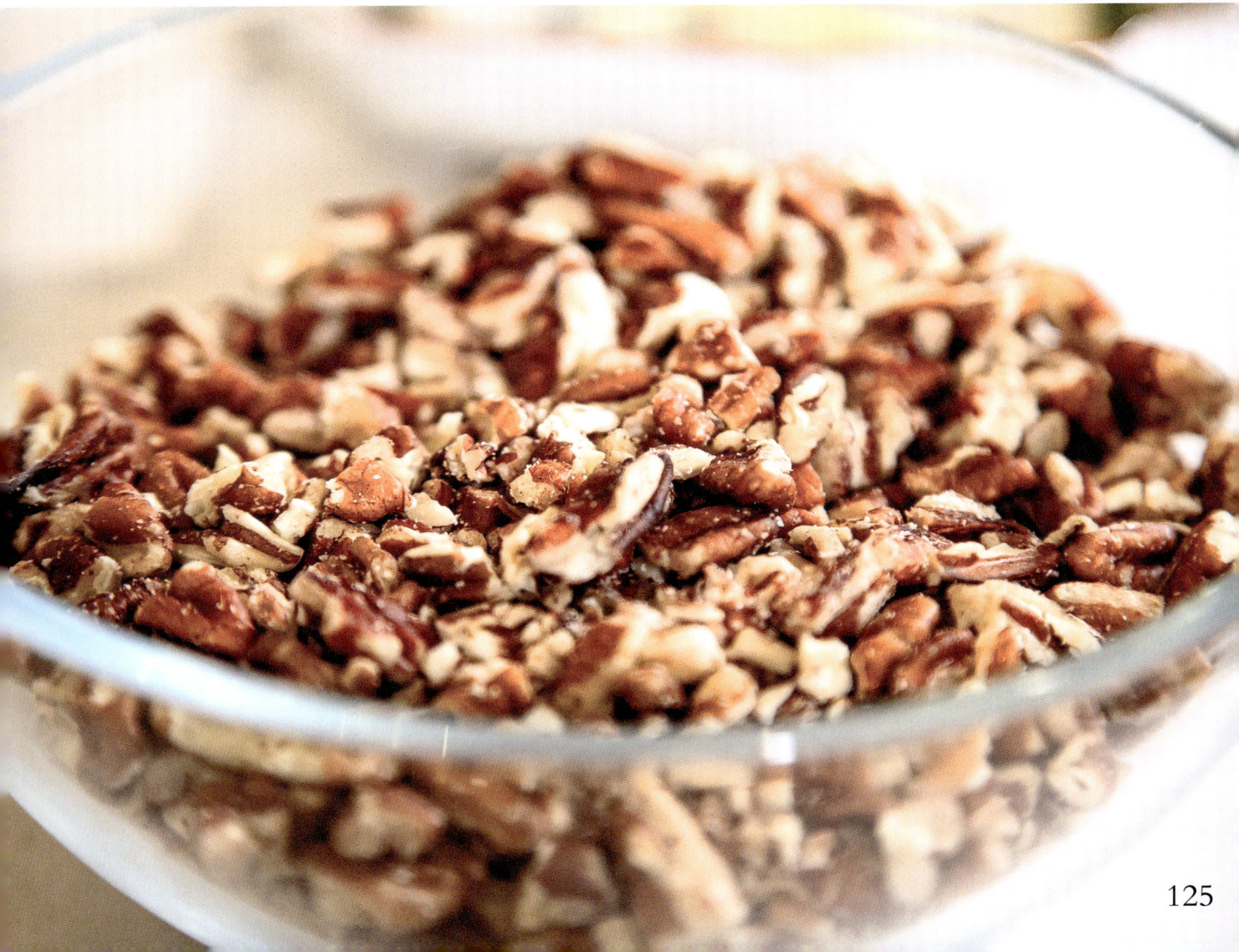

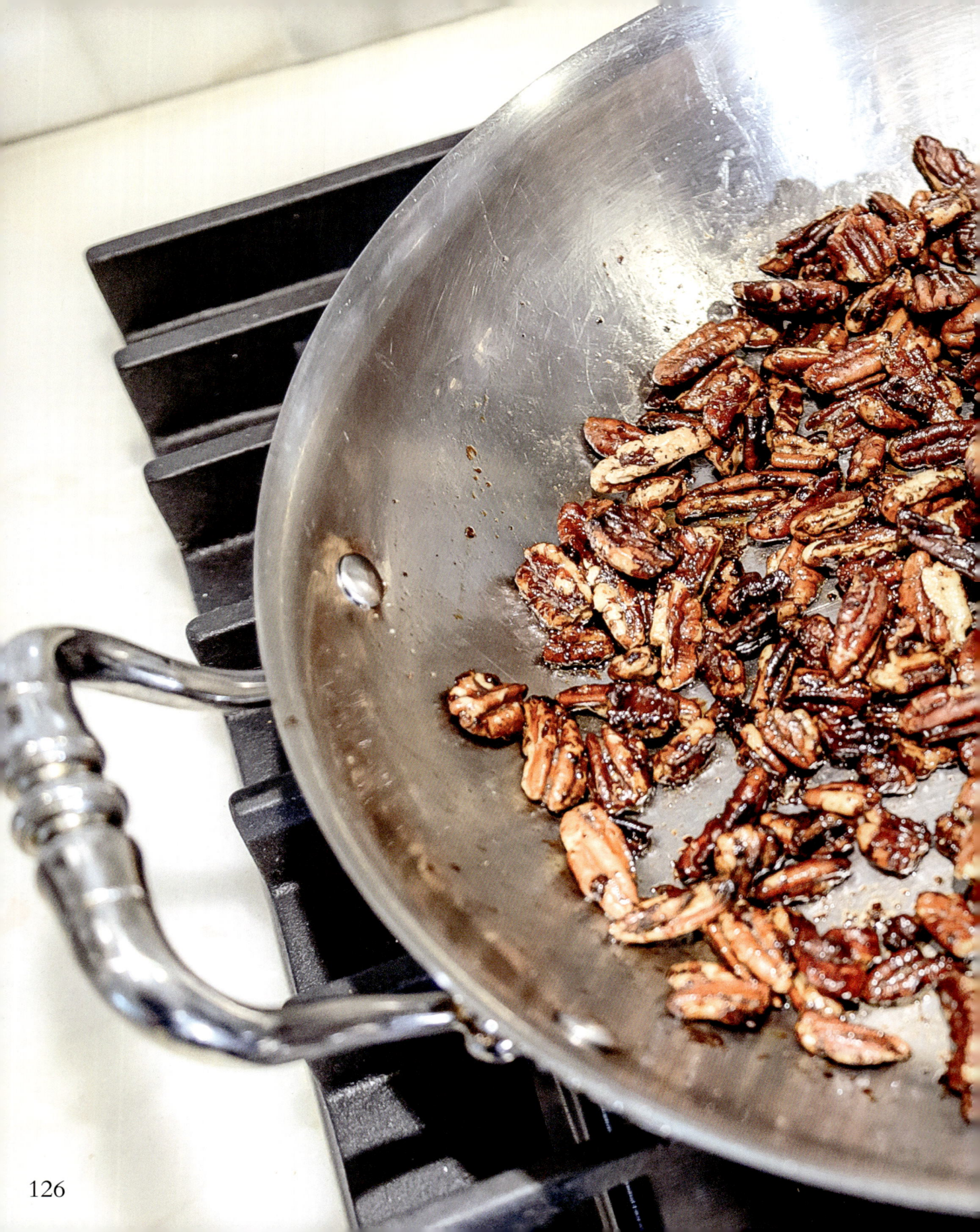

"During the filming of this recipe, the smell of the honey toasted pecans was so tantalizing, that my students and I lost all restraint and began eating them before we could even get them into the recipe!"

(Learn more about my 7-Week Digital Healthy Cooking Course on page 12)

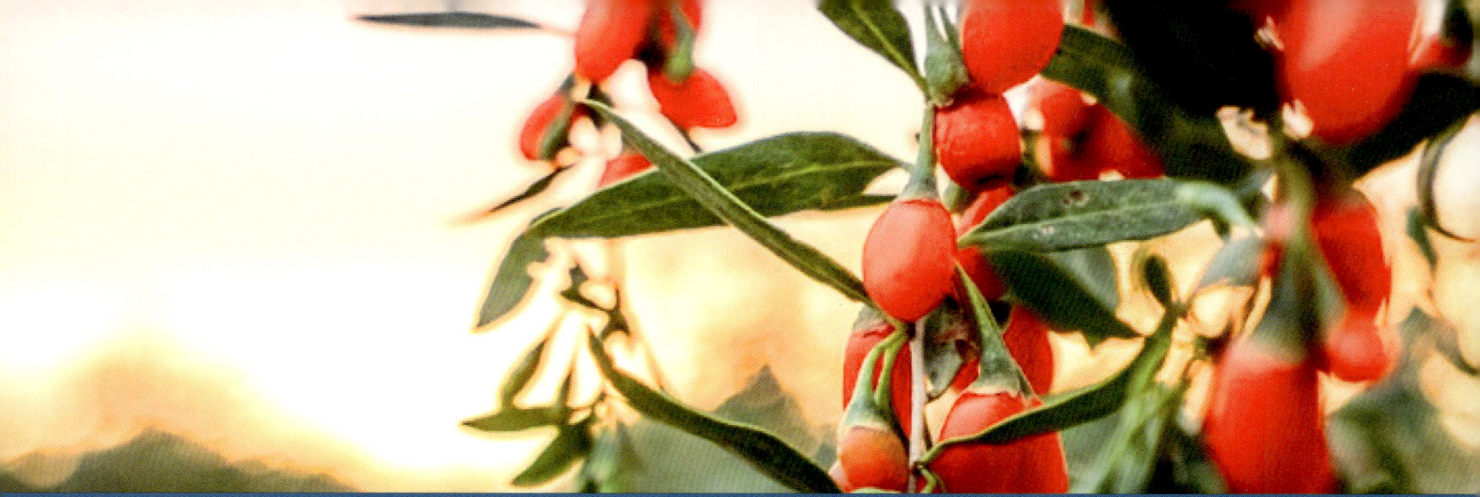

NINGXIA RED PARFAIT

Ingredients
Creates 6 Amazing Portions!

Parfaits

1 cup NingXia Red juice

3 cups unsweetened red juice or
red juice blend of your choice

3 packets unflavored vegan gelatin

2 Tbsp agave nectar (optional)

Topping

Whipped cream or whipped
coconut cream
(see recipe)

1 cup fresh organic blueberries
and organic raspberries

Zest of lemon or orange

"Be sure to take time to find organic vegetarian gelatin. It makes the texture so much smoother without being hard."

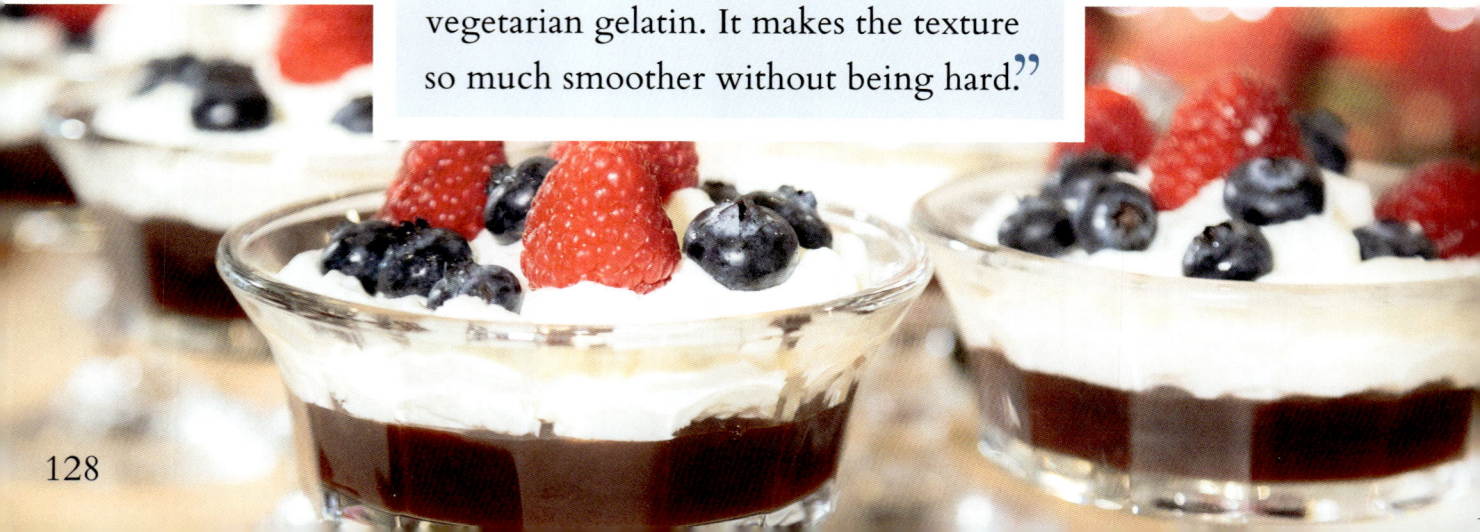

1. Pour all packets of the dry gelatin into a mixing bowl. Stir in the NingXia Red juice. Allow to stand for a minute or so until it thickens.

2. Warm 3 cups of unsweetened red juice or red juice blend in a saucepan—do not boil. Add agave nectar, if desired.

3. Pour the warmed red fruit juice blend into the Ningxia Red and gelatin mixture. Stir until completely blended, 3-5 minutes.

4. Pour equal portions into 6 parfait glasses. Cover each glass with plastic wrap and place in refrigerator until set, about 3 hours.

5. To serve, top with whipped cream (or whipped coconut cream), fresh berries, and grated lemon or orange zest.

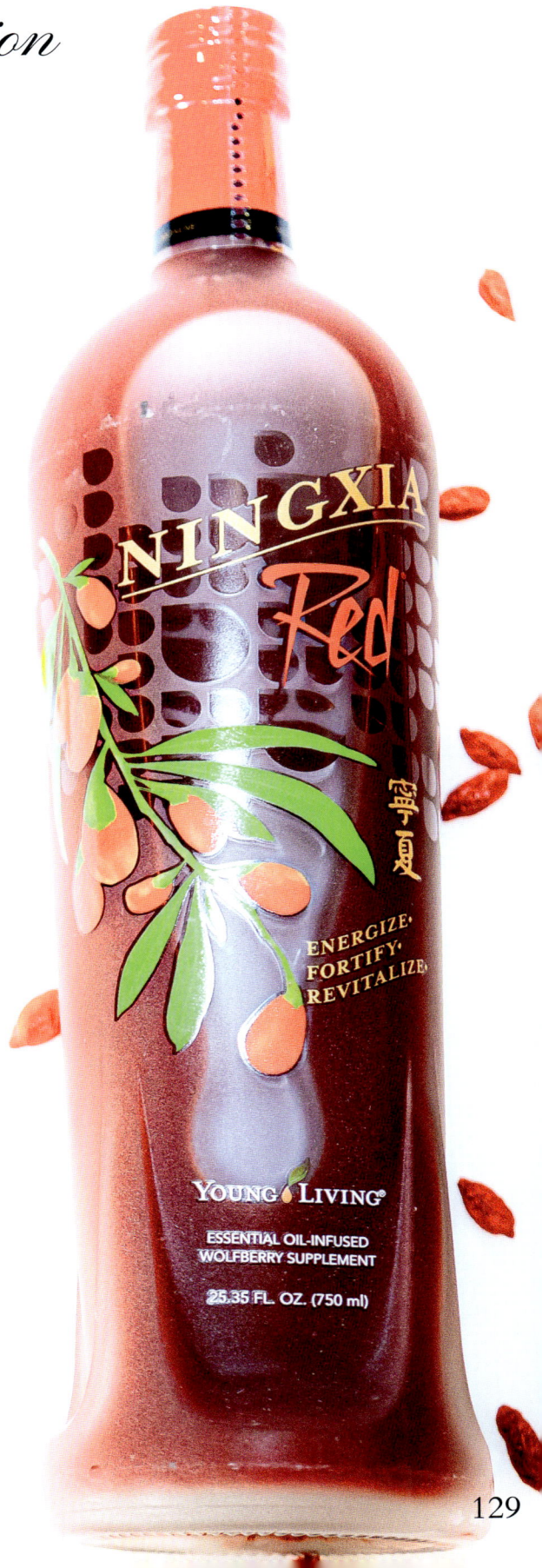

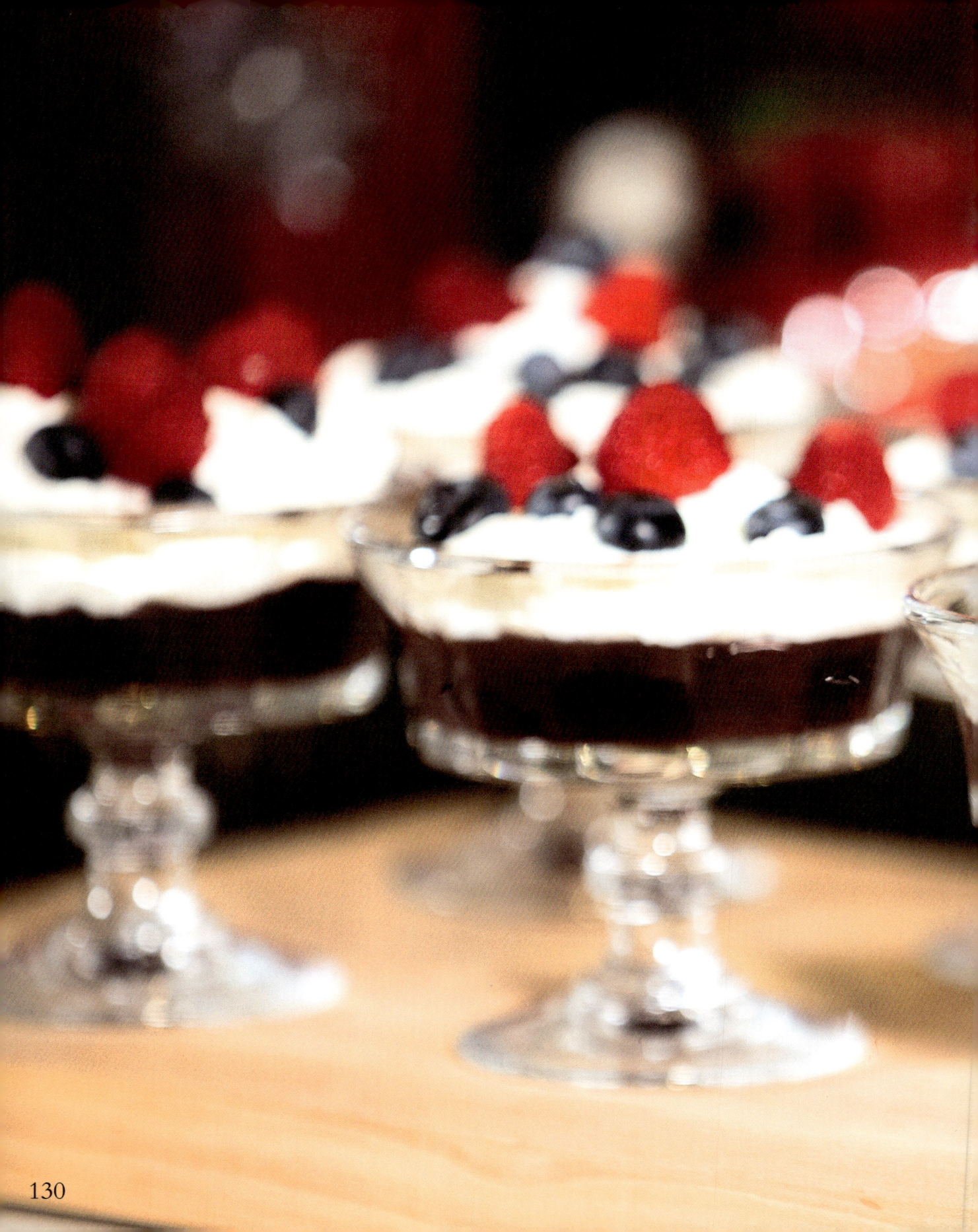

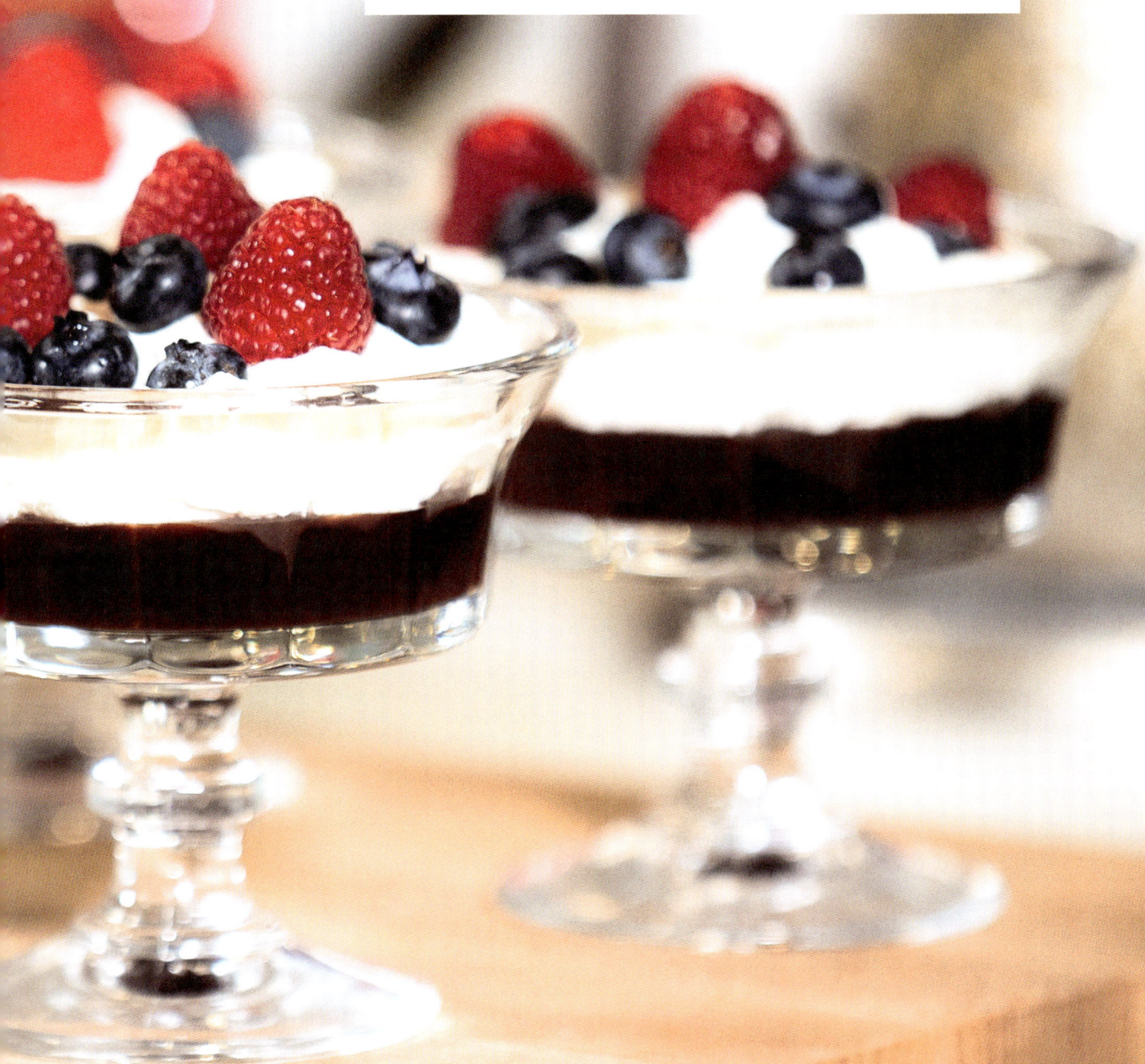

Help! I don't have time to cook!

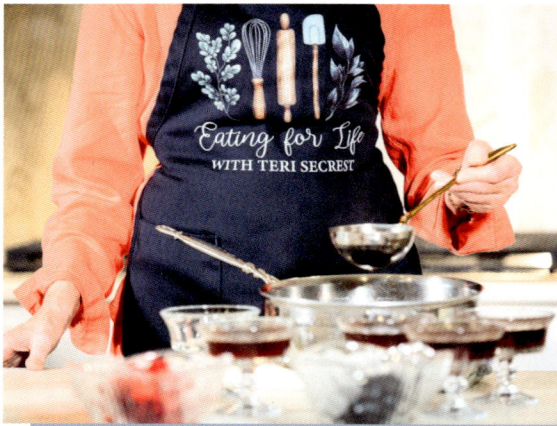

One of the most frequent comments I hear as a wellness coach is, "Teri, everything you teach is great, but we are two working parents and we don't have time to prepare healthy meals!" If you are looking for something to fill in the nutritional gaps in your daily menu, especially during the busy times in of life, I'd like to introduce you to one of the most nutrient dense foods in my household, NINGXIA RED!

You just learned how to make the NingXia Red Parfit, developed by my good friend and restaurateur, Melinda Powers! The best part? It reduces stress significantly to improve mental well-being!

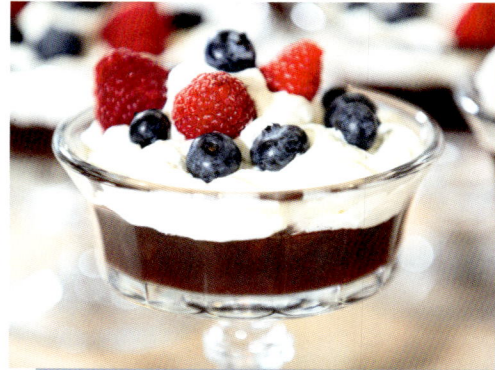

For the last 20 years, our family has enjoyed a daily dose of Ningxia Red and this powerhouse juice continues to support our overall health fully. The ingredients in Ningxia Red are so full of life that the very cells of your body seem to come alive with each daily dose. We find this juice supports our physical energy levels, improves our sleep patterns, reduces our daily stress, supports our healthy vision and more! Best yet, all of these benefits are clinically proven! So if you are a family on the move, NingXia is the way to go!

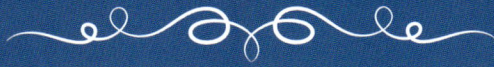

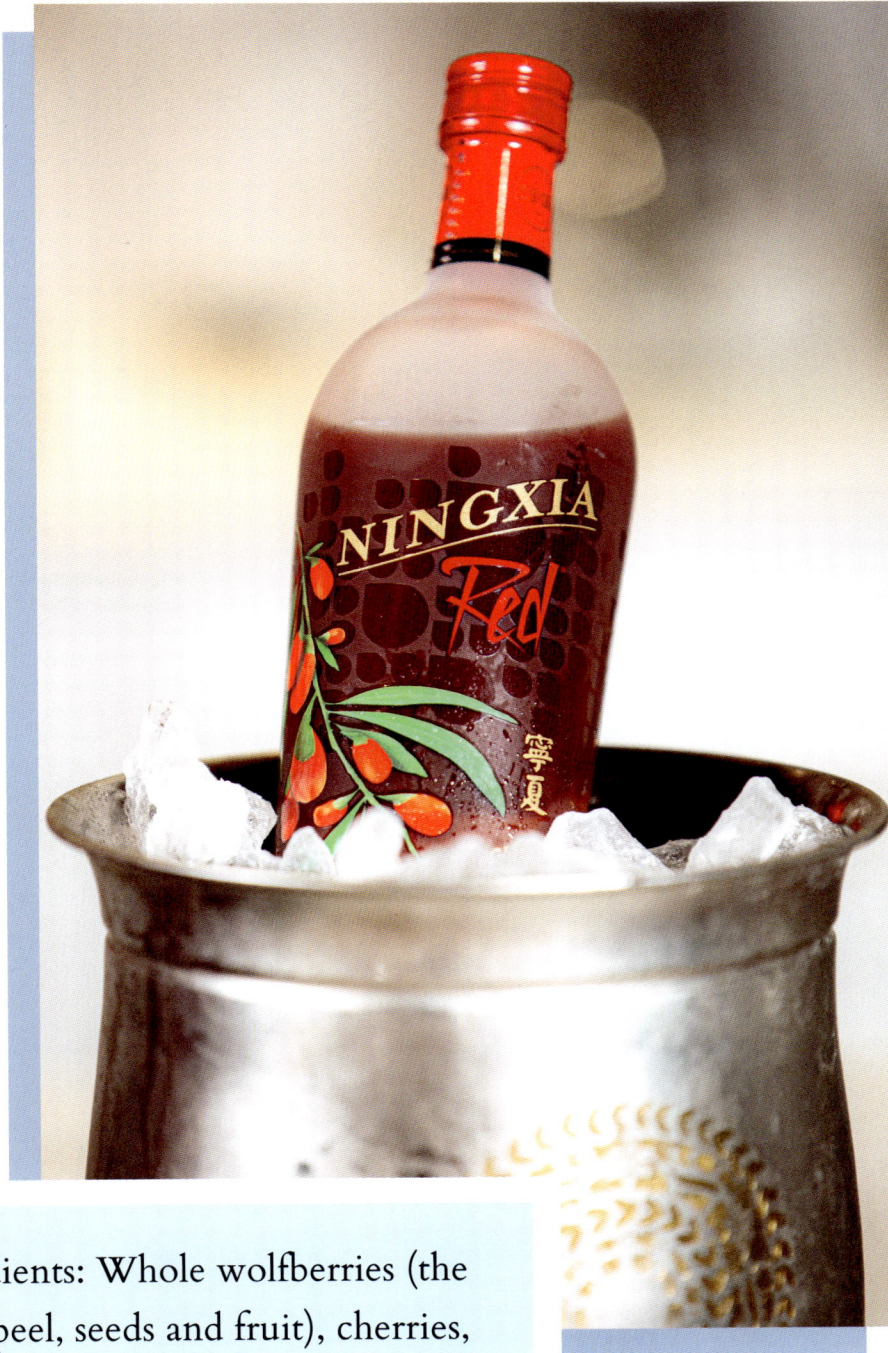

Ingredients: Whole wolfberries (the juice, peel, seeds and fruit), cherries, blueberries, pomegranate, plums, aronia berries, essential oils of Orange, Lemon, Tangerine, Yuzu and Stevia.

To learn more scan QR Code

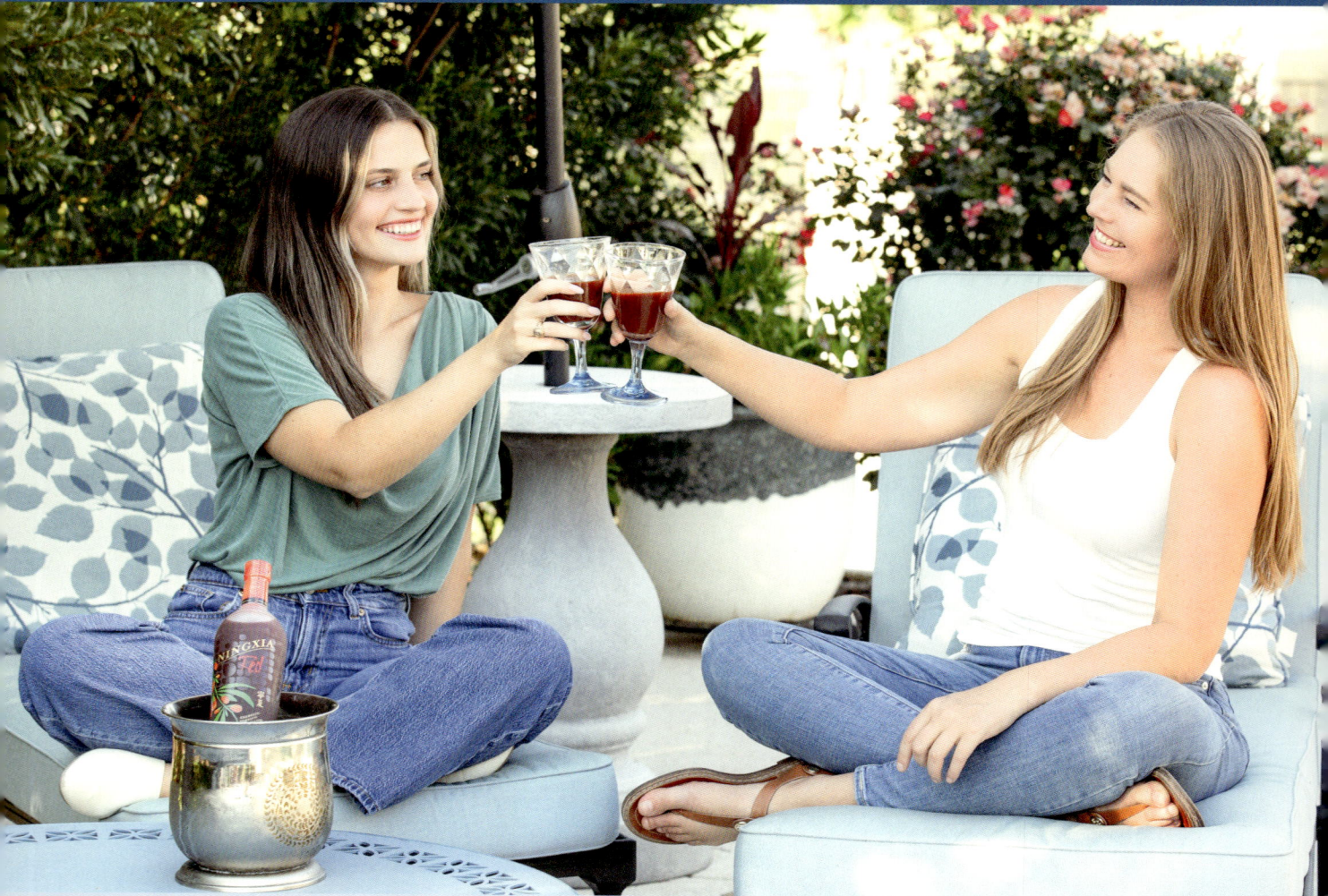

Let's celebrate these life giving ingredients!

134

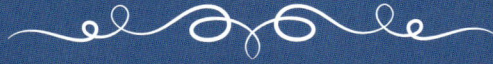

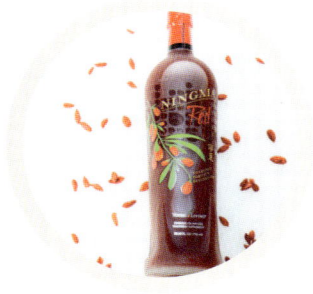

NingXia Red

- High in antioxidants, especially anthocyanins
- Protects cells from damage by free radicals
- Supports cardiovascular health
- High in vitamins C, A, B6, and E
- Contains potassium, and amino acids
- Boosts immune function
- Promotes healthy aging
- Provides sustained energy and vitality
- Supports eye health

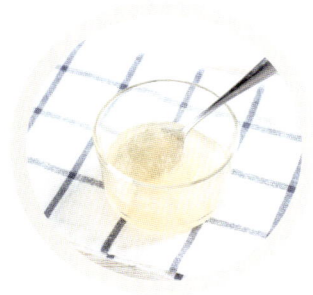

Unflavored Vegan Gelatin

- Rich in protein and essential amino acids.
- Supports joint health
- Great for skin elasticity, and hair and nail strength, due to its collagen content.
- Beneficial to gut bacteria growth
- Reduces inflammation

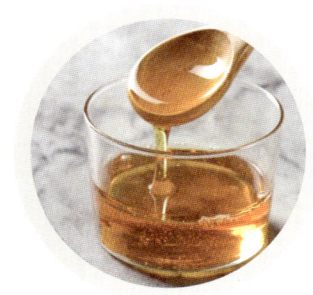

Agave Nectar

- Low glycemic index
- Contains polyphenols, which protect cells from damage.
- Healthier option for those watching their sugar intake

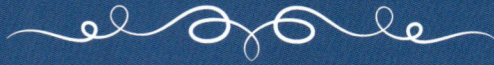

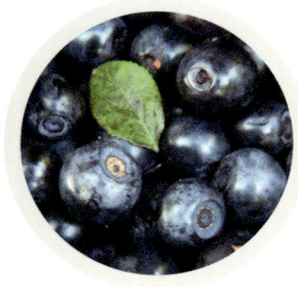

Organic Blueberries

- Packed with antioxidants, particularly anthocyanins
- Protect cells from oxidative damage
- Reduce inflammation
- Great source of vitamins, including vitamin C and vitamin K
- Essential for immune function and bone health

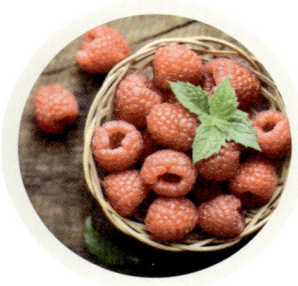

Organic Raspberries

- High in vitamin C, supporting immune function and skin health
- High in fiber
- Antioxidants like ellagic acid and quercetin combat inflammation and oxidative stress
- Aids digestion
- Low calorie and carbohydrate content, suitable for weight management
- Including vitamin K, manganese, and potassium
- Aids in blood clotting
- Supports healthy heart function

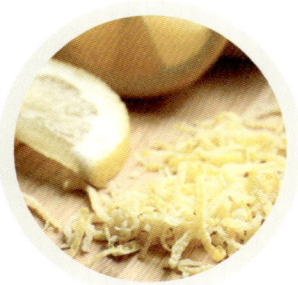

Lemon Zest

- Rich in essential oils and natural compounds
- Vitamin C for immune function and skin health
- Contains antioxidants like limonene and flavonoids
- Helps reduce inflammation and protect cells from oxidative damage

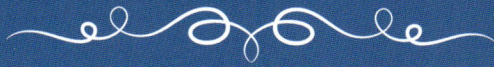

"As you become more confident in using essential oils in your recipes, I encourage you to try a few drops of YL Vitality Orange or Tangerine oil in this fun dessert."

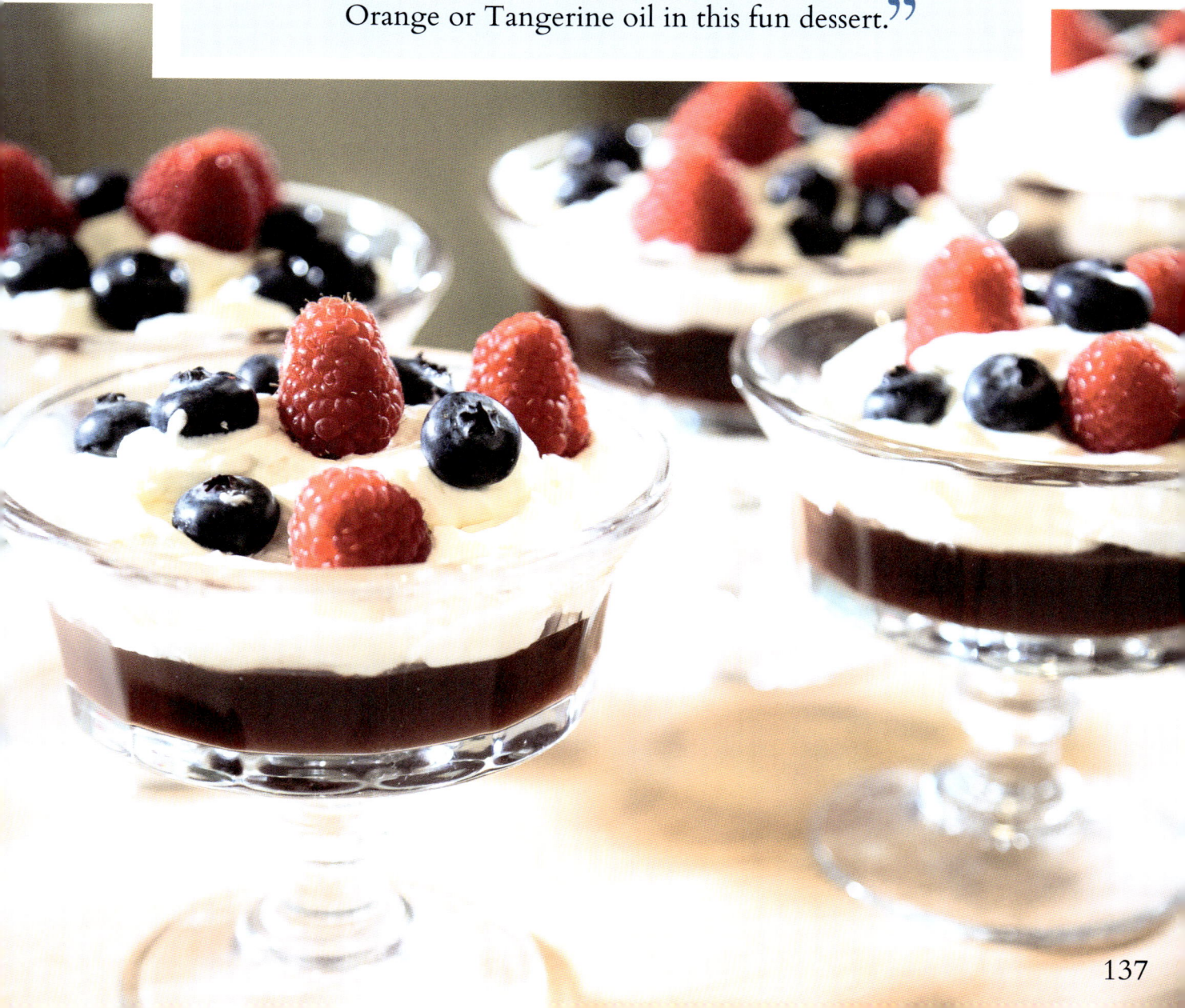

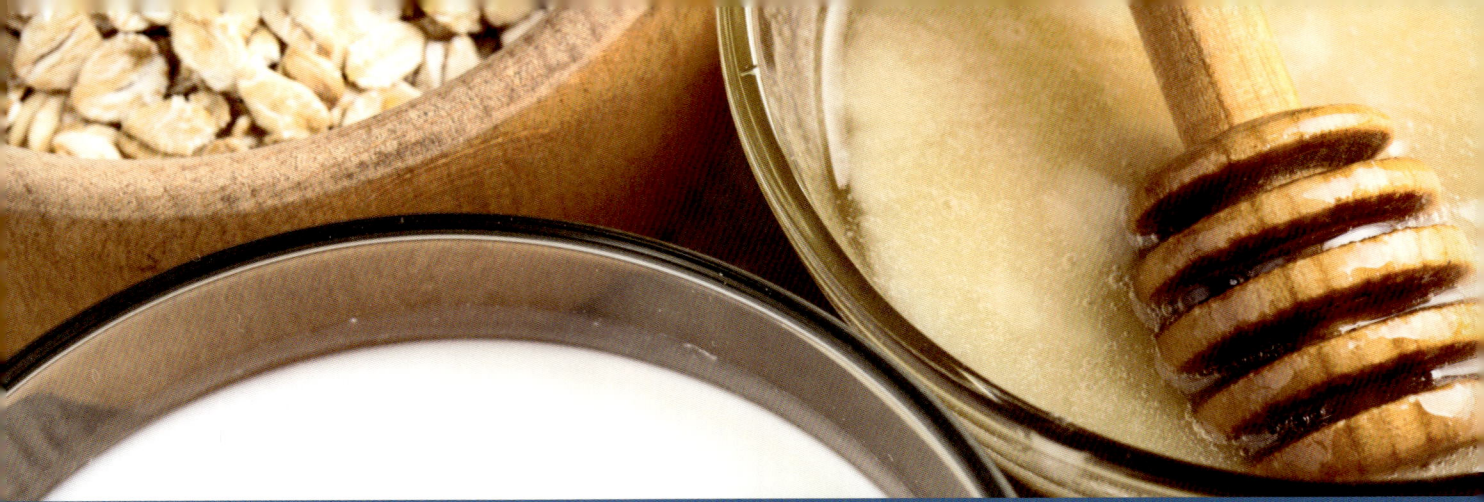

WHIPPED CREAM/COCONUT CREAM

Ingredients

1-2 tsp raw, unfiltered honey

1/2 tsp vanilla

1pt organic heavy whipping cream

1 – 13.5 oz can organic coconut cream

2 drops YL Vitality Orange or

YL Vitality Tangerine Oil
(Order YL Vitality Essential Oils on page 39)

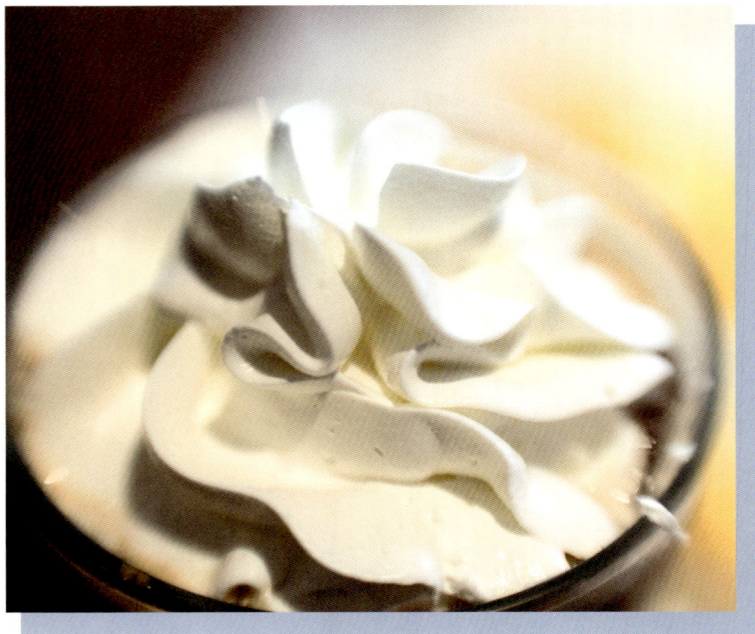

Organic Whipped Cream

1. Place the ingredients into a chilled stainless steel or glass bowl. Pro Tip: add essential oils
2. Using a small hand mixer, beat on high speed until you see nice peaks. Adjust the honey to taste.

Organic Non-Dairy Coconut Whipped Cream

1. Chill coconut cream for several hours or overnight.
2. Scoop out all of the white coconut solids and place them into a chilled stainless steel or glass bowl. Add remaining ingredients. Pro Tip: add essential oils at this step
3. Using a small hand mixer, beat on high speed until you see nice peaks. Adjust the honey to taste.

"Over the years, it has been so much fun adding food grade essential oils such as tangerine, orange or lemon to my whipping cream. Guests are amazed with the flavors and can't wait to try it at home."

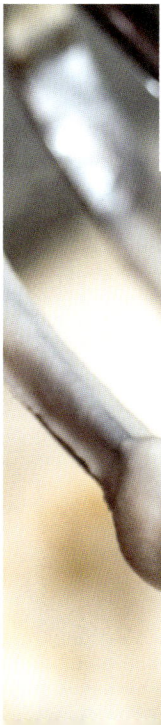

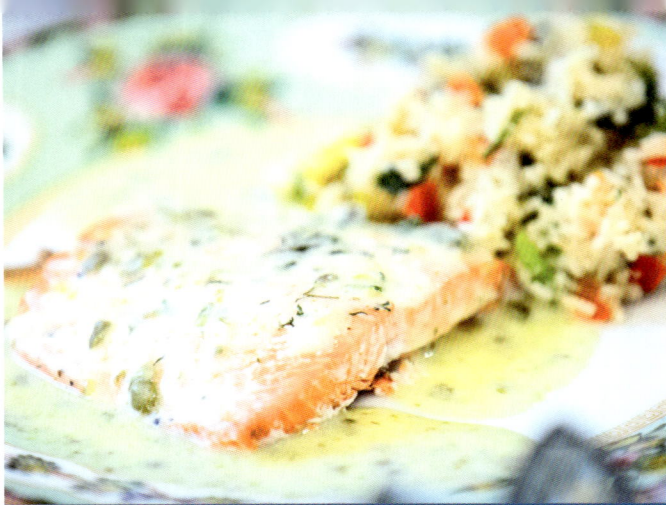

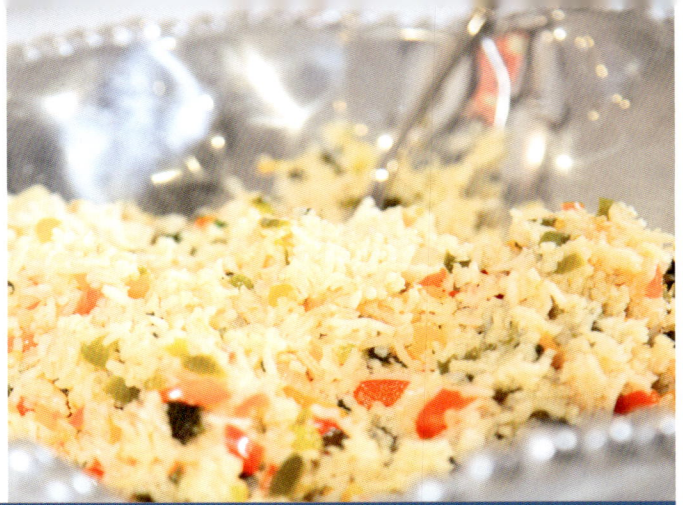

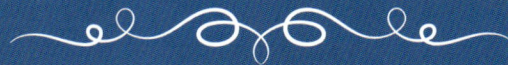

Week 4
Full Menu Shopping List

Produce

1 bunch fresh dill

4 lemons

1 orange

1 red bell pepper

1 green bell pepper

1 yellow bell pepper

1 onion

2 cloves garlic

1 bunch fresh cilantro

1 head of organic butter lettuce

2 ripe pears

2 ripe avocados

1 cup fresh organic blueberries

1 cup fresh organic raspberries

Baking & Spices

Lemon pepper seasoning

Olive oil

Arrowroot powder

Tony Chachere's Creole Seasoning (Blue label)

Raw, unfiltered honey

3 packets natural unflavored vegan gelatin

Agave nectar (optional)

Soup

2 cartons organic chicken broth

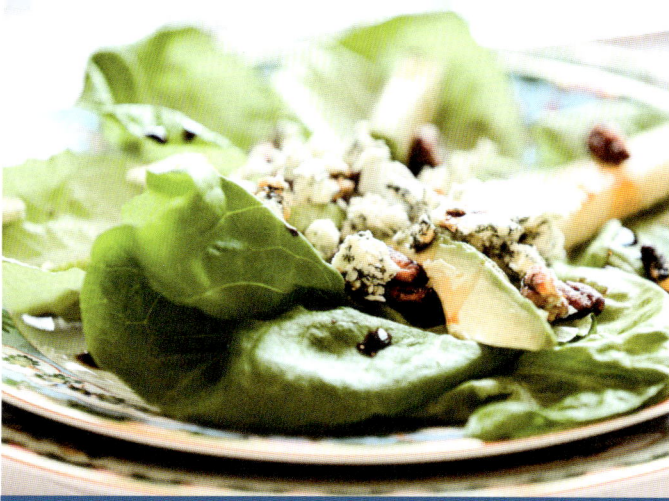

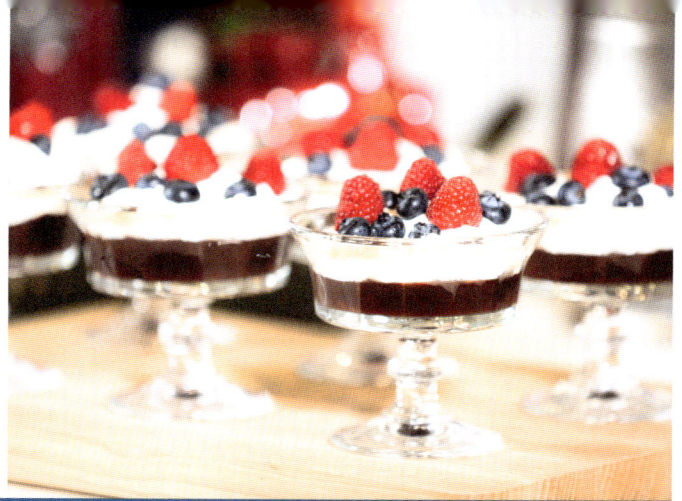

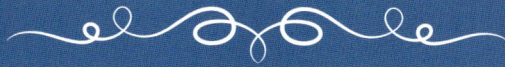

Full Menu Shopping List continued

Dairy

Butter

1pt organic heavy whipping cream

Soft Blue Cheese (optional Feta)

Dry Goods

1 cup basmati rice

1/2 cup raw pecans

International
(Non-Dairy Option)

1 - 13.5oz can organic Coconut cream

Seafood

Wild-caught salmon, 6 to 8 ounces per person

Condiments

Capers

High quality balsamic vinegar reduction such as Aged Balsamic Vinegar of Modena

Juice

3 cups unsweetened red juice or red juice blend of your choice

Wine

White wine for sauce (optional)

From Young Living*

NingXia Red Juice

SEE PAGE 133 FOR ORDERING DETAILS

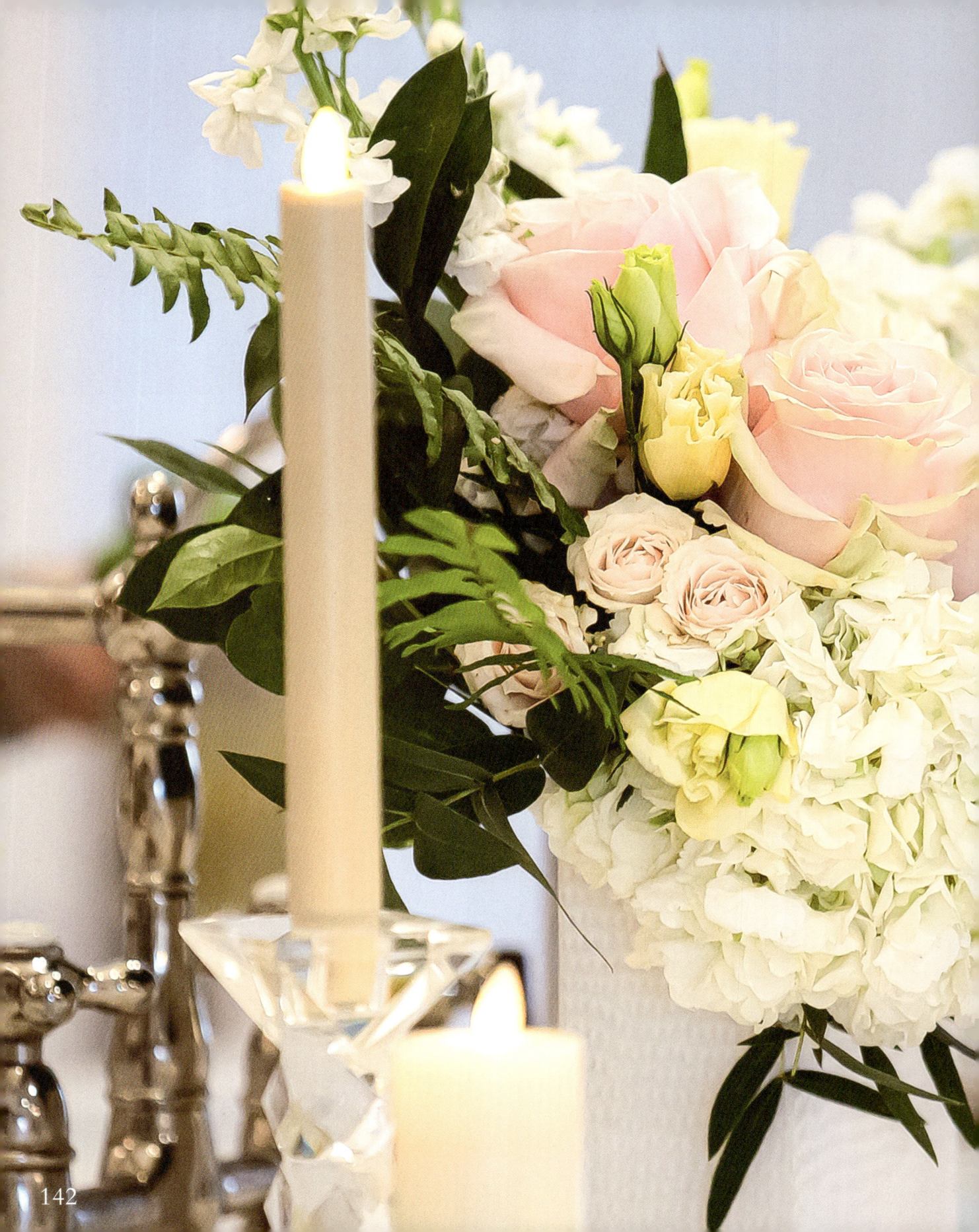

EATING FOR
Life
TERI SECREST

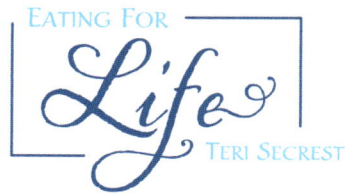

WEEK *Five* MENU

Almond Pecan Pie Crust

❀

Organic Beef & Broccoli Pie

❀

Garlic Roasted Carrots

❀

Bountiful Basic Salad

❀

Healthy Ranch Dressing

❀

143

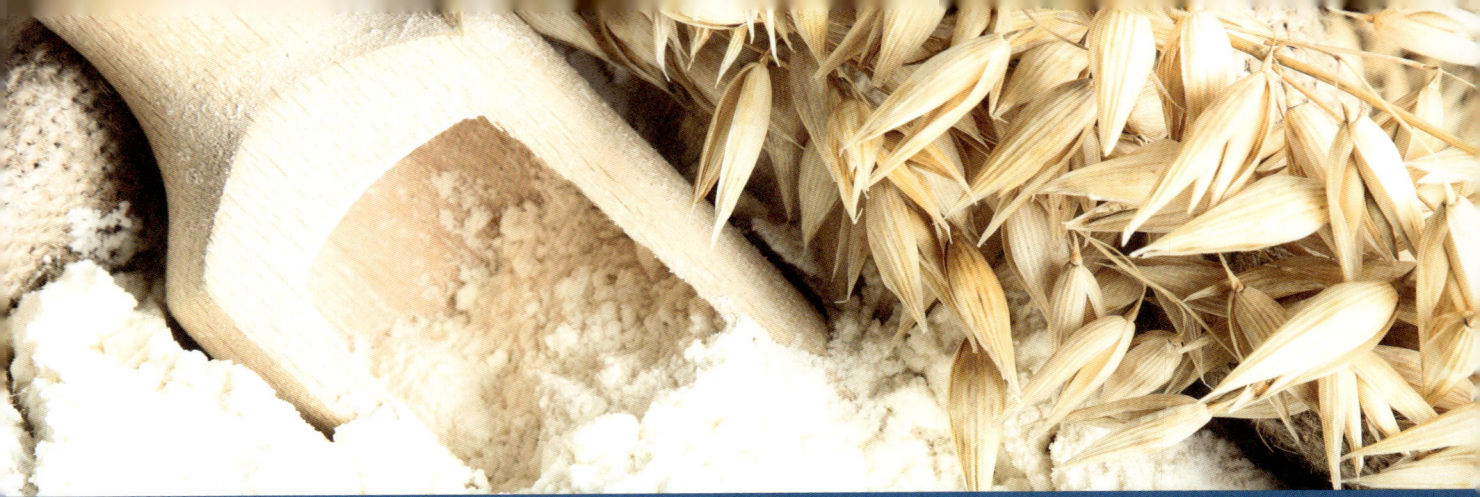

ALMOND PECAN PIE CRUST

Ingredients

Makes One 9 inch Pie Crist

3⁄4 cup raw almond and raw
pecan blend (1/2 raw almonds
1/2 raw pecans)
4 Tbsp softened butter, cut
into small pieces
1/2 cup organic unbleached
all-purpose flour
½ cup Young Living
Einkorn Flour
Dash of salt
3-5 Tbsp ice water

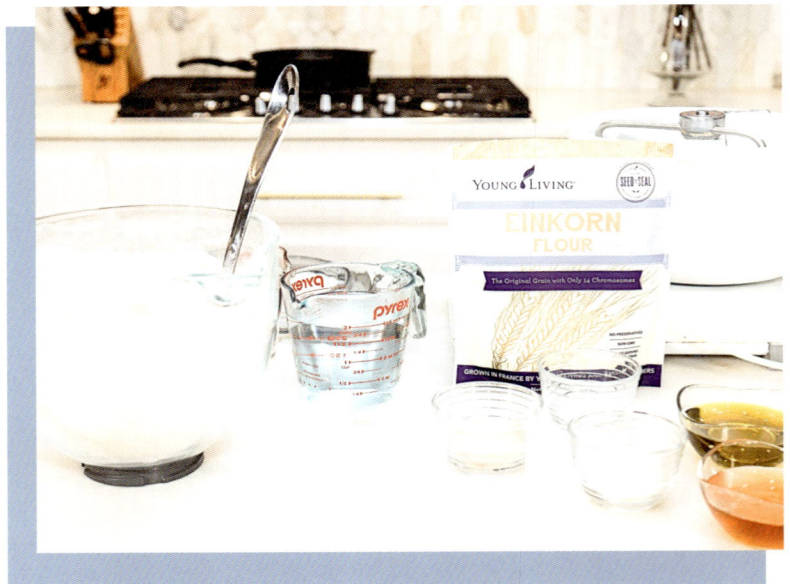

Preparation

1. Butter a 9" pie pan and dust with flour.

2. Place nuts in your food processor. Pulse until nuts are finely minced (just this side of ground.) Place minced nuts, softened butter, flour, and salt in a bowl. Using a pastry cutter, work the mixture until it is uniform and resembles a coarse cornmeal. PRO TIP: I actually love to mix up these ingredients in my hands.

3. Remove the cubes from the ice-cold water. Gradually drizzle in the water and begin mixing with fork, pushing the dough onto itself in the center of the bowl. When the dough adheres to itself, you've added enough water. Form the dough into a round ball.

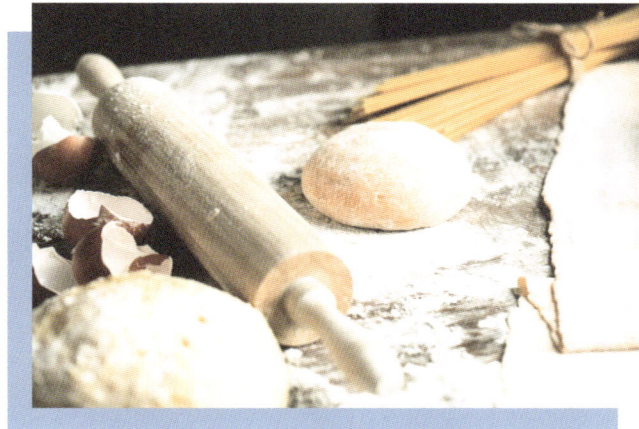

4. Put a piece of waxed paper on your countertop, place your round ball of dough onto the wax paper, gently push down and flatten it a bit, then place another piece of was paper on the top. With your rolling pin, roll out the dough from the middle out on one half, then go back to the middle and roll out the other direction, then go back to the middle and roll up, and finally go back to the middle and roll down. Once it is about one inch bigger than the diameter of your pie pan, you are ready for the next step.

5. Remove the top layer of wax paper. Flip your buttered pie pan upside down onto the rolled-out dough. Put your hand underneath the bottom wax paper and gently flip the dough into the pan. Remove the wax paper and gently push the dough evenly in the pie pan. Flute the edges. You now have a beautiful crust!

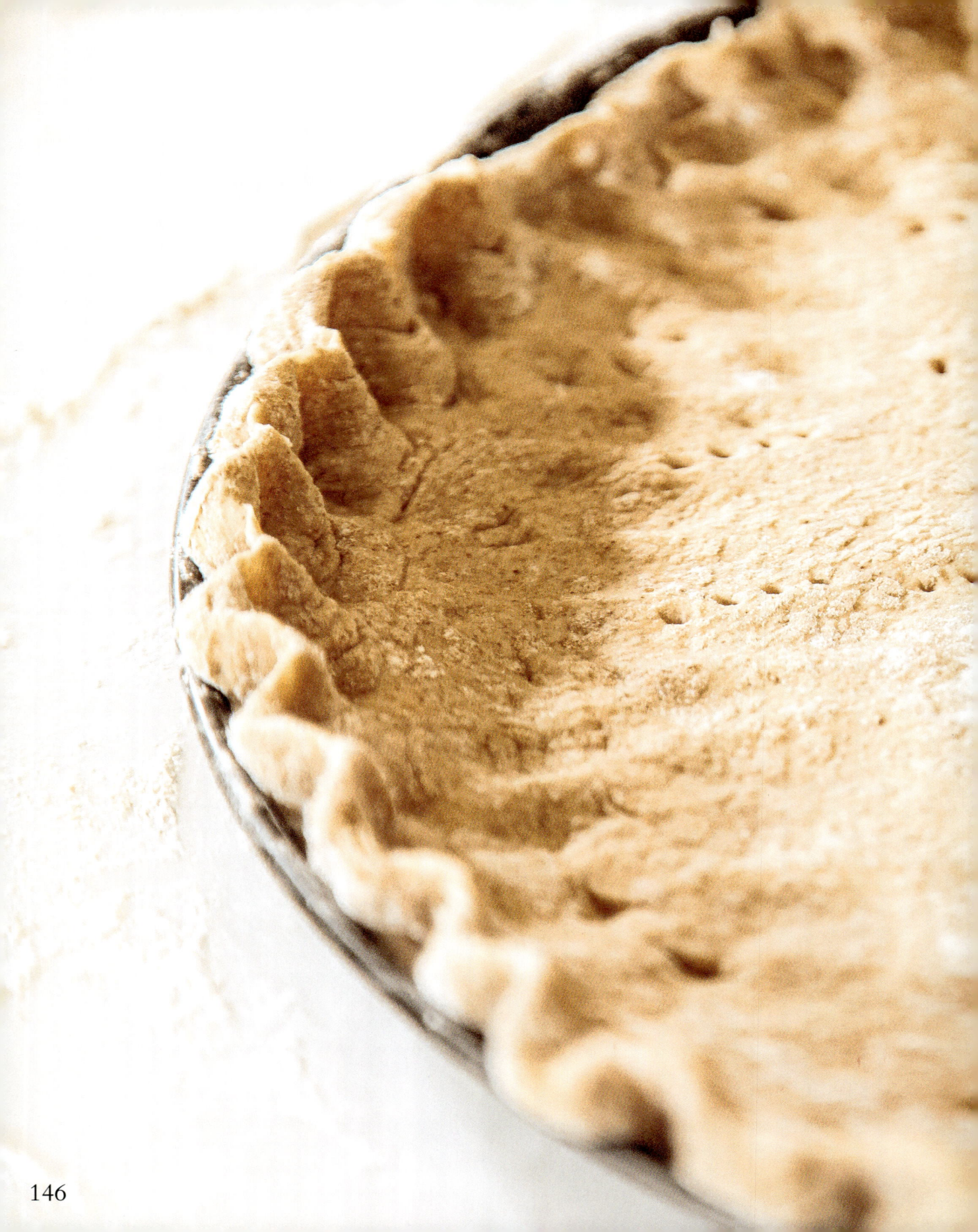

"I love making this Almond Pecan Pie Crust for both savory, main course pies and dessert pies! It is full of texture and nutty, buttery flavor."

Why I Love Cooking with Einkorn Grain

"Oh beautiful for spacious skies, for amber waves of grain"

…when I imagine a field of ripe wheat in the early days of America, my mind sees a bountiful land with luscious golden stalks of wheat waving in a gentle breeze.

Suddenly I am brought into the reality of today where a third of my health clients say they are sensitive to wheat. With bread being the staff of life for centuries, I'm pondering, *what has happened to our bread?*

Traveling to France and hearing about the research being done on Einkorn, one of the oldest grains in civilization has brought great hope to my heart. Young Living is pioneering this research and together with some of the most knowledgeable French farmers, are spearheading the growing of this remarkable ancient grain.

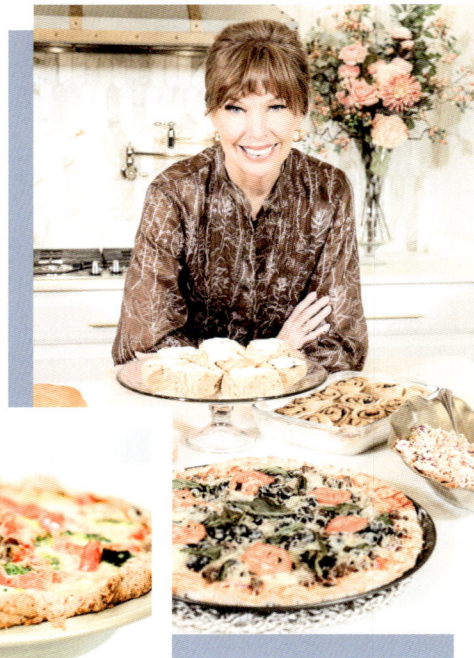

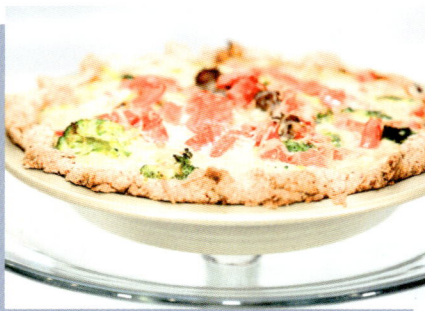

What is the difference between Einkorn and the majority of modern wheat? Einkorn has only 14 chromosomes compared to modern wheat's 42, making it easier to digest, especially for those sensitive to modern hybridized wheat.

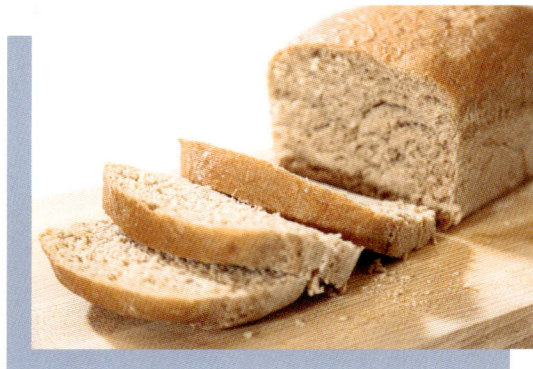

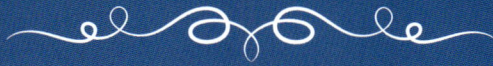

The results speak for themselves. Einkorn is being celebrated for its exceptional nutritional profile and natural integrity.

During this "Eating for Life" book, we will incorporate Einkorn flour into Week 5, for our delicious Almond Pecan Pie Crust and in Week 6, for our bountiful bread, our organic Cinnamon Rolls and our Pizza Crust with Pizzazz! I'm so excited to share my love of Einkorn with you!

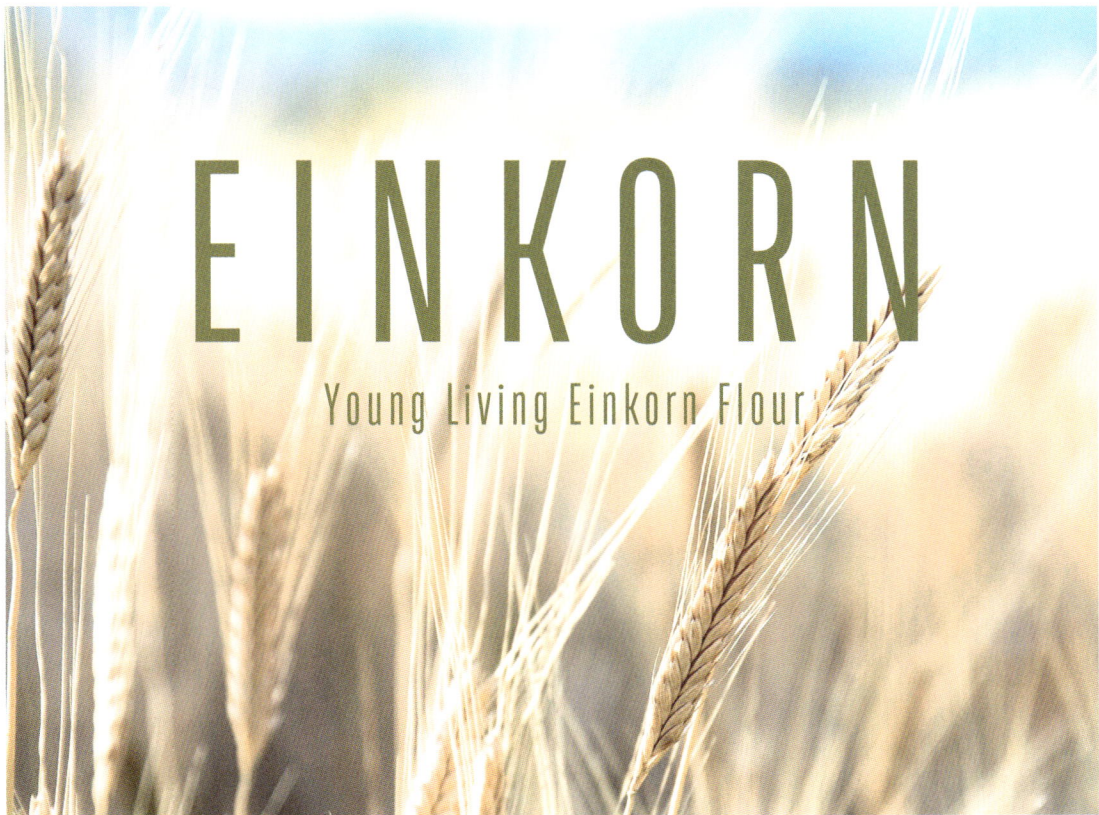

EINKORN
Young Living Einkorn Flour

To learn more scan QR Code

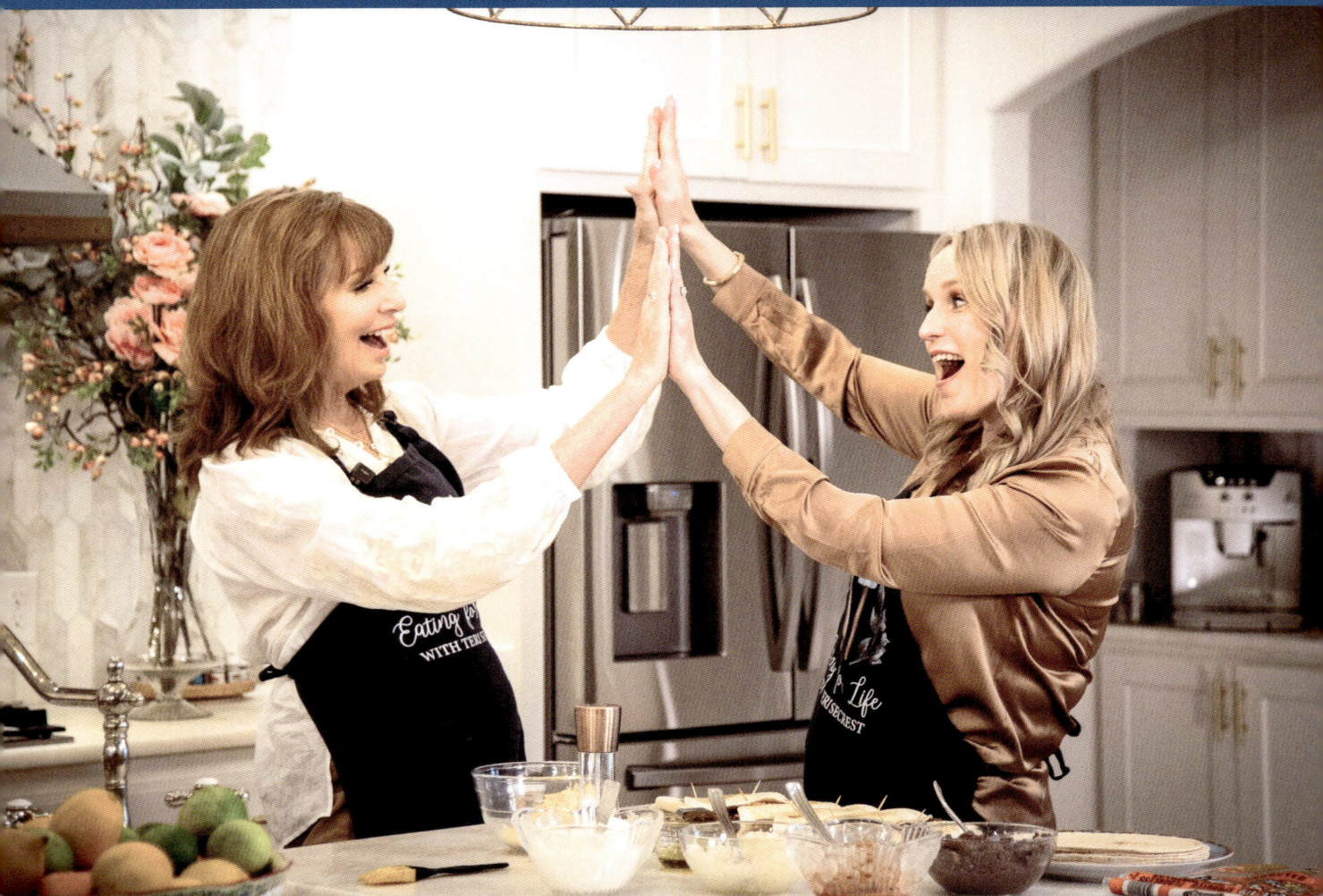

Let's celebrate these life giving ingredients!

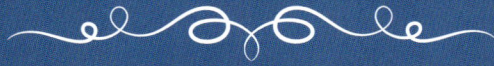

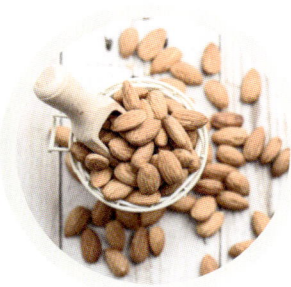

Almonds

- High in plant-based protein
- Source of healthy fats
- Helps lower bad cholesterol levels
- High fiber content supports digestive health
- Helps regulate blood sugar levels
- Smart choice for weight management and diabetes prevention
- Reduces inflammation in the body

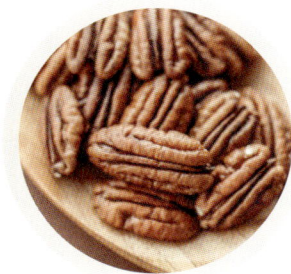

Pecans

- Minerals like calcium, magnesium, and potassium
- Helps maintain healthy blood pressure levels
- Helps balance cholesterol levels
- Good source of fiber
- Aids in digestion
- Helps regulate blood sugar levels

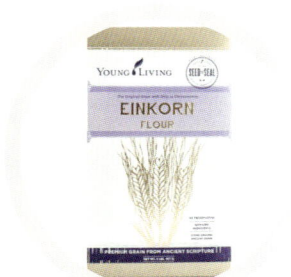

Young Living Einkorn Flour

- Contains protein, iron, dietary fiber, and essential B vitamins
- Contains the antioxidant lutein
- Rich in antioxidant content
- Einkorn has only 14 chromosomes compared to most modern wheat's 42, making it easier to digest, especially for those sensitive to modern hybridized wheat.

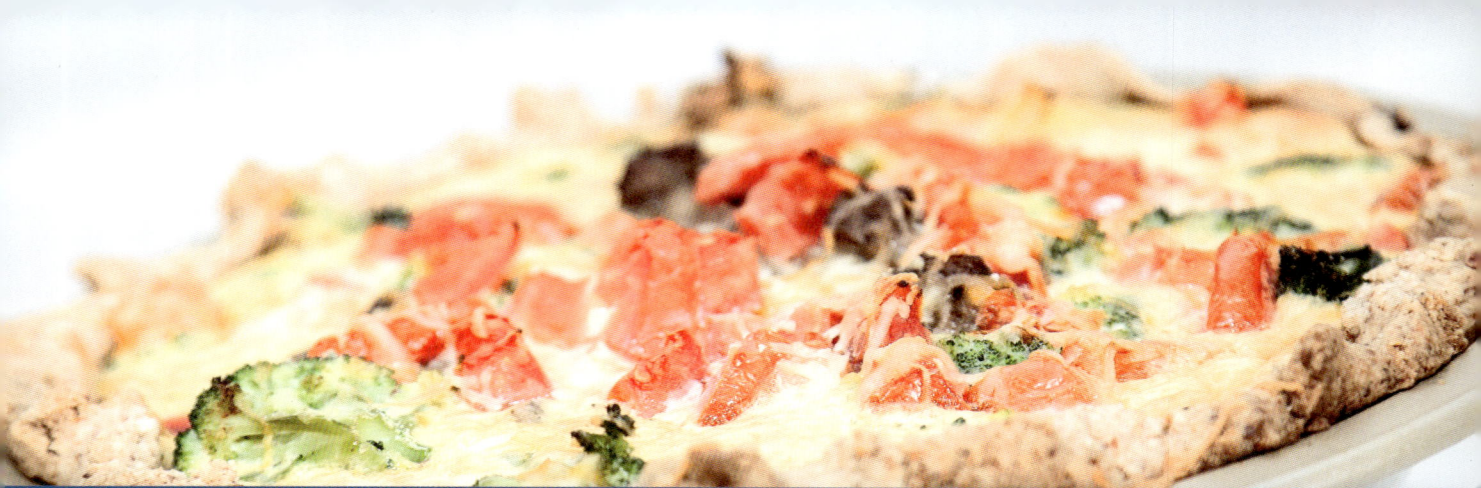

ORGANIC BEEF & BROCCOLI PIE

Ingredients
Makes One 9 inch Pie Crust

1 Almond Pecan Pie Crust, unbaked *(page 144)*

1lb organic ground beef

1 small yellow onion, finely chopped

1 bunch organic broccoli florets cut into bite size pieces

1 ripe tomato, seeded, drained and chopped

1 ½ cups organic cheddar cheese, grated and divided

Dash of Worcestershire sauce

1 cup whole milk or unsweetened non dairy milk

1 ½ Tbsp organic, all-purpose flour

3 large organic eggs

2 drops YL Vitality Oregano oil

2 drops YL Vitality Thyme oil

2 drops YL Vitality Black Pepper oil

(Order YL Vitality Essential Oils on page 39)

½ tsp sea salt

¼ tsp dry mustard

2 tsp tamari sauce

Parmesan cheese, shaved, optional

Preparation

1. In your blender or food processor blend whole milk or non dairy milk, flour, large organic eggs, YL Vitality Oregano oil, YL Vitality Thyme oil, YL Vitality Black Pepper oil, sea salt, dry mustard, tamari sauce, and Worcestershire sauce. Set aside.

2. In a large skillet, brown meat and onion together. Drain grease very well.

3. In a sauce pan, steam the broccoli florets until al dente, for only 3-4 minutes.

4. Now, assemble your award-winning pie! Start by evenly sprinkling ½ of the cheddar cheese on the bottom of the Almond Pecan Pie Crust.

5. Spread ½ of your beef and onion mixture evenly over the chedder cheese.

6. Layer ½ of the steamed broccoli and ½ of the chopped tomato over the beef and onion.

7. Layer again using steps 5 and 6

8. Next, pour the blender mixture over meat and vegetables and top with the chopped tomato OPTIONAL: Sprinkle shaved Parmesan cheese over the top. Avoid covering up all the colorful vegetables.

9. Back at 350° for one hour. Allow to cool for 10-15 minutes before cutting and serving. Enjoy!

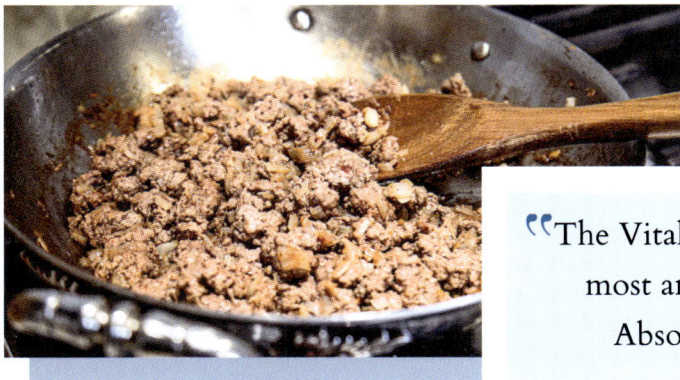

> "The Vitality Oils in this pie give the most amazing Ba-boom flavor! Absolutely to-live-for taste!"
> -Susan McGinnis

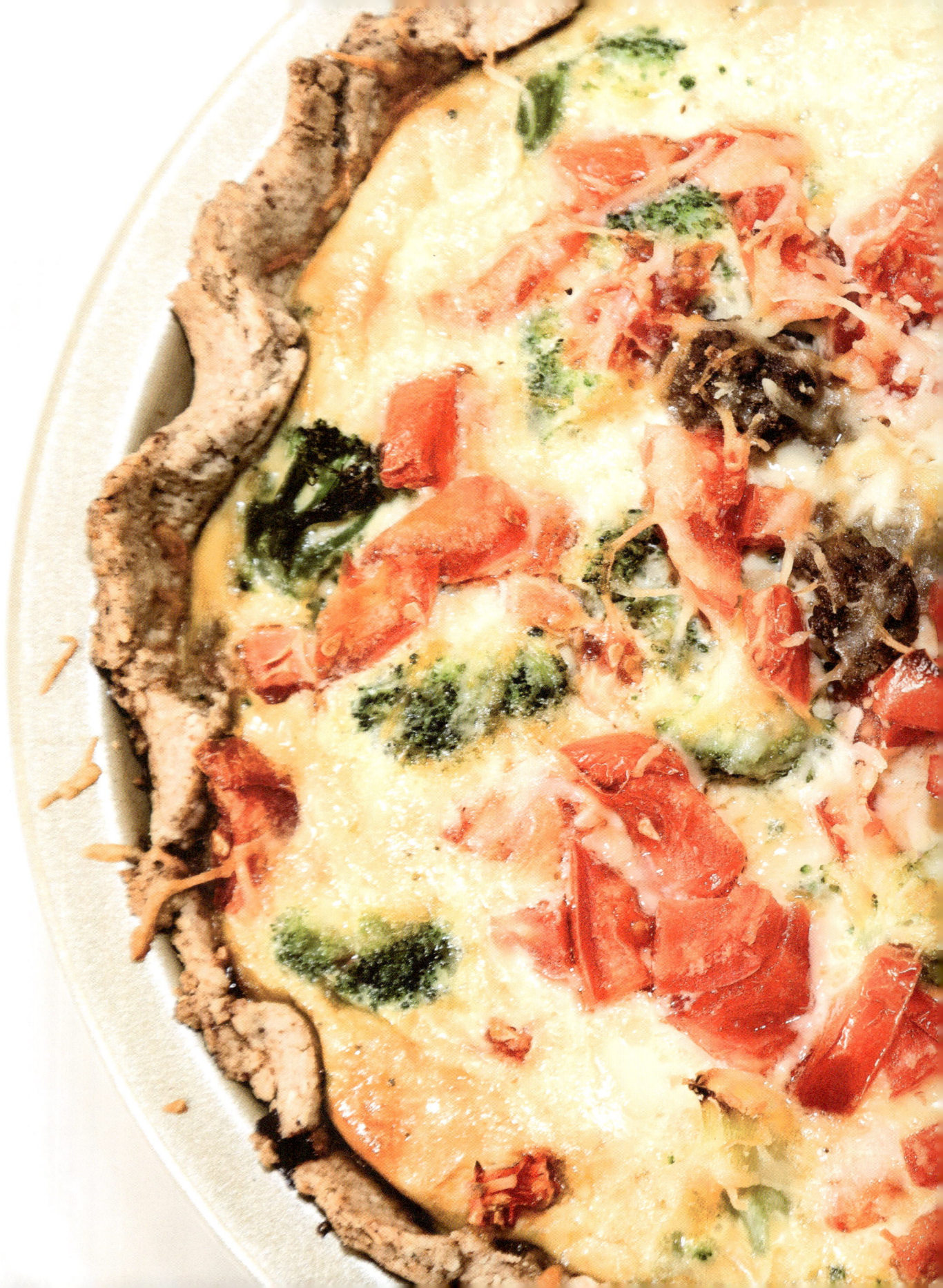

ORGANIC BEEF & BROCCOLI PIE NUTRITIONAL BENEFITS

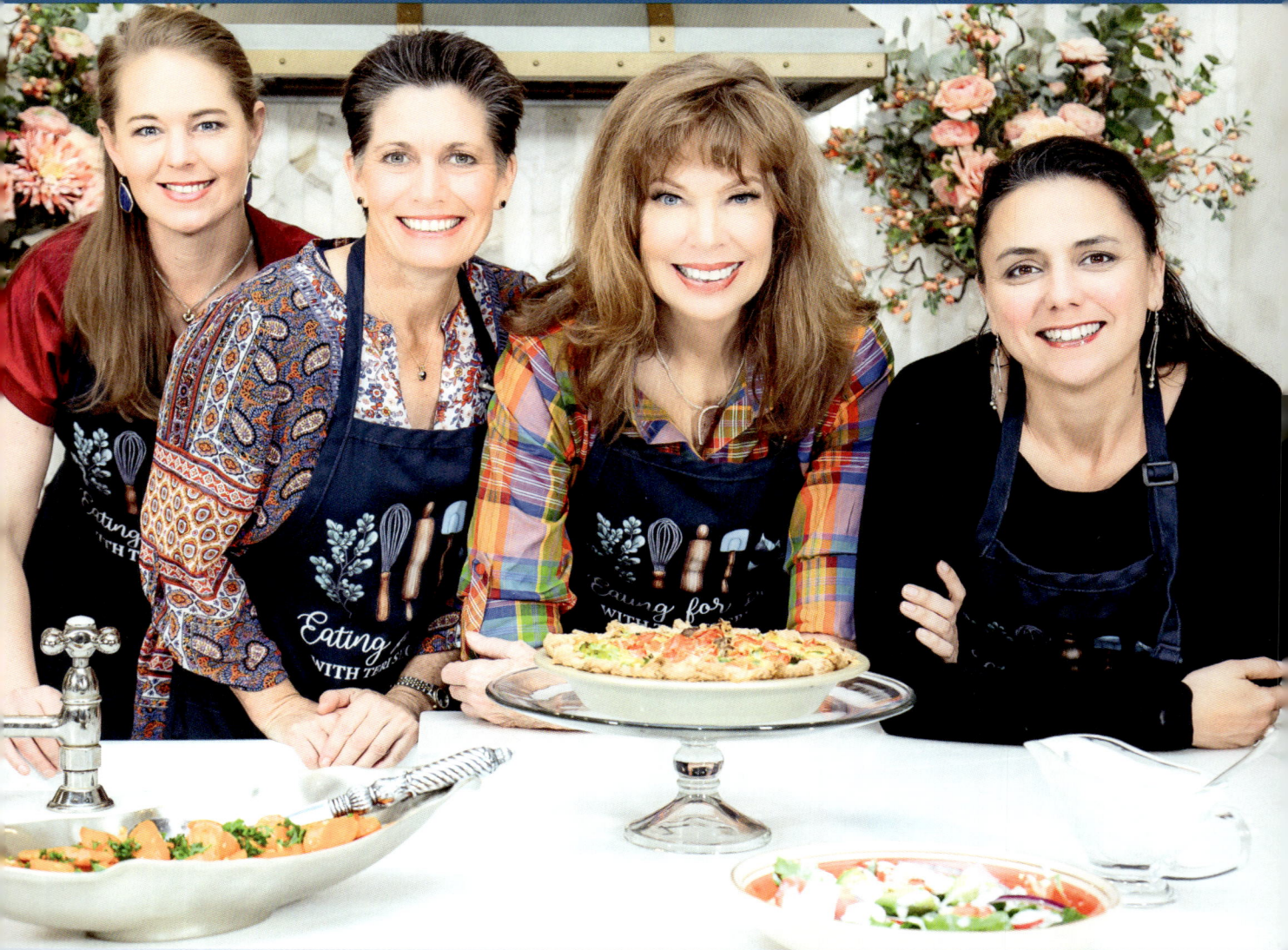

Let's celebrate these life giving ingredients!

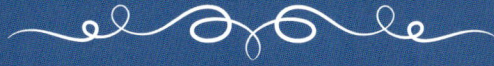

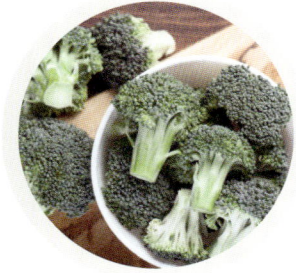

Broccoli

- Rich in vitamins C, K, and folate, supporting the immune system and overall health
- Contains powerful antioxidants like sulforaphane, offering anti-cancer properties
- High fiber content aids digestion and may assist in weight management
- Excellent source of calcium and vitamin D, promoting bone health

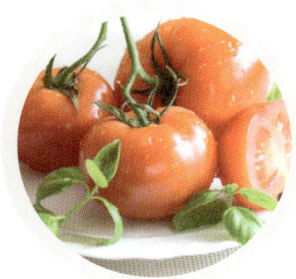

Tomatoes

- Includes vitamin C, potassium, and folate
- Supports the immune system
- Rich in antioxidants like lycopene
- Promotes heart health
- Fiber content aids in digestion
- Contributes to weight management

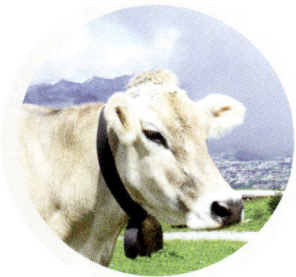

Organic Beef from Happy Cows

- Leaner than conventional beef
- Rich in heart-healthy omega-3 fatty acids
- Contains antioxidants such as Vitamin E
- High in muscle-building protein

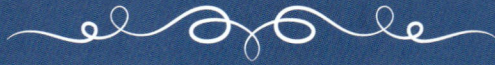

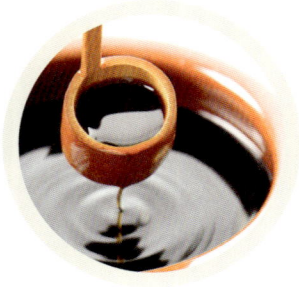

- Gluten-free alternative to soy sauce
- Rich in essential amino acids
- Good plant-based protein
- Contains healthy phytonutrients
- Antioxidants
- Contains the minerals iron, manganese, potassium

Tamari Sauce

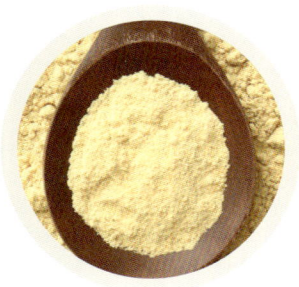

- Contains antioxidants
- Anti-inflammatory
- Promotes digestion
- Boosts metabolism

Dry Mustard

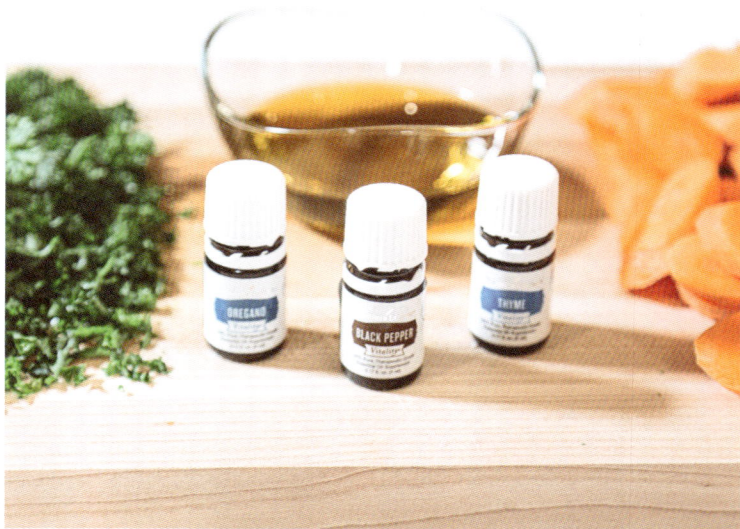

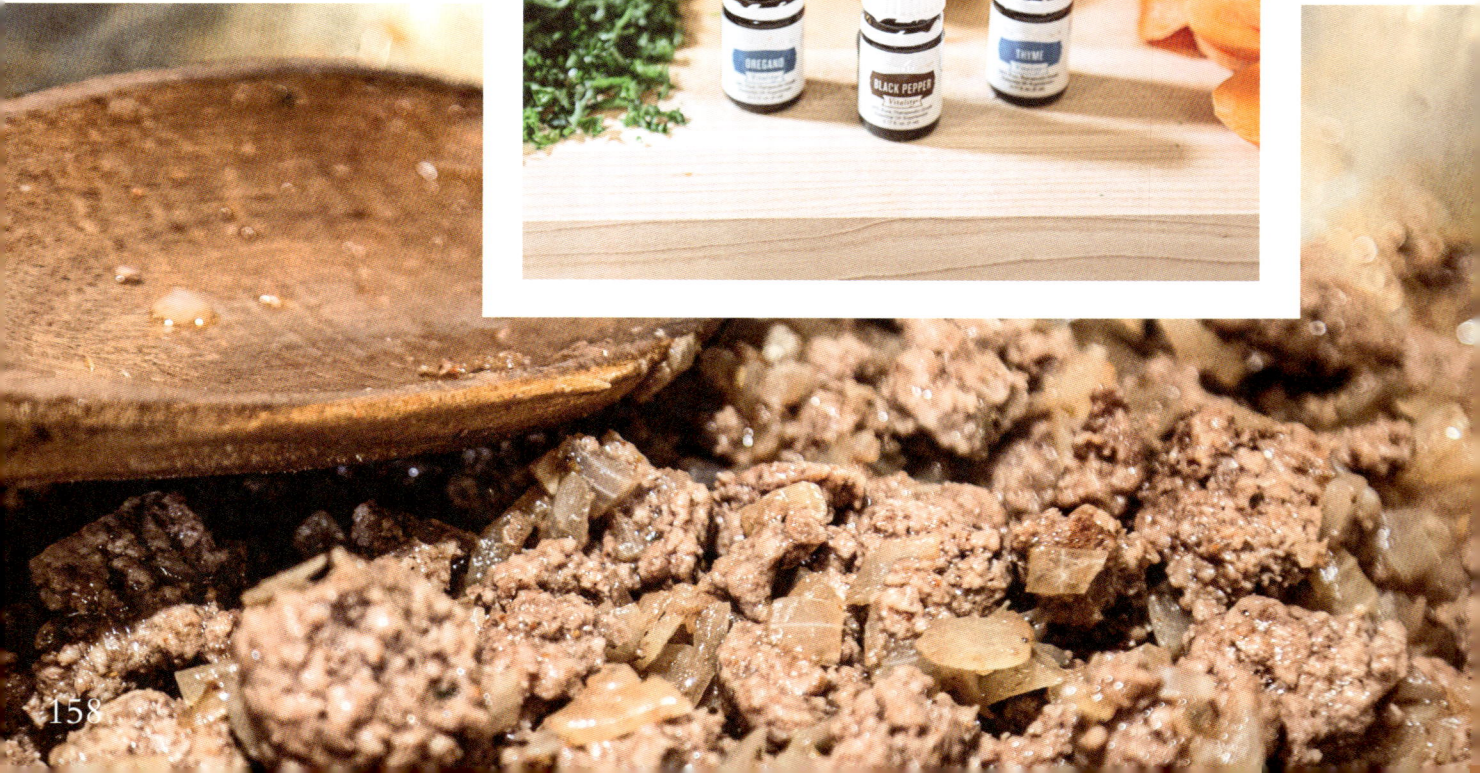

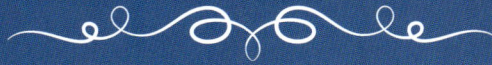

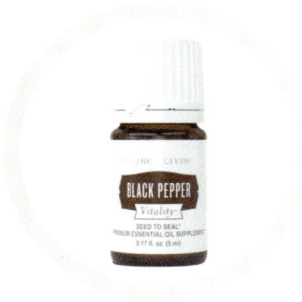

- Aids in digestive health
- Promotes secretion of enzymes
- Helps alleviate digestive discomfort
- Invigorates the mind
- Boosts alertness

YL Vitality Black Pepper Oil

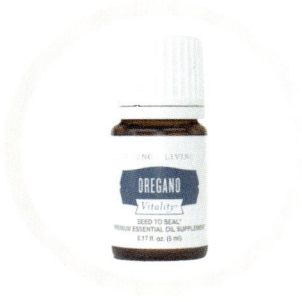

- Rich in antimicrobial compounds like carvacrol and thymol
- High in antioxidants
- Supports digestion
- Provides respiratory support

YL Vitality Oregano Oil

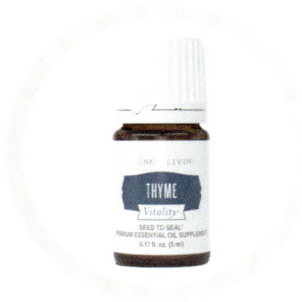

- Rich in thymol which is antimicrobial
- Contains antioxidants
- Supports respiratory health

YL Vitality Thyme Oil

"Add a layer of exotic flavor to this already delicious pie with the YL Vitality Essential Oils of Oregano, Thyme and Black Pepper."

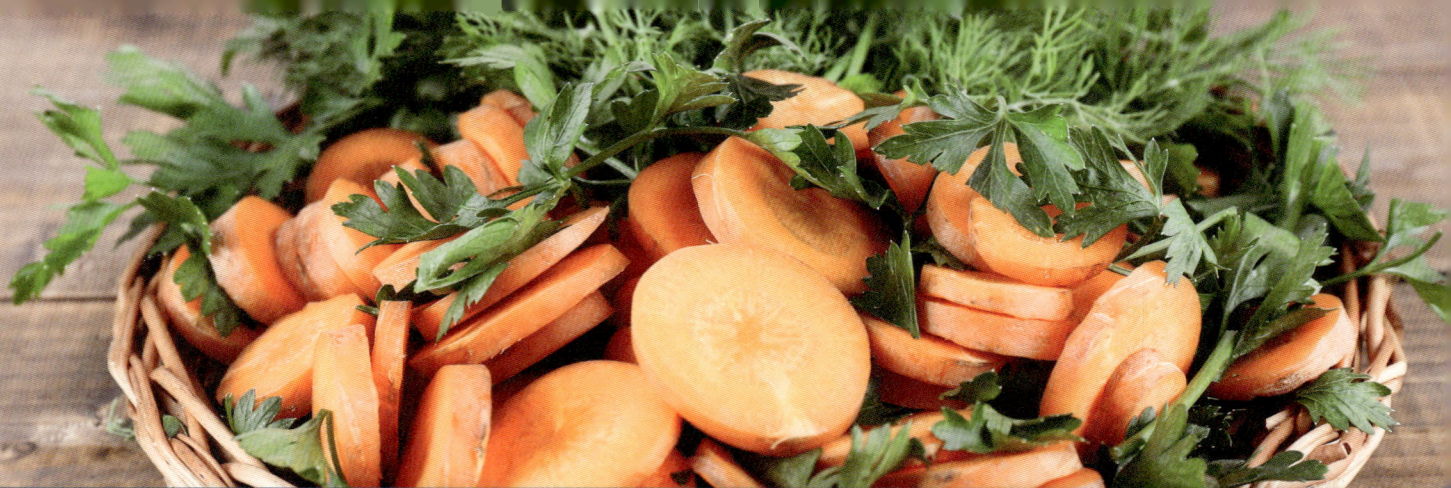

GARLIC ROASTED CARROTS

Ingredients

Makes 4 Savory Servings

1 lb organic carrots, washed

3 Tbsp olive oil

3 cloves garlic, finely chopped

1 drop YL Vitality Oregano oil

1 drop YL Vitality Thyme oil

1 drop YL Vitality Black Pepper oil

(Order YL Vitality oils on page 39)

¼ tsp sea salt or to taste

2 Tbsp fresh organic parsley, finely chopped

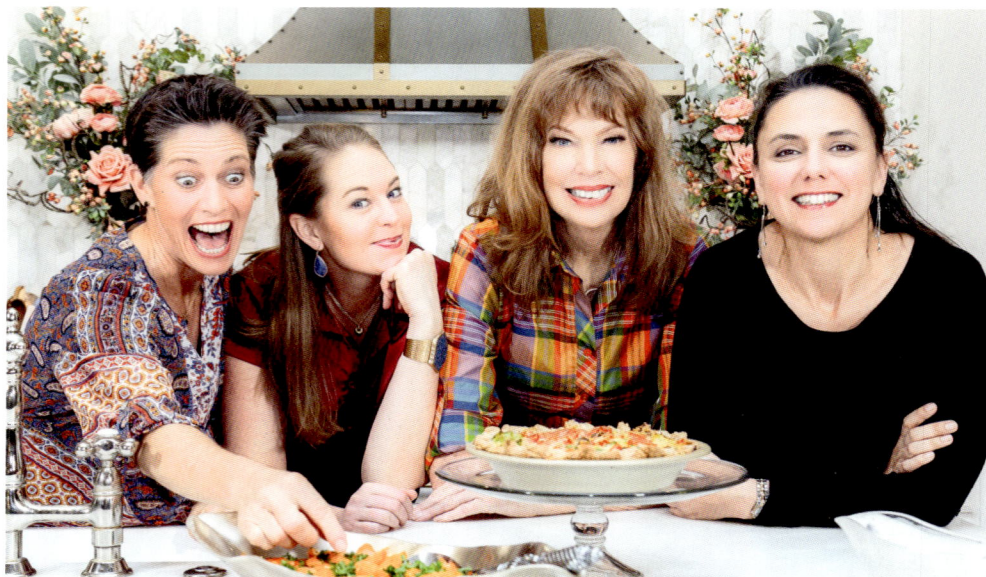

Preparation

1. Preheat oven to 350°.
2. Cut carrots into ¼" slices on the diagonal
3. In a small bowl whisk together the olive oil, essential oils, minced garlic, and salt.
4. Place carrots in a gallon size ziploc bag. Pour olive oil mixture over carrots and shake well making sure all the carrots are covered with the oil mixture.
5. Arrange the carrots on the sheet pan.
6. Bake at 350° for 40 minutes. Check to make sure they are done to your liking.
7. Sprinkle the finely chopped parsley and serve.

"The carrots, roasted to perfection, were beautifully enhanced by the simple yet powerful blend of olive oil, minced garlic and essential oils. Cooking with Teri's recipes bring joy to the kitchen and makes me excited to create wholesome meals!"

-Anthoney Teague

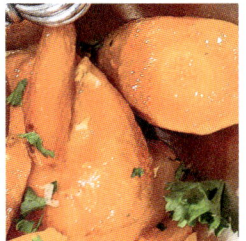

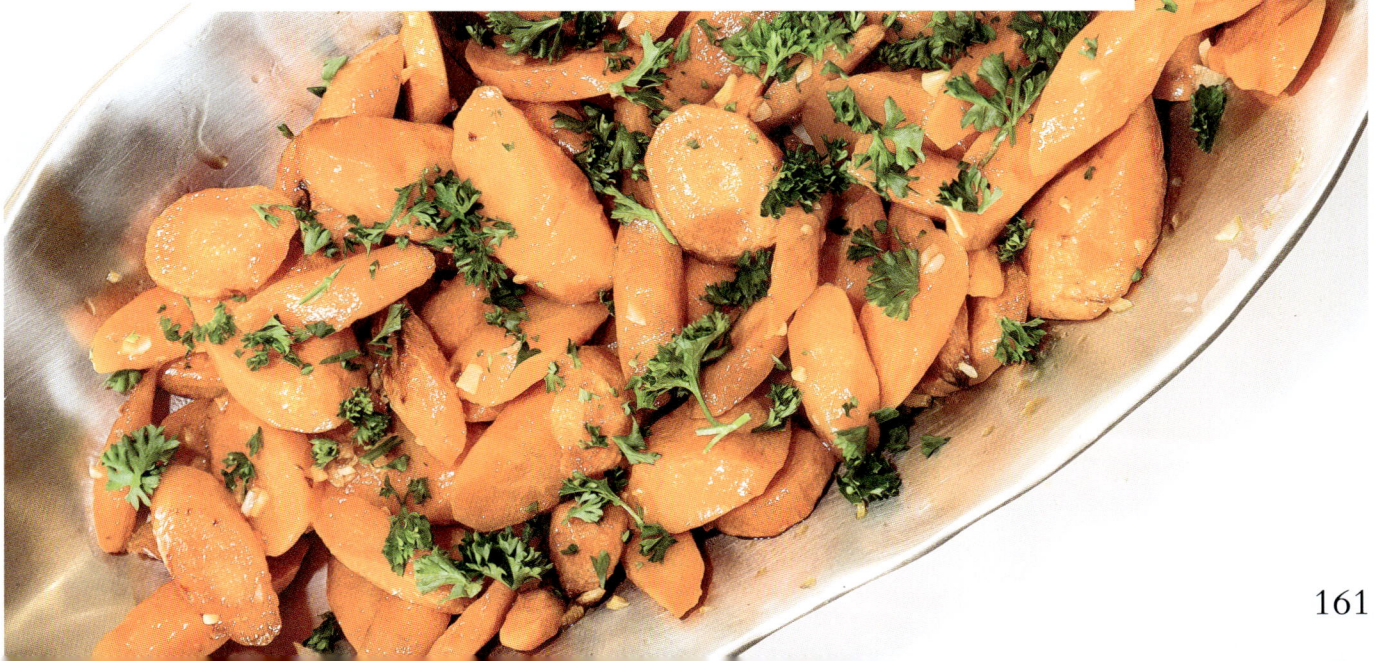

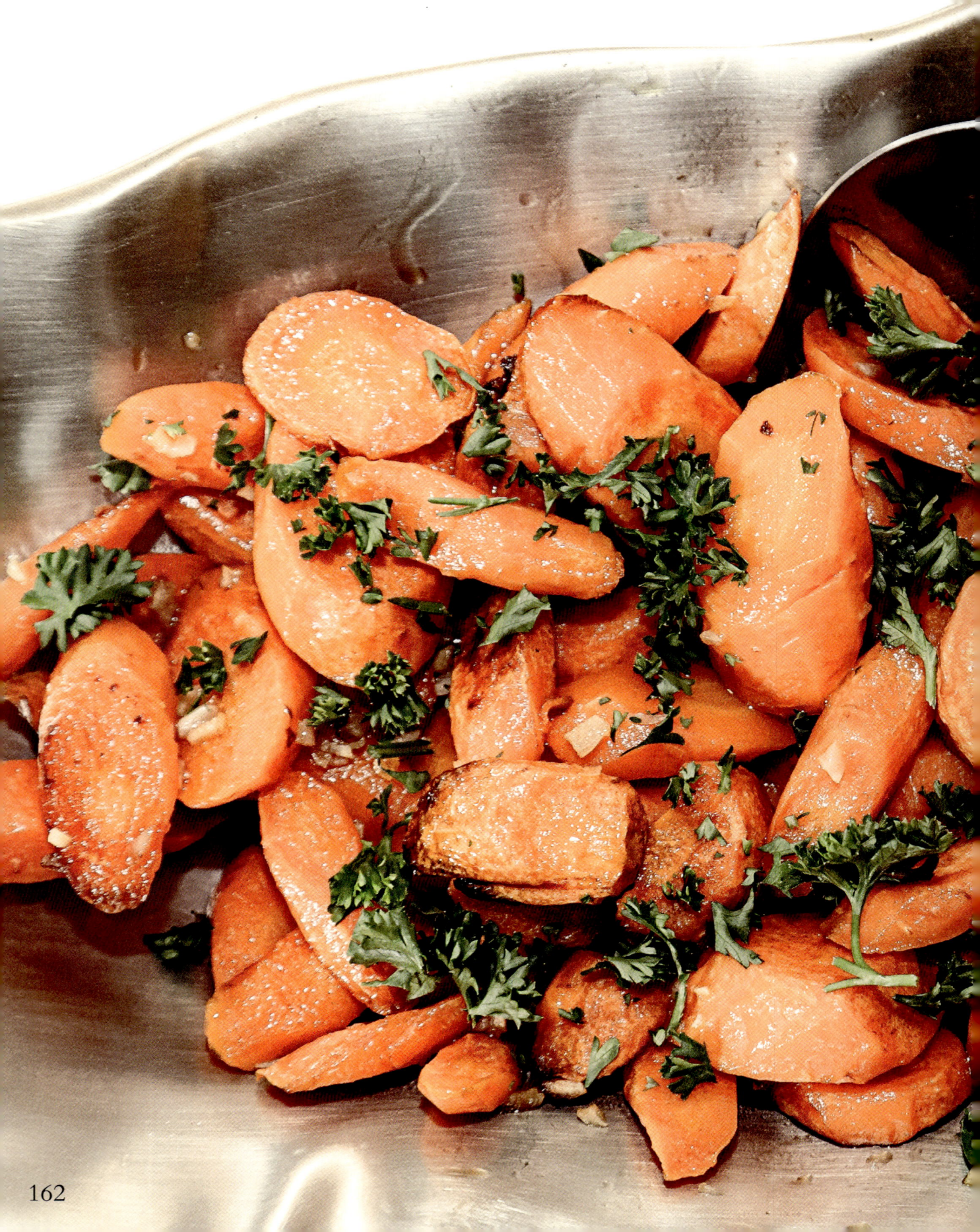

"Recently, when I made these carrots for our cooking class, the men could not wait until they were served and began eating them right out of the oven!"

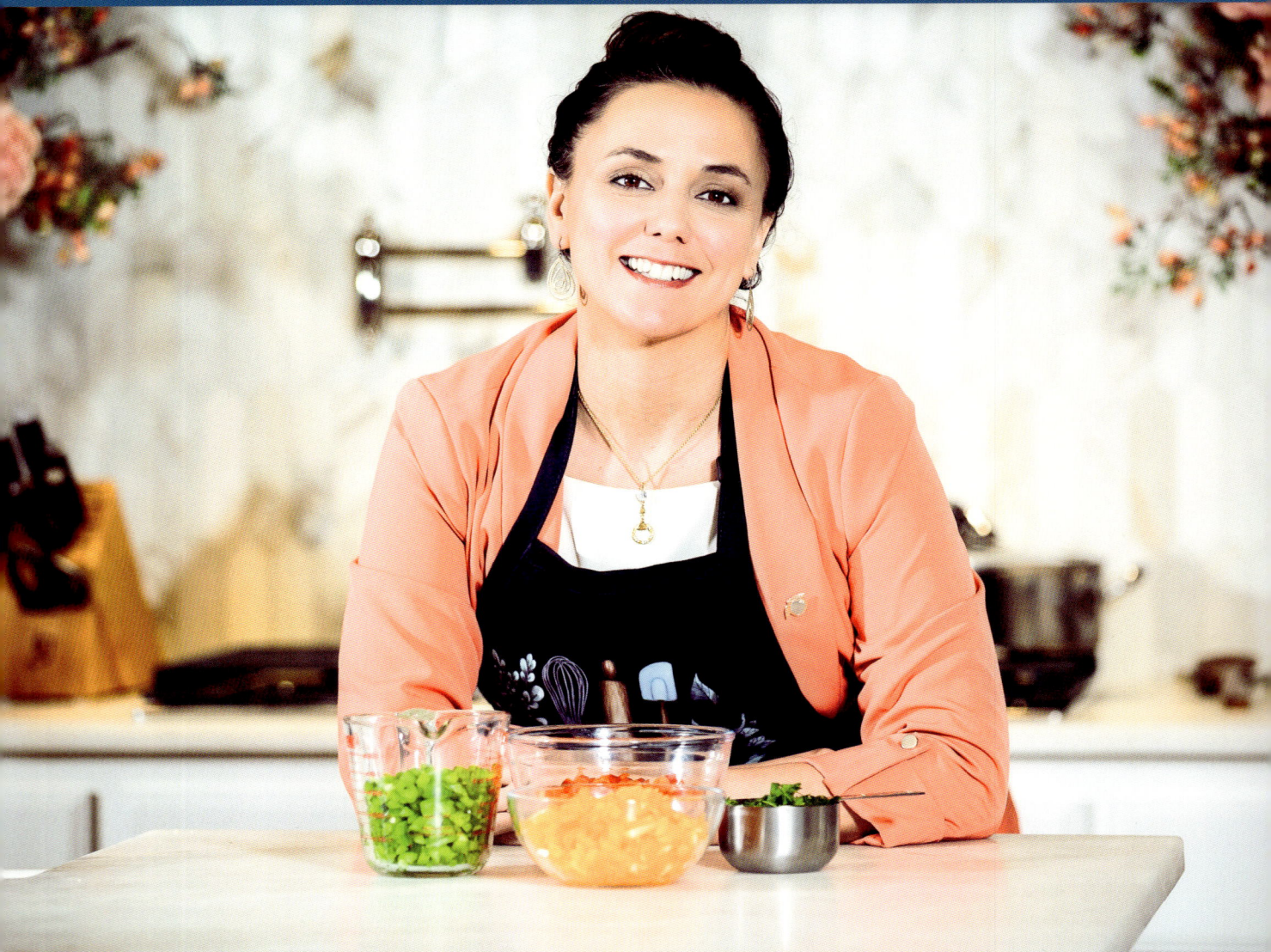

Let's celebrate these life giving ingredients!

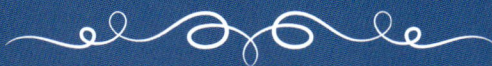

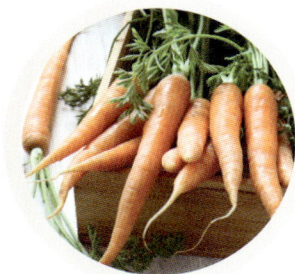

Carrots

- Packed with beta-carotene
- Supports vision health
- Boosts immune system
- Great for skin health
- Contains antioxidants like vitamin C and lutein
- High fiber supports digestive health
- Promotes feelings of fullness

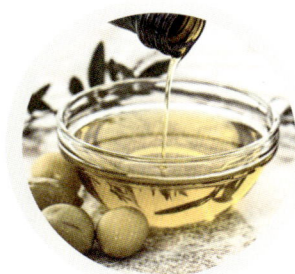

Olive Oil

- Rich in monounsaturated fats
- Heart-healthy choice
- Lowers bad cholesterol levels and reduce the risk of heart disease
- Packed with antioxidants like vitamin E and polyphenols
- Protects cells from damage caused by free radicals and oxidative stress
- Reduces the risk of Alzheimer's

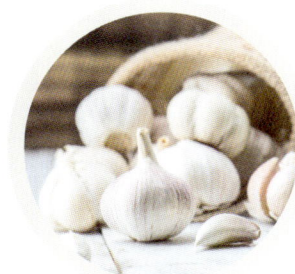

Garlic

- Renowned for natural antibiotic and antimicrobial properties
- Helps combat infections and boosts the immune system
- Rich in antioxidants, including allicin
- Well-documented support for heart health
- Lowers blood pressure and improves cholesterol levels
- Reduces the risk of cardiovascular diseases
- Anti-inflammatory properties

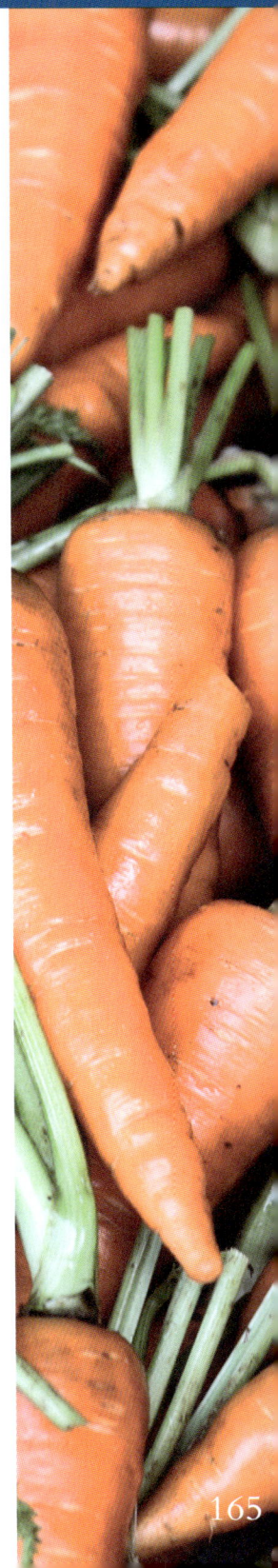

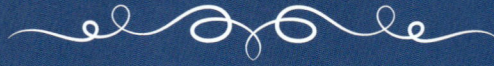

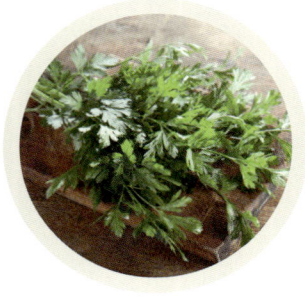

Parsley

- Excellent source of vitamin K. – crucial for blood clotting and bone health
- Contains vitamin C
- Supports immune function and collagen production
- Promotes skin health and wound healing
- High antioxidant content, including flavonoids and carotenoids
- Supports heart health by lowering blood pressure and cholesterol levels

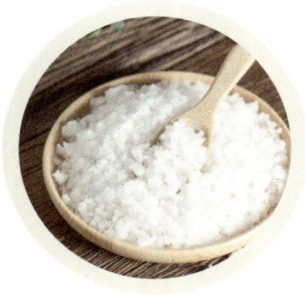

Sea Salt

- Retains natural minerals like magnesium, calcium, potassium which are essential for bone health, muscle function, hydration, and nerve transmission.
- Lower-sodium than table salt

"Friend, here is a challenge for you... take one commercially raised carrot and one organic carrot, cut them into pieces and do a taste test with your family. I think you will be amazed at the profound difference in the flavor between the two carrots!"

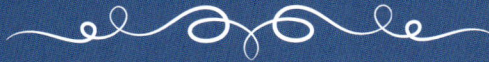

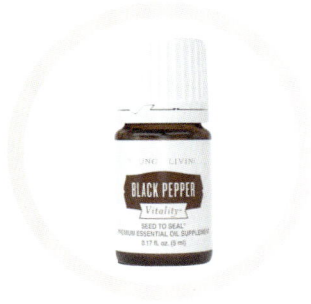

- Aids in digestive health
- Promotes secretion of enzymes
- Helps alleviate digestive discomfort
- Invigorates the mind
- Boosts alertness

YL Vitality Black Pepper Oil

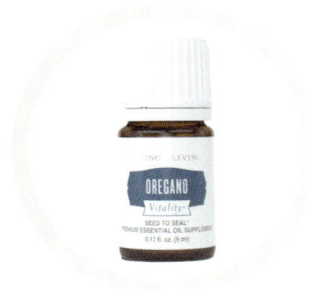

- Rich in antimicrobial compounds like carvacrol and thymol
- High in antioxidants
- Supports digestion
- Provides respiratory support

YL Vitality Oregano Oil

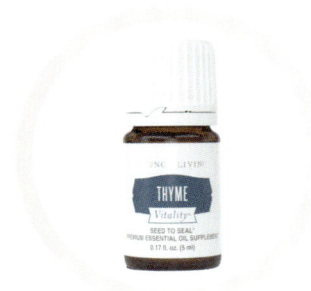

- Rich in thymol, which is antimicrobial properties
- Contains antioxidants
- Supports respiratory health

YL Vitality Thyme Oil

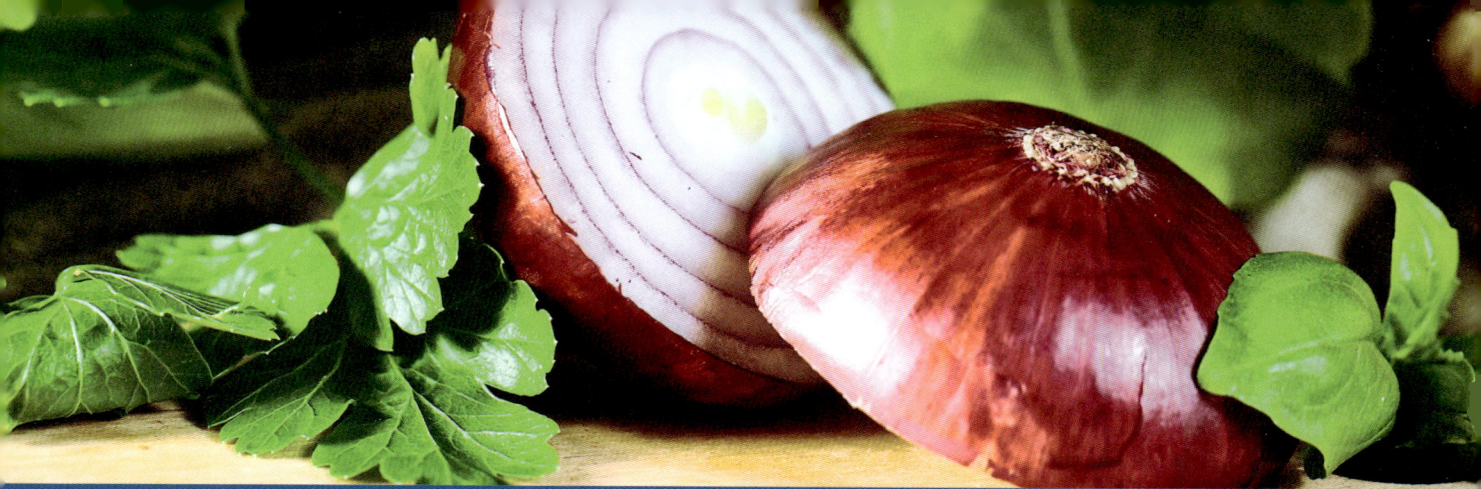

BOUNTIFUL BASIC SALAD

Ingredients

Makes 4 Servings

1 head of organic butter lettuce

1 small red onion

1-2 organic cucumbers
depending on size

2 avocadoes

2 small ripe tomatoes

4-6 red radishes

OPTIONAL: feta cheese

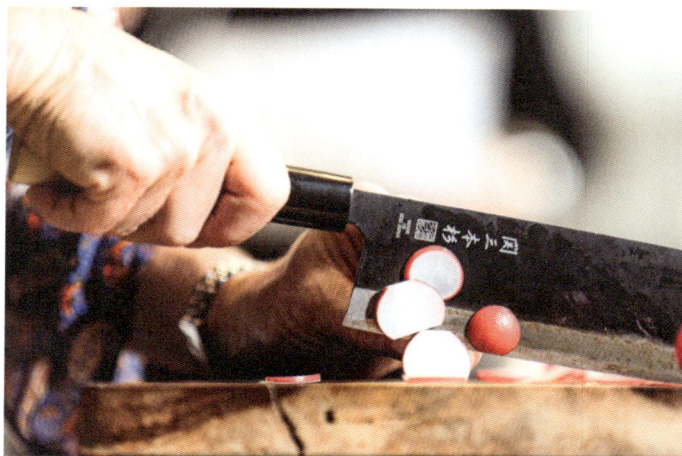

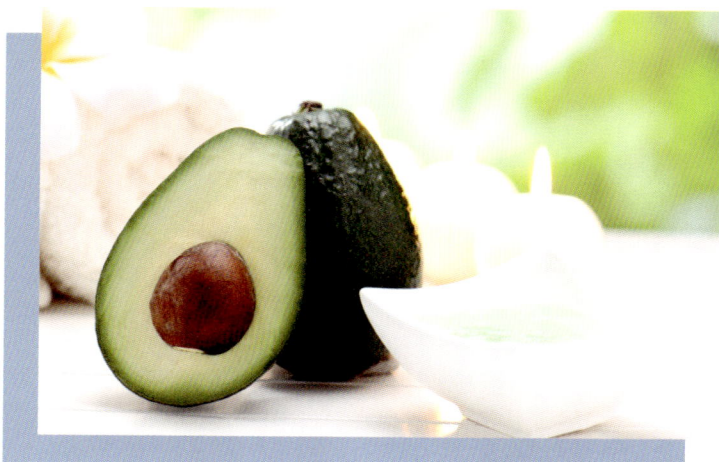

Preparation

1. Wash and dry lettuce well. I recommend using a lettuce spinner. It's a very valuable tool in your kitchen.
2. Tear lettuce gently into bite-sized pieces; avoid cutting lettuce with a knife.
3. Place lettuce in the bottom of your favorite salad bowl.
4. Using your French-style chef's knife, cut very thin slices of red onion Add to the lettuce.
5. Cut avocados into nice, bite-sized pieces and add.
6. Remove the seeds from your tomatoes, cut in wedges then add to the salad.
7. Slice cucumber into 1/4 inch coins and add.
8. Cut radishes very thin and add.
9. Add your dressing of choice and gently toss, making sure the dressing coats all of the vegetables.
10. Sprinkle Feta cheese all over top of salad, optional.

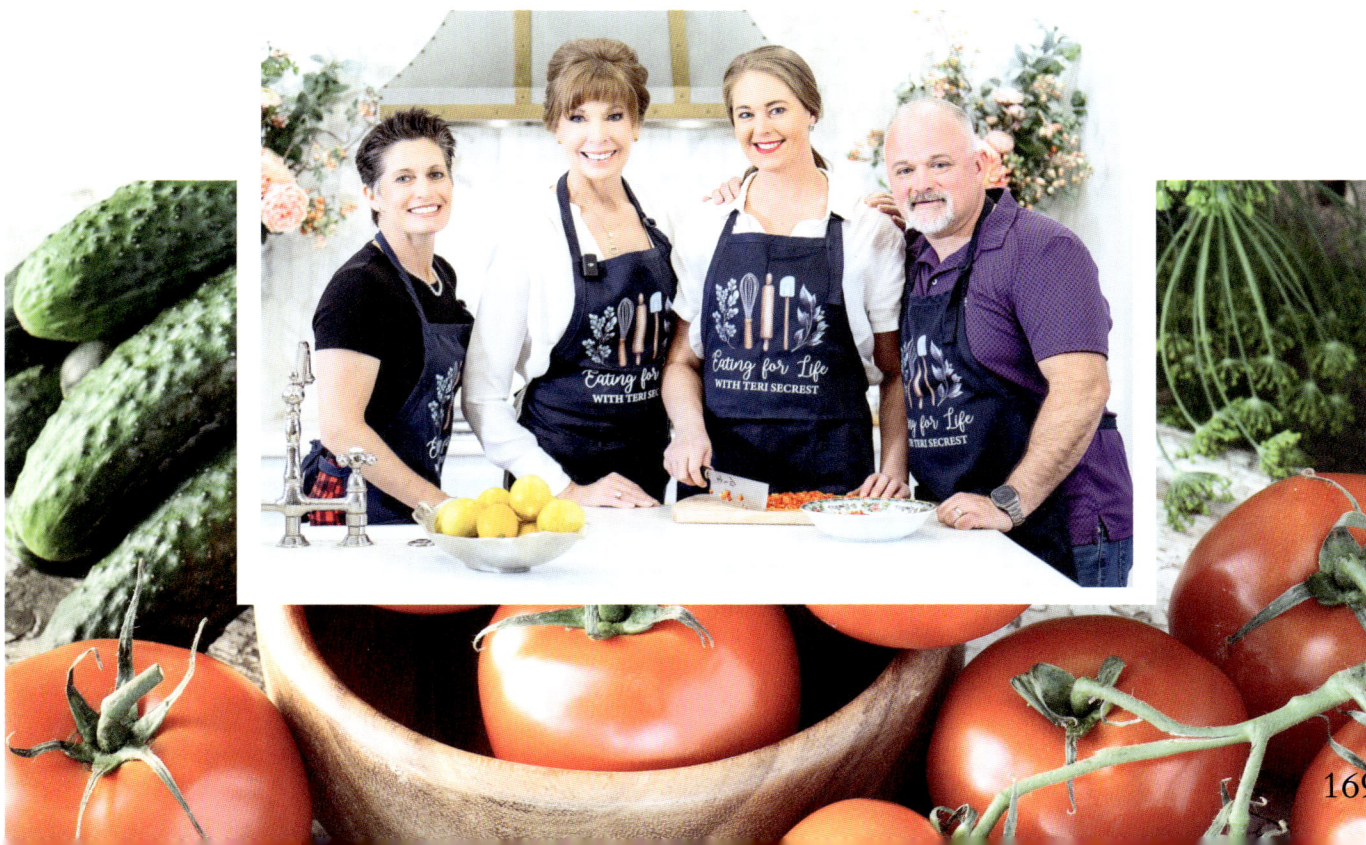

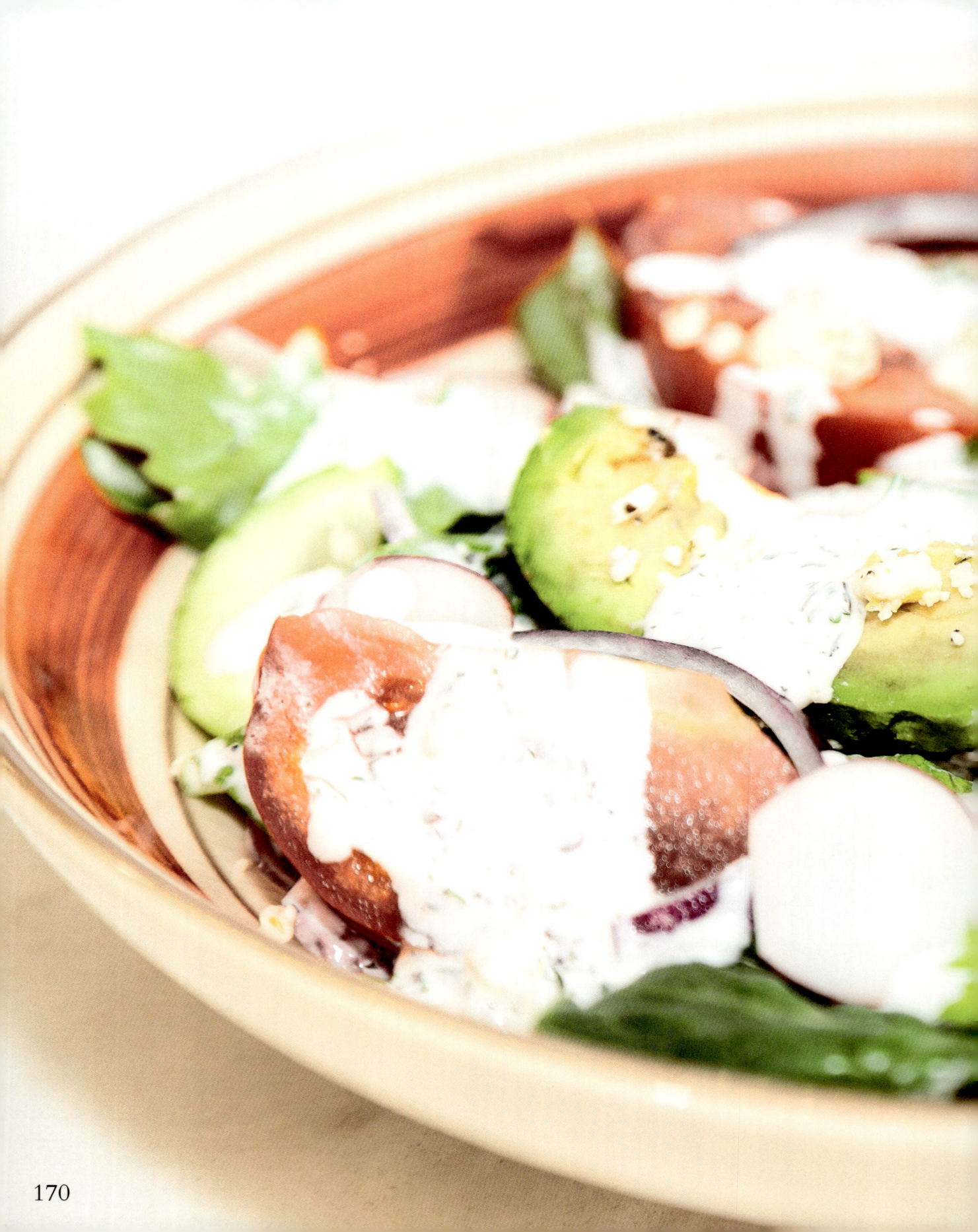

"One night my neighbors came over to have salmon on the grill. One of my dear friends walked in with the biggest smile on her face. She surprised me and made the Bountiful Basic Salad with my Healthy Ranch Dressing. It was delicious and everyone loved it!"

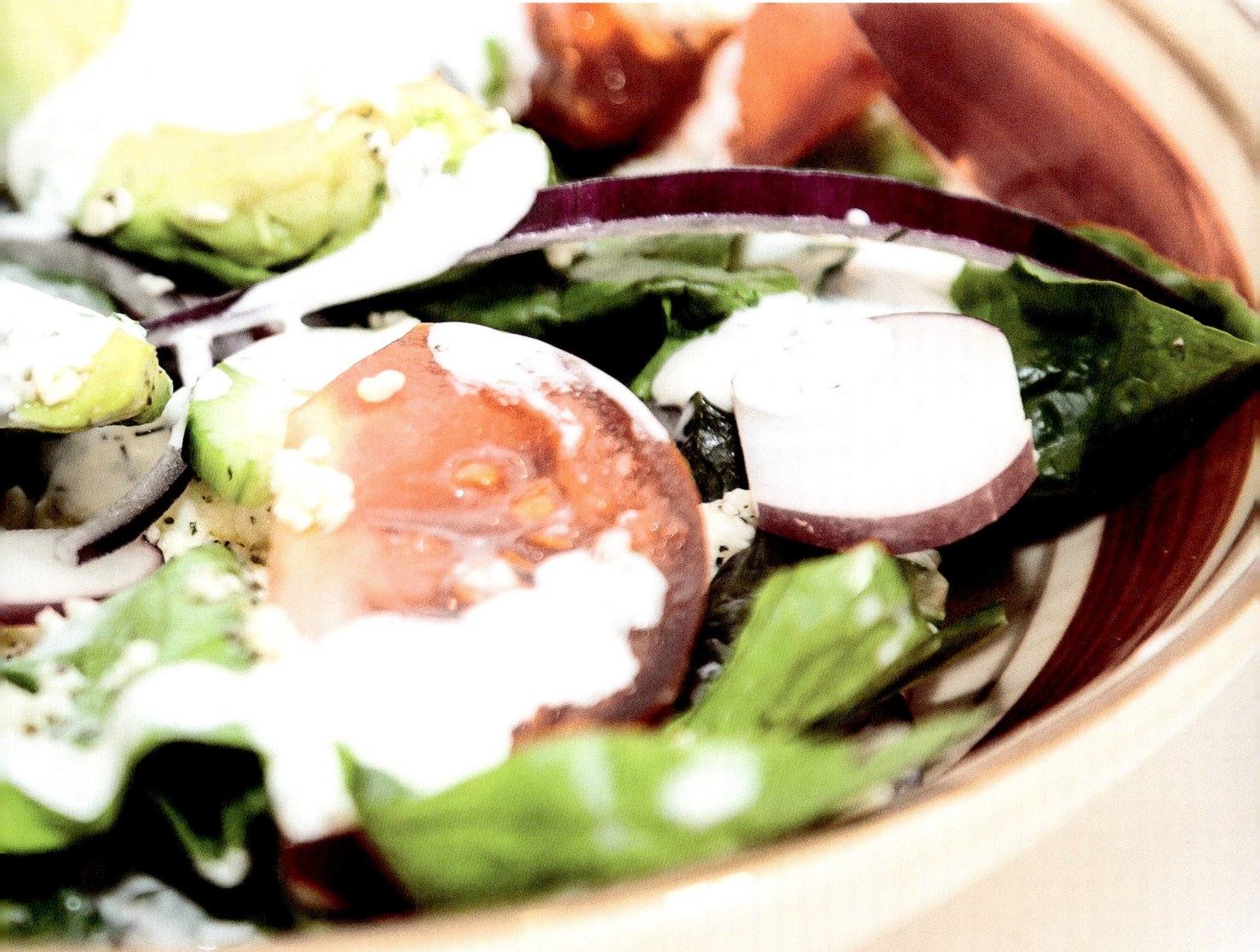

Let's celebrate these life giving ingredients!

ating for Life
WITH TERI SECREST

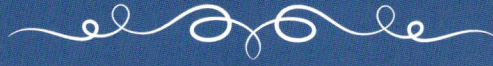

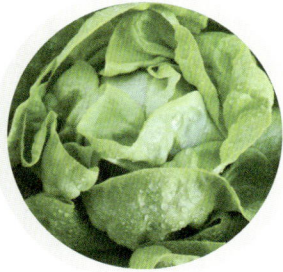

Butter Lettuce

- Excellent source of vitamins A and K for eye health, immune function, and bone strength
- Contains folate, important for cell division and DNA synthesis
- Provides small amounts of vitamin C, potassium, and iron
- High water content helps keep you hydrated and promotes feeling of fullness

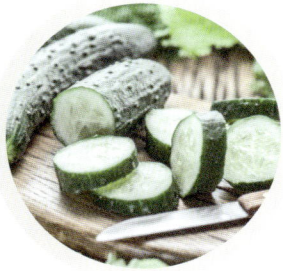

Cucumbers

- Promotes healthy skin.
- Vitamins K and vitamin C
- Contains potassium, and manganese, which support bone health, immune function, and electrolyte balance.
- Contains beta-carotene and flavonoids
- High fiber

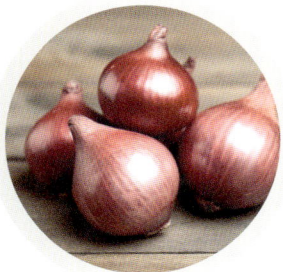

Red Onion

- Antioxidants such as flavonoids and anthocyanins, which help combat oxidative stress and inflammation
- Contains quercetin which is great for lowering inflammation
- Rich in vitamin C

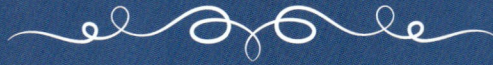

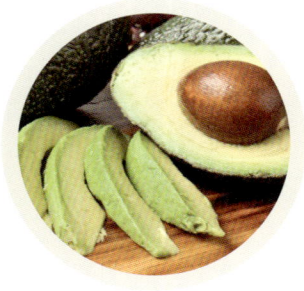

Avocados

- Packed with heart-healthy monounsaturated fats
- Helps lower bad cholesterol and raise good cholesterol levels
- Loaded with fiber for digestion and weight management
- Source of vitamins E and K for skin health, blood clotting, and bone strength
- Provides potassium, folate, and vitamin C

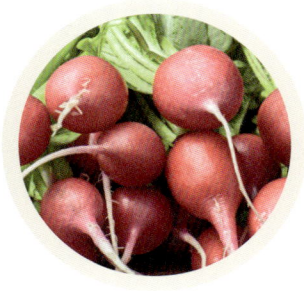

Radishes

- Rich in vitamin C, supporting a healthy immune system and skin
- Provide essential minerals like potassium and folate contributing to heart health and overall well-being
- Contain antioxidants
- Good source of dietary fiber

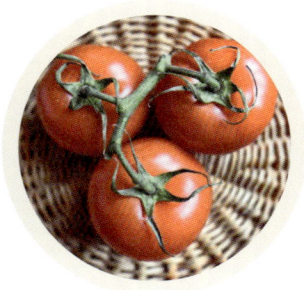

Organic Tomatoes

- Includes vitamin C, potassium, and folate
- Supports the immune system
- Rich in antioxidants like lycopene
- Promotes heart health
- Fiber content aids in digestion
- Contributes to weight management

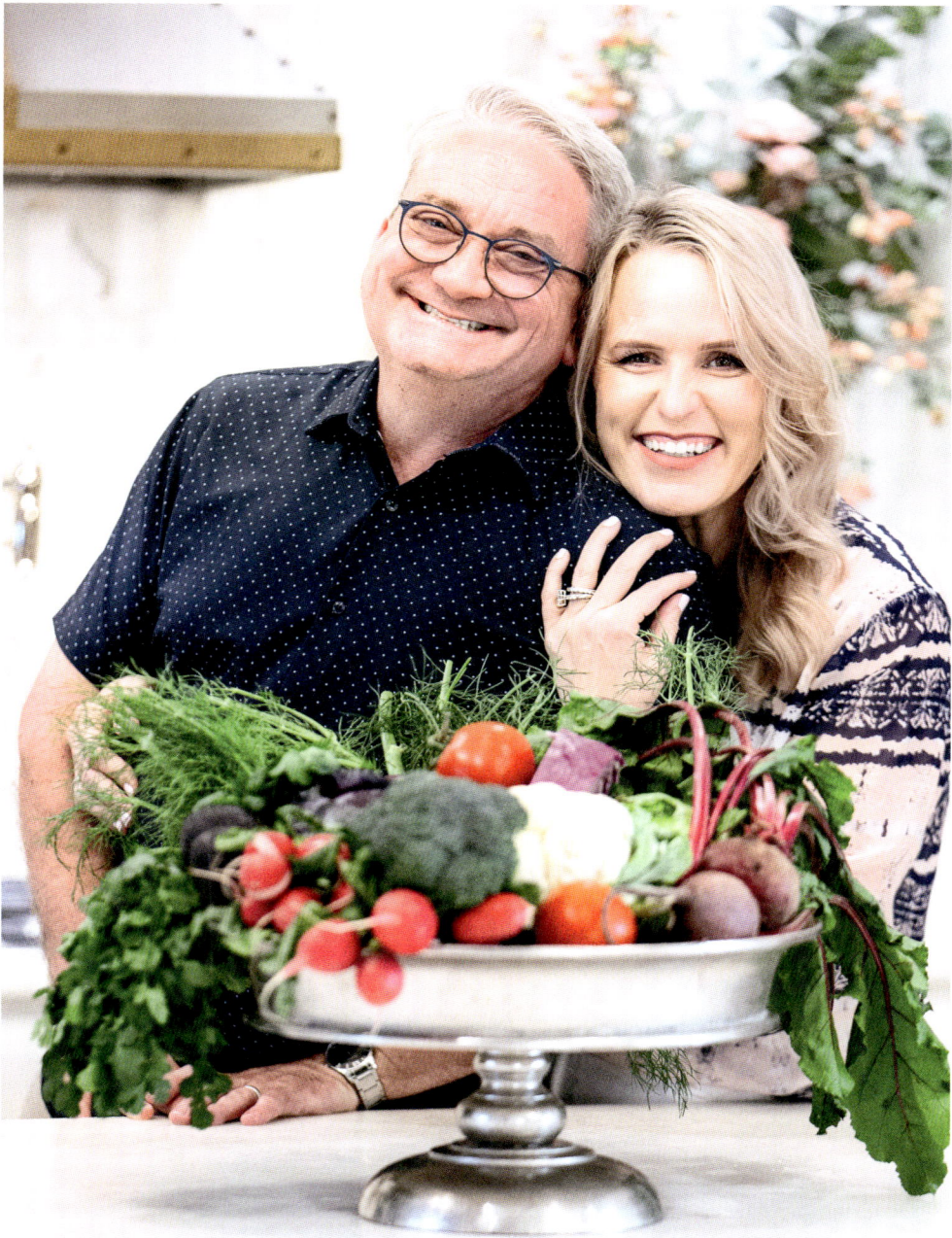

HEALTHY RANCH DRESSING

Ingredients

Creates 1 1/2 cups of zesty dressing!

½ cup good-quality organic mayonnaise

½ cup organic sour cream

½ cup buttermilk

3 Tbsp fresh parsley, minced

½ tsp dried dill and

1 drop YL Vitality Dill oil *(Order YL Vitalty Essential Oils on page 39)*

½ tsp apple cider vinegar

½ tsp Worcestershire sauce

2 cloves garlic, pressed with garlic press

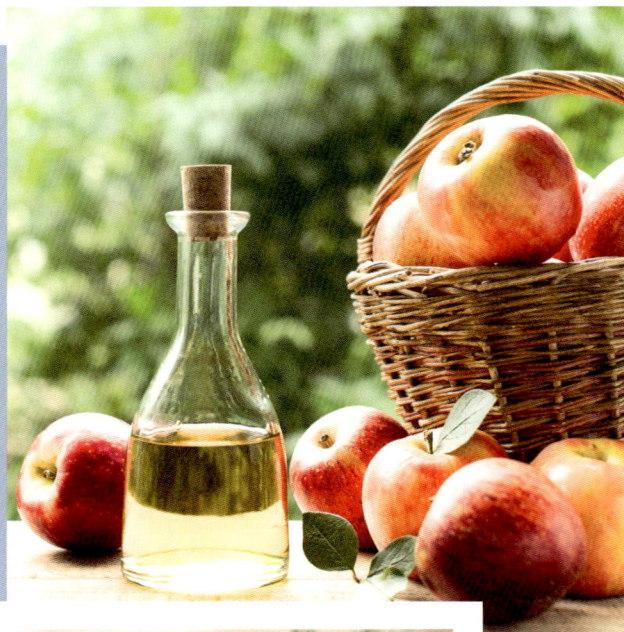

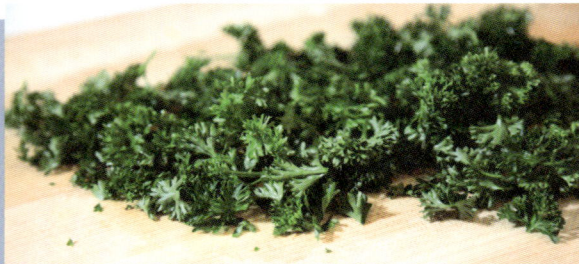

Preparation

Add all ingredients to a medium-sized mixing bowl and gently combine with a wire whisk. Adjust the seasoning to your liking, take a lettuce leaf and give it a taste. Add more salt or any other desired flavor. Use as a salad dressing or a yummy veggie dip!

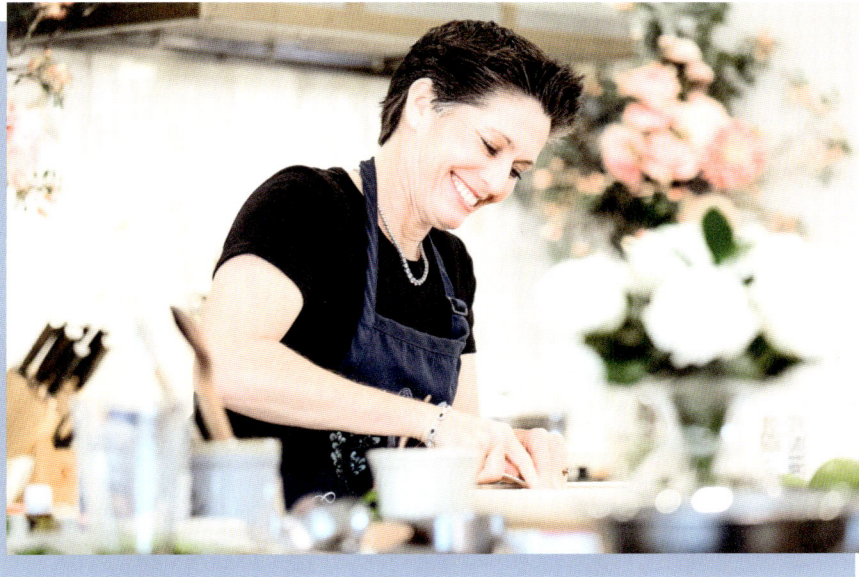

"I absolutely love this healthy ranch dressing! It makes me feel so good to know I can enjoy a healthy and tasty ranch without all the unhealthy ingredients you get in store bought dressings. This will be my new go-to-ranch recipe!"

-Lisa Carpenter

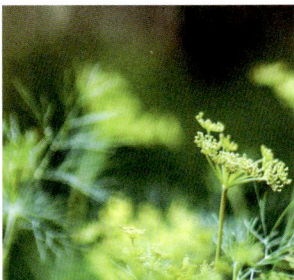

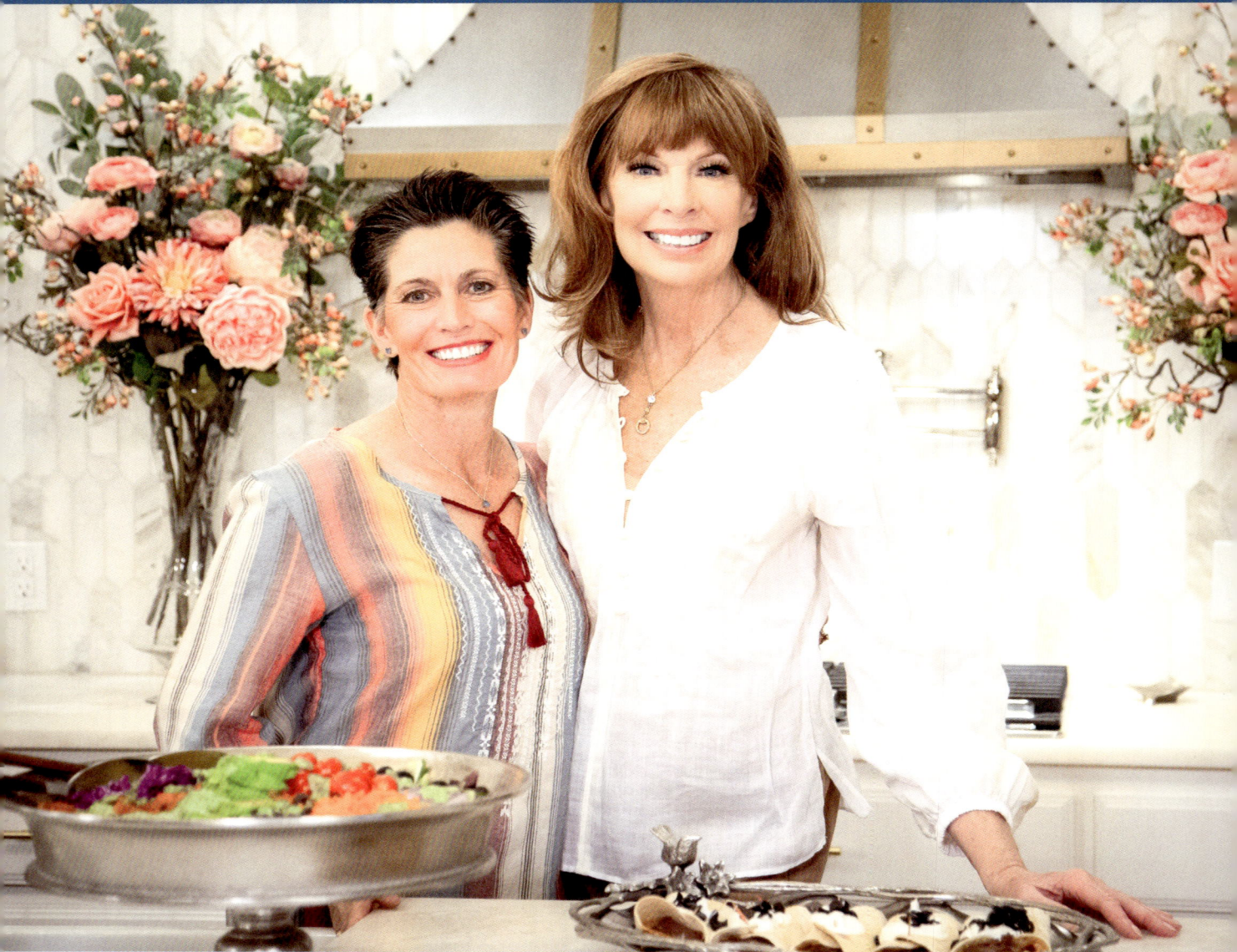

Let's celebrate these life giving ingredients!

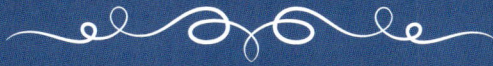

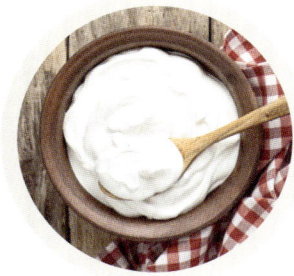

- Rich source of healthy fats
- Contains folate
- Provides probiotics

Organic Sour Cream

Why make your own ranch dressing?

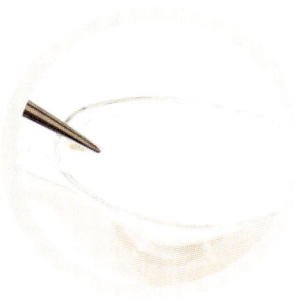

- Reduce additives and preservatives
- You can use organic ingredients
- Customizable flavors to suit taste preferences
- The apple cider vinegar aids in digestion and gut health
- Essential oils will take your dressing from ordinary to extravagant.

Healthy Ranch Dressing

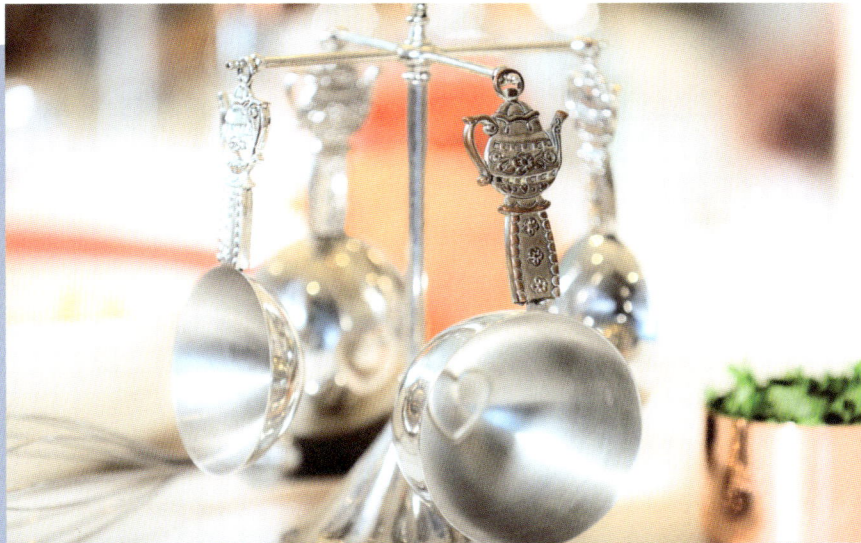

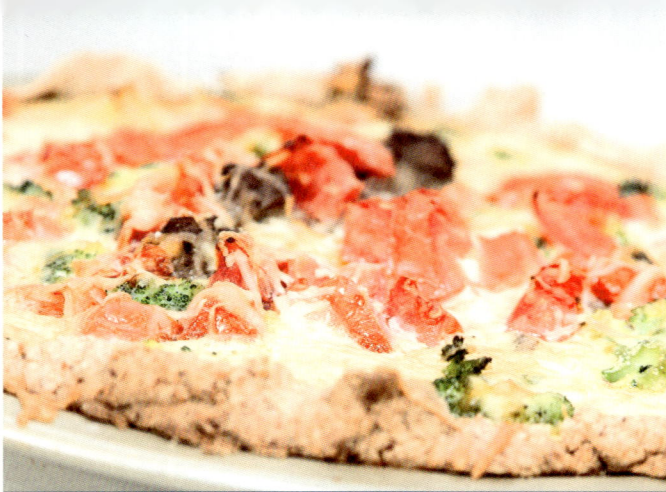

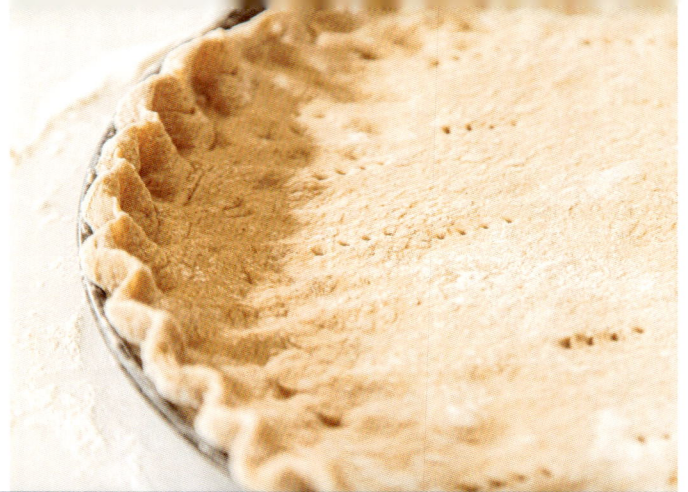

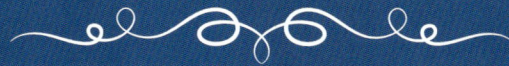

Week 5
Full Menu Shopping List

Produce

1 small yellow onion

1 bunch organic broccoli

1 ripe tomato

1 lb organic carrots

5 cloves garlic

1 bunch fresh organic parsley

1 head of organic butter lettuce

1 small red onion

1-2 organic cucumbers depending on size

2 avocados

2 small ripe tomatoes

4-6 Red radishes

Baking & Spices

Organic unbleached all-purpose flour

Sea salt

Dry mustard

Tamari sauce

Worcestershire sauce

Olive oil

Apple cider vinegar

Meat

1 lb organic ground beef

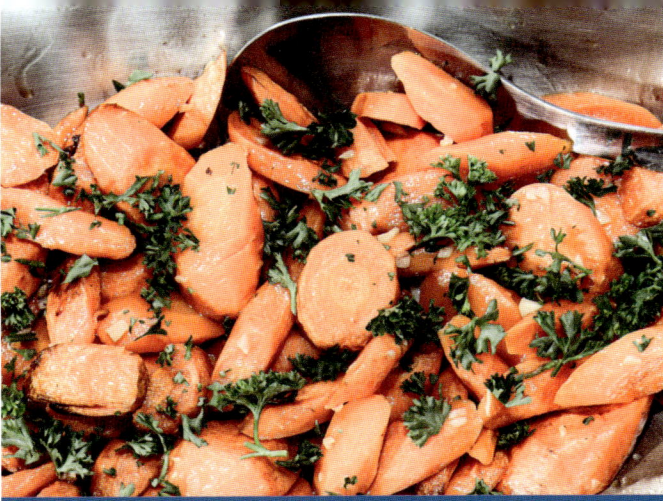

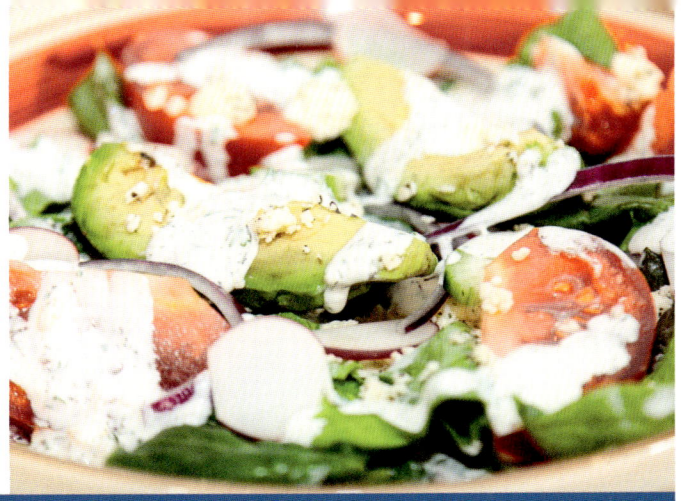

Full Menu Shopping List continued

Dairy

1 ½ cups grated organic cheddar cheese

1 cup whole milk or non dairy milk

3 large organic eggs

Butter

1 sm container organic sour cream

1 pt buttermilk

OPTIONAL; Parmesan cheese, shaved

OPTIONAL; feta cheese

Dry Goods

3⁄4 cup raw almonds and raw pecans blend (1/2 raw almonds and 1/2 raw pecans)

Condiments

1 jar good-quality organic mayonnaise

From Young Living*

YL Vitality Oregano oil

YL Vitality Thyme oil

YL Vitality Black Pepper oil

YL Vitality Dill oil

Young Living Einkorn Flour

SEE PAGE 39 FOR ORDERING DETAILS

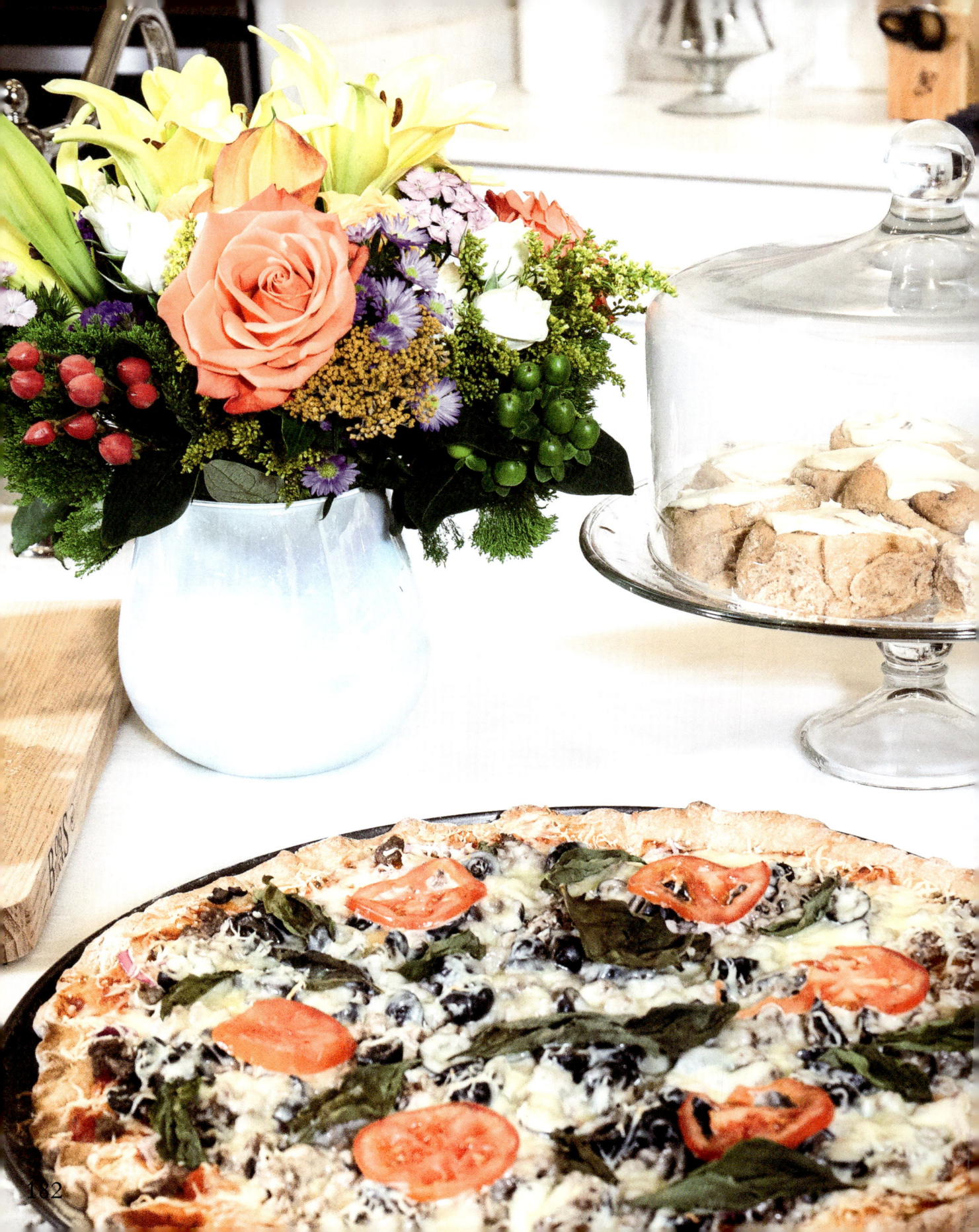

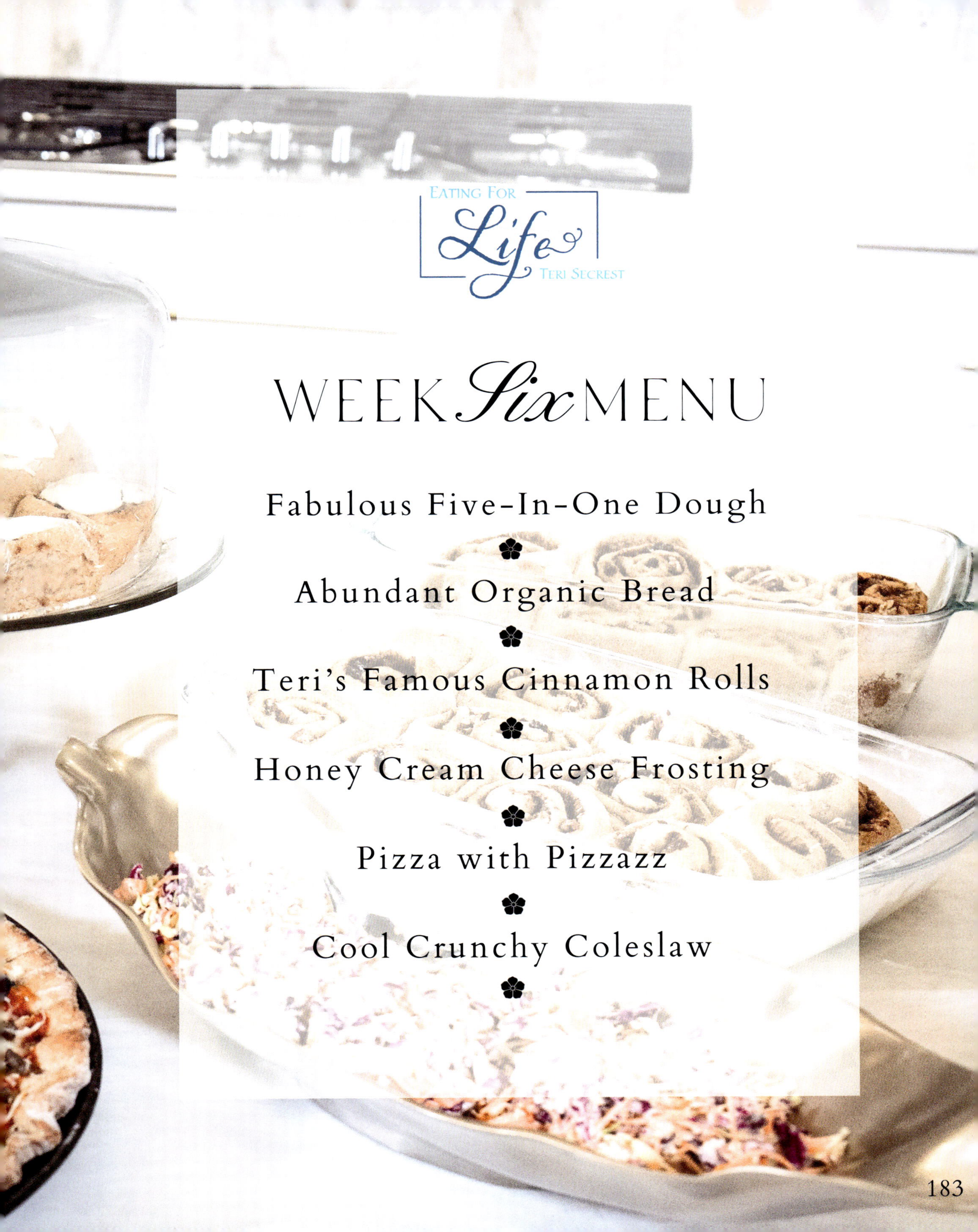

WEEK *Six* MENU

Fabulous Five-In-One Dough

❀

Abundant Organic Bread

❀

Teri's Famous Cinnamon Rolls

❀

Honey Cream Cheese Frosting

❀

Pizza with Pizzazz

❀

Cool Crunchy Coleslaw

❀

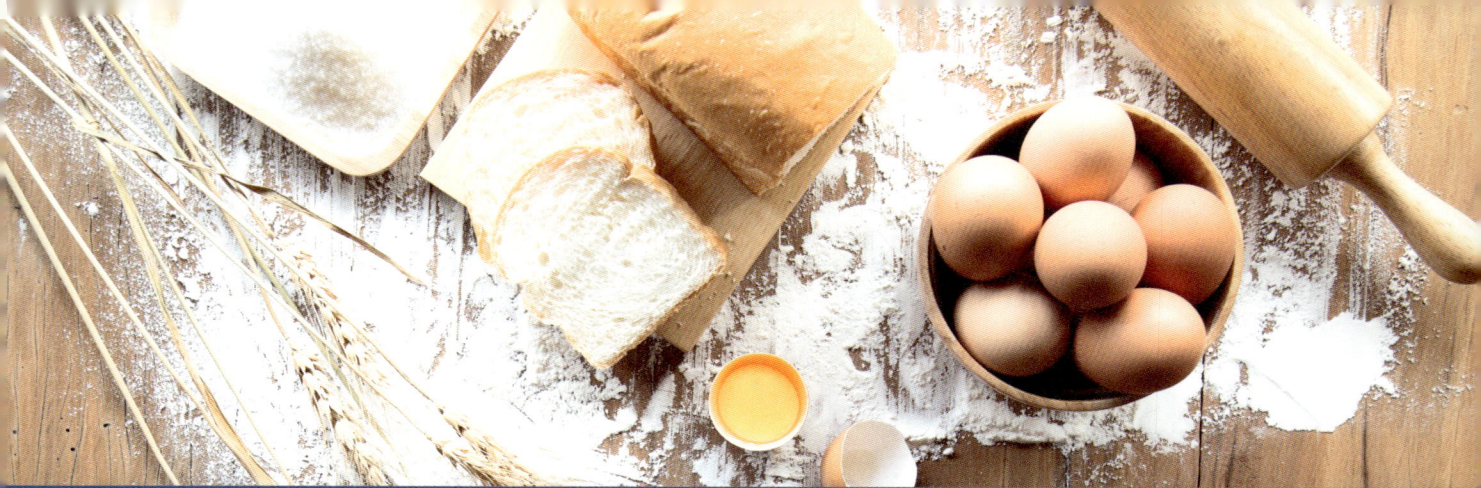

FABULOUS FIVE-IN-ONE DOUGH

Ingredients

5 cups warm water

1/2 cup raw, unfiltered honey

1/2 cup olive oil

1 heaping Tbsp salt

1 Tbsp dough enhancer
(Most grocery stores don't
carry it! I get mine from Amazon)

6 cups of Young Living
Einkorn Flour
(Order YL Einkorn Flour
on page 149)

6 cups organic Non-GMO
bread flour

3 heaping Tbsp active dry
yeast

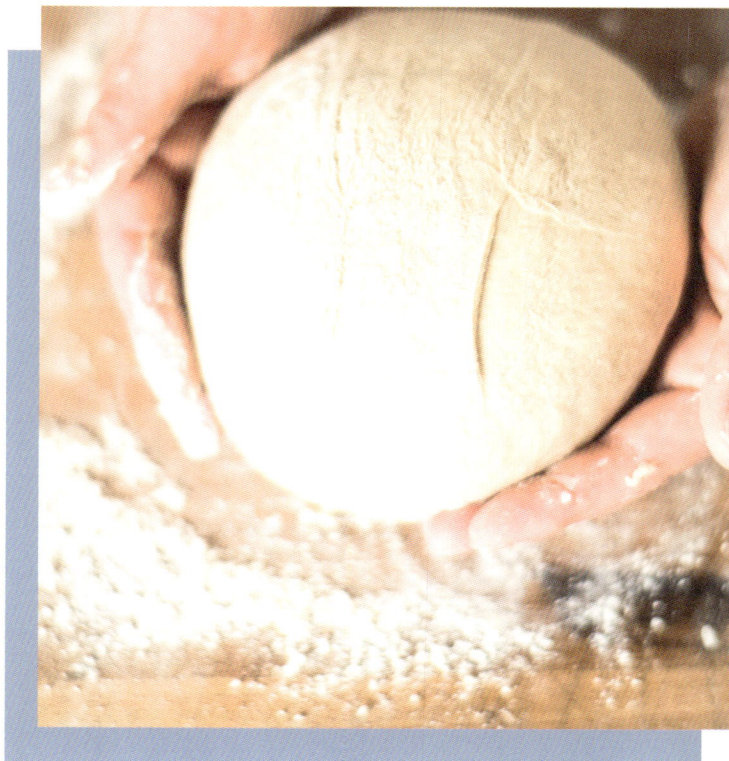

Preparation

1. Use a heavy-duty mixer with a dough hook. Add to the mixer bowl the warm water, honey, oil, salt, and dough enhancer. Mix on low speed until well combined.

2. In a separate mixing bowl, combine the Einkorn flour and the organic bread flour. Whisk together well.

3. Continue on low speed. Add your flour one cup at a time until you have incorporated 6 cups.

4. Add the yeast.

5. Slowly add 5 additional cups of flour, one cup at a time, until fully combined.

6. As you begin to add your final cup, pay very close attention to how your dough is looking. You may not need the entire amount. Continuing on low speed, once you see the dough pull away from the sides of the bowl you are done adding flour.

7. Allow the dough to mix on low for 5 full minutes (this kneads the dough.)

8. Flour your countertop and remove the dough from the mixer. Divide into five equal portions. Each portion will create one of the following recipes.

"This dough continues to create some of our family's favorite foods every year including cinnamon rolls, pizza dough and bountiful bread. It's your choice! This dough makes enough to create 5 recipes. For example, you can make 2 loaves of bread, 2 pans of cinnamon rolls, and one large pizza dough. Mix and match for your family fun!"

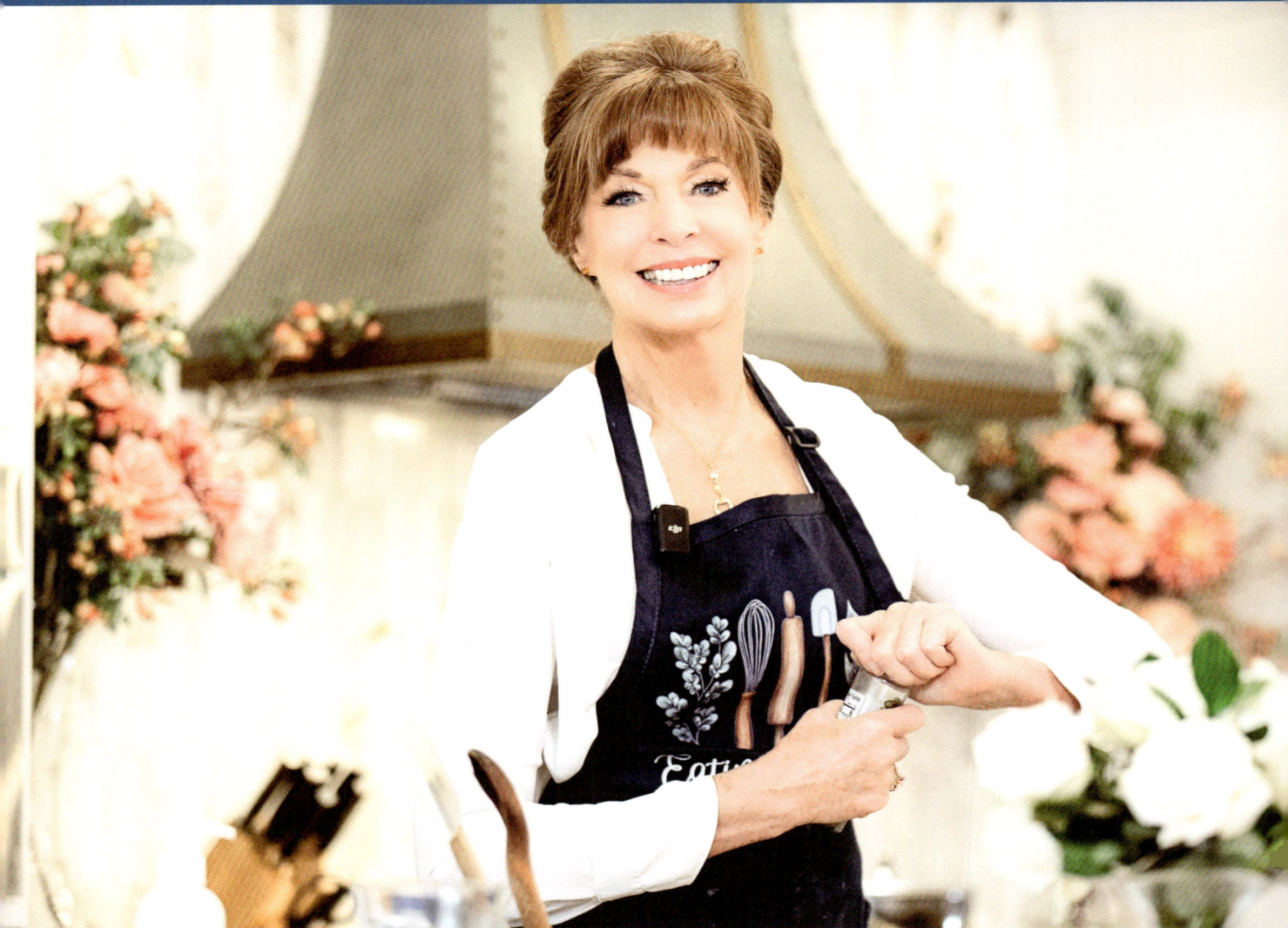

Let's celebrate these life giving ingredients!

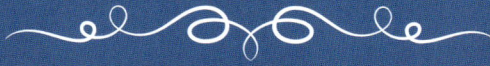

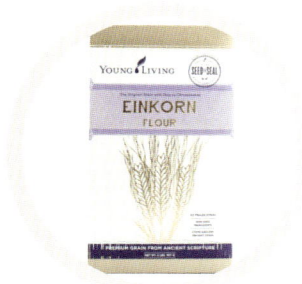

Young Living Einkorn Flour

- Known as an ancient grain and is considered one of the first crops to be domesticated
- Higher levels of protein, essential fatty acids, phosphorus, and beta-carotene than modern wheat varieties
- It is genetically closer to wild grasses than more modern, hybridized wheat varieties
- Contains iron, dietary fiber, and essential B vitamins
- Contains lutein which is great for eye health
- Einkorn has only 14 chromosomes compared to modern wheat's 42, making it easier to digest.

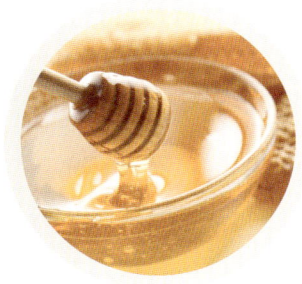

Raw Organic Honey

- Rich in antioxidants, vitamins, and minerals
- Contains flavonoids and phenolic acids
- Has immune-boosting properties
- Used for centuries as a natural remedy for sore throats, coughs, and wounds
- Antimicrobial properties to inhibit the growth of bacteria
- Effective topical treatment for minor cuts and burns
- Natural energy source

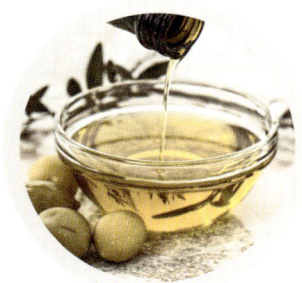

Olive Oil

- Rich in monounsaturated fats
- Heart-healthy choice
- Lowers bad cholesterol levels and reduce the risk of heart disease
- Packed with antioxidants like vitamin E and polyphenols
- Protects cells from damage caused by free radicals and oxidative stress
- Reduces the risk of Alzheimer's

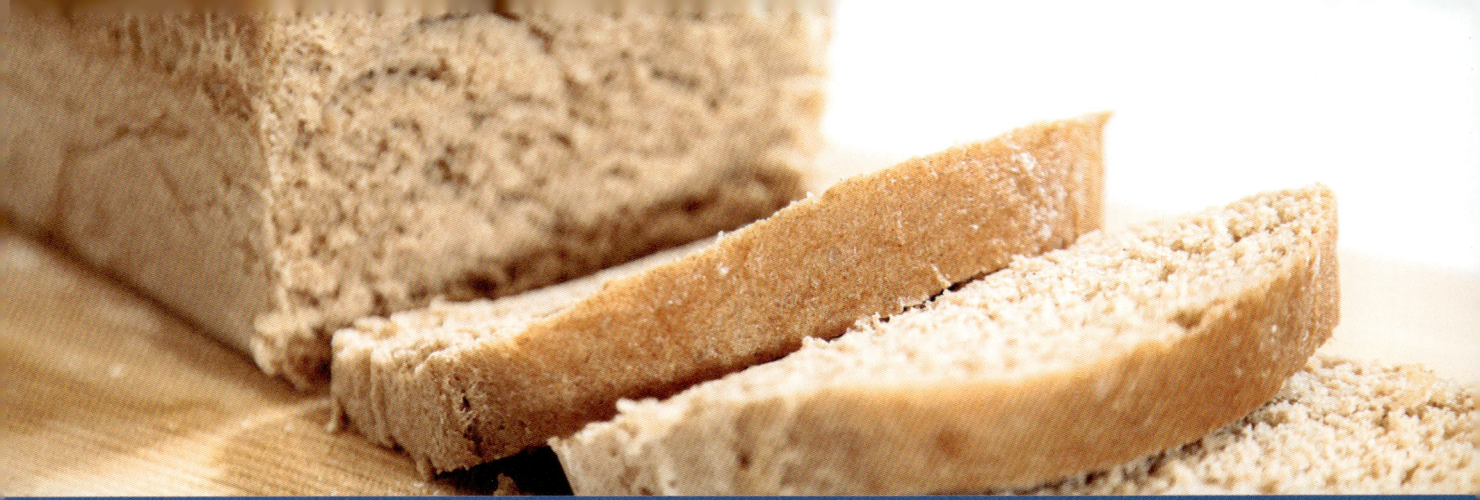

ABUNDANT ORGANIC BREAD

Ingredients

Makes 1 Loaf

1 portion of Teri's Five-In-One Dough
Butter and flour for your bread pan

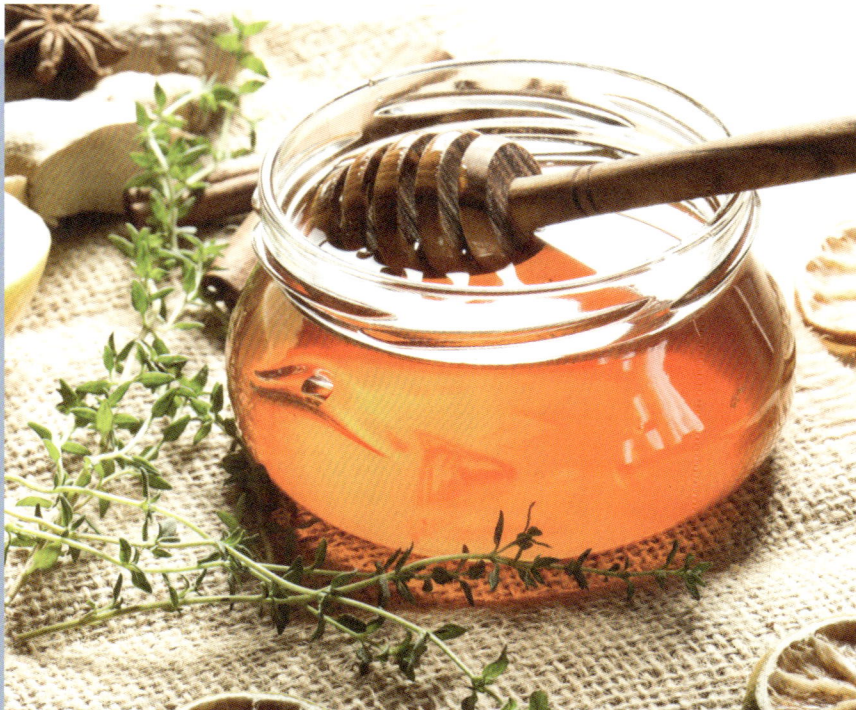

Preparation

1. Butter and flour your bread pan.
2. Gently pick up the portion and form the dough into the bread pan without pushing down.
3. Set your bread pan aside and cover with wax paper to rise. Allow your bread to rise to the top of the pan (this is when I start prepping cinnamon rolls if that is one of your choices.)
4. Preheat your oven to 375° while your bread is rising.
5. Once the dough reaches the top of the pan (20-30 minutes) place it on the middle rack of the oven and bake for about 20 minutes or until golden brown.
6. Remove from oven and let rest for 2 minutes. Then, gently turn out onto a cooling rack and allow it to cool completely.

"This is a wildly popular bread and it is a really fun gift to give someone for a special occasion! It is delicious toasted with butter!"

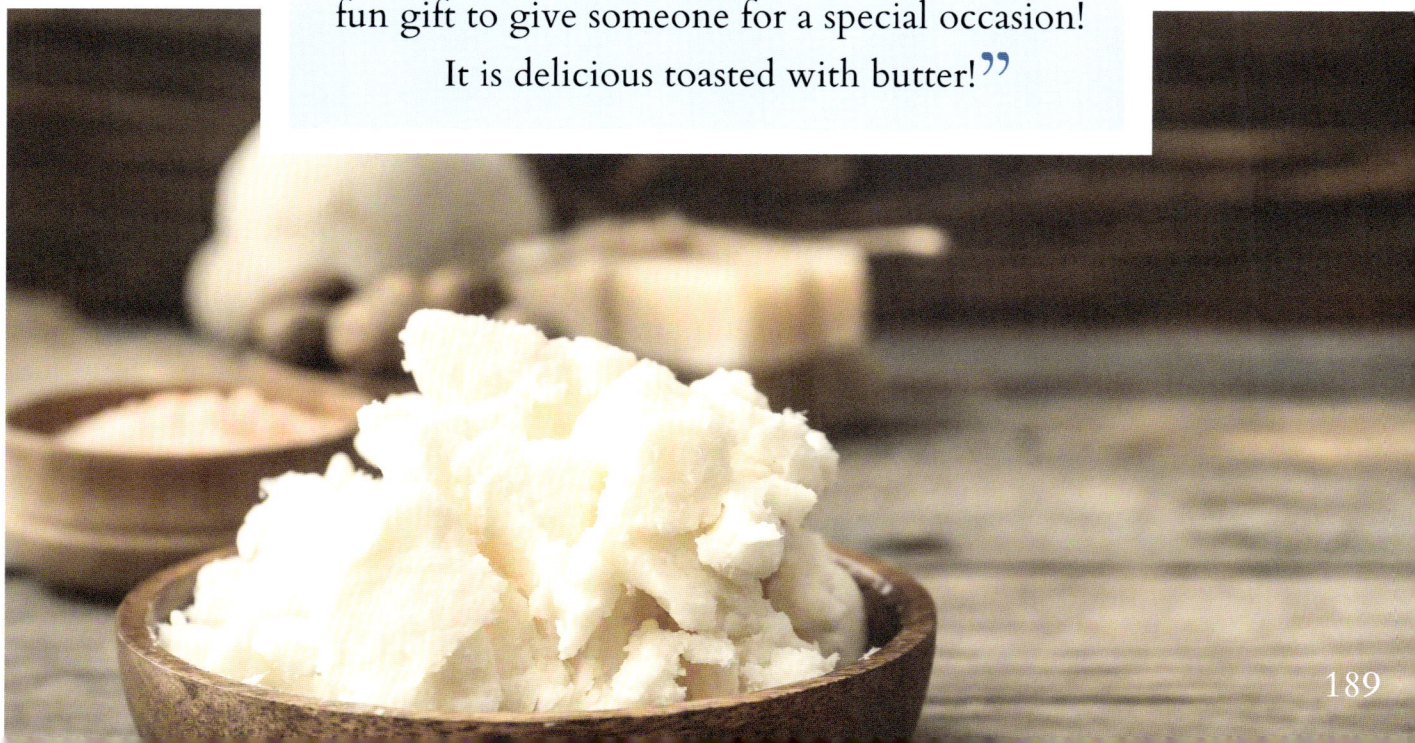

Let's celebrate homemade bread!

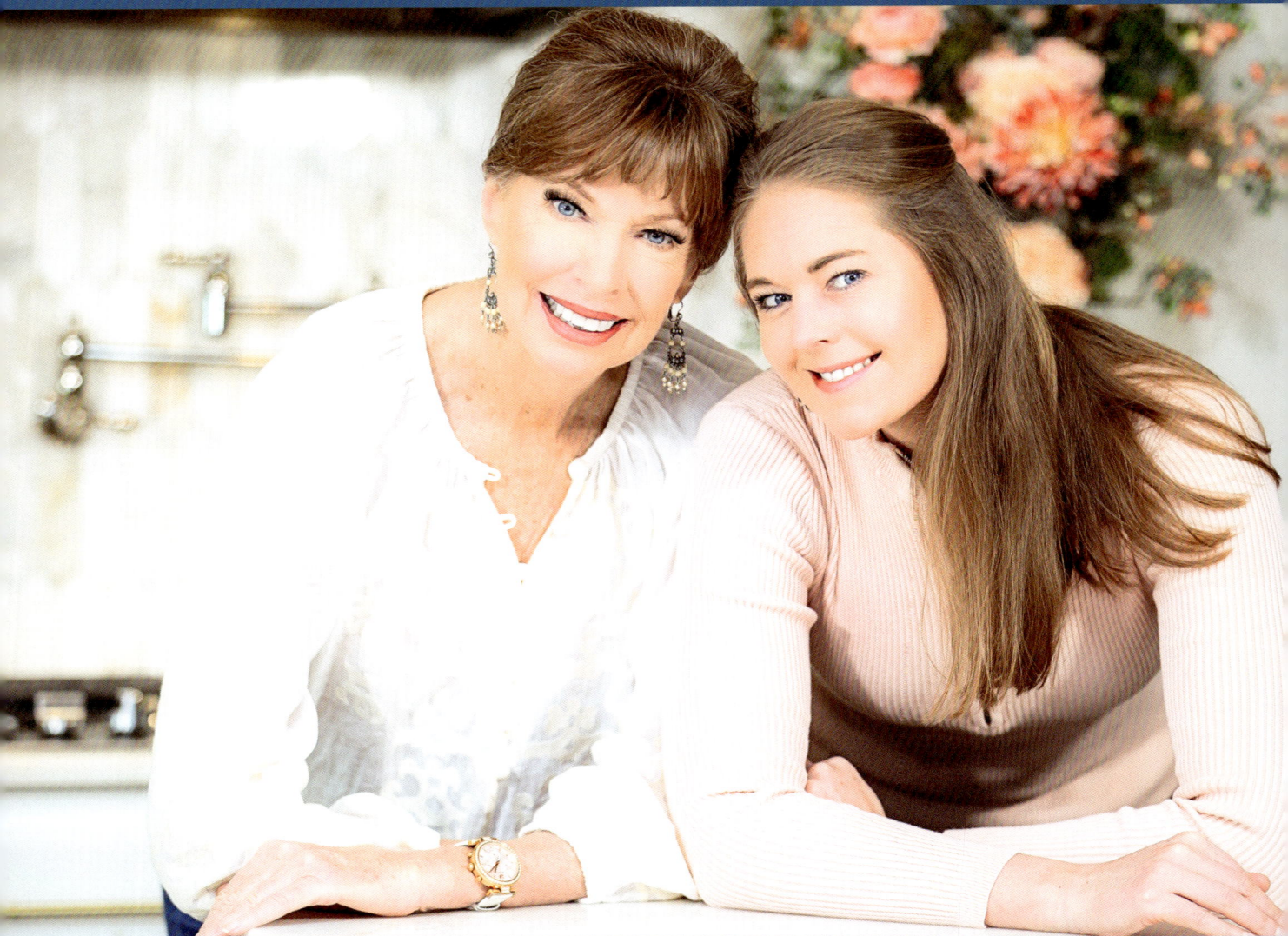

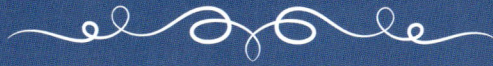

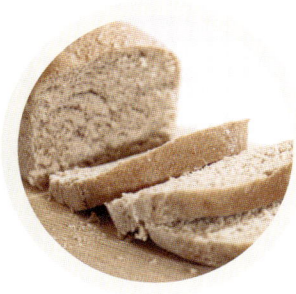

Abundant Bread

Why Make Bread at Home?

- Control over ingredients: avoid unnecessary additives, preservatives, and artificial ingredients You can use organic ingredients.
- Whole grains: use whole grain flours over refined flours
- No added sugars
- Freshness: store bought bread may be sitting on shelves for days.
- Experiment with different types of flours, seeds, nuts, and other mix-ins to create unique flavors and textures.
- Family activity: baking bread at home can be a fun family activity, helping to teach children about cooking and nutrition.
- Cost-effective
- The aroma of bread baking in the oven is unbeatable and can make a house feel more like a home.

"Ever since Mom started baking with Einkorn Flour, I have noticed a very positive response in my digestive system."

- Elizabeth Rose

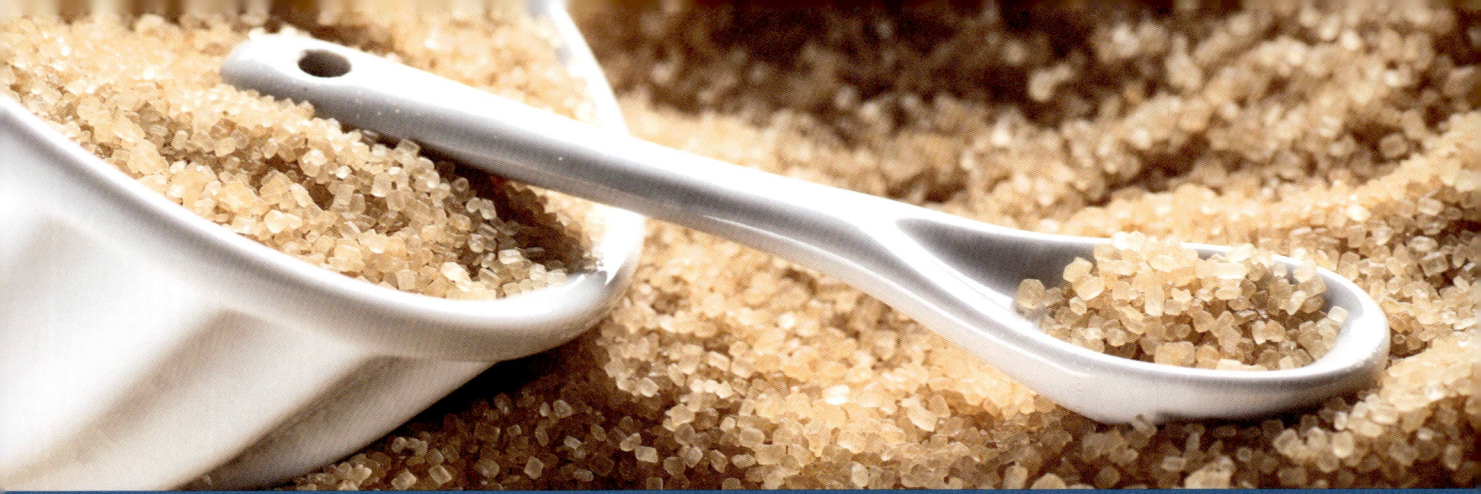

TERI'S FAMOUS CINNAMON ROLLS

Ingredients

1 portion of the Fabulous Five-in-One Dough

1/4 cup organic brown sugar

1/4 cup raisins

1/4 cup raw pecans, chopped

2 tsp ground cinnamon

1/4 cup butter

2 drops YL Vitality Cinnamon Bark oil

(Order YL Vitality Essential Oils on page 39)

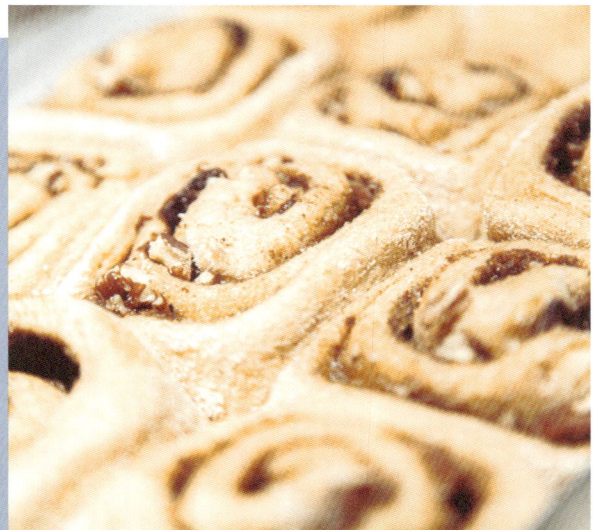

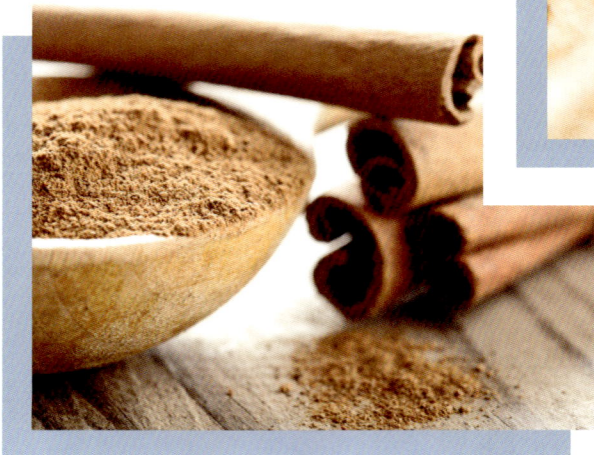

Preparation

1. Preheat your oven to 375°. Butter and flour an 9 x 13" baking pan.

2. Lightly flour your counter top and place one portion of your Fabulous Five-in-One dough. Roll out and shape into a rectangle. Take your time working from the center out.

3. In a small saucepan, melt the butter. Remove from heat. Then, stir in 2 drops of YL Vitality Cinnamon Bark oil.

4. Add your toppings to the dough as follows: First, using a pastry brush, spread melted butter all around the dough. Second, evenly sprinkle the brown sugar, raisins, pecans, and ground cinnamon on the dough and to the edges.

5. Third, roll up the long side of the dough into a log. Pinch the dough closed where the seam meets the log. Turn over the log so it's seam side down.

6. Using unflavored dental floss, cut dough into 12 equal rolls. Then, place slices onto your prepared pan, spiral side up.

7. Give your cinnamon rolls time to rise. Place your cinnamon rolls on top of the stove, cover with wax paper and let them rise until they reach the top of the pan (30-45 minutes.)

8. Bake for 15 minutes until they're a little brown, but do not overbake.

9. Once they cool, transfer them to your favorite cake plate and frost them with our delicious organic cream cheese frosting. They are to live for!

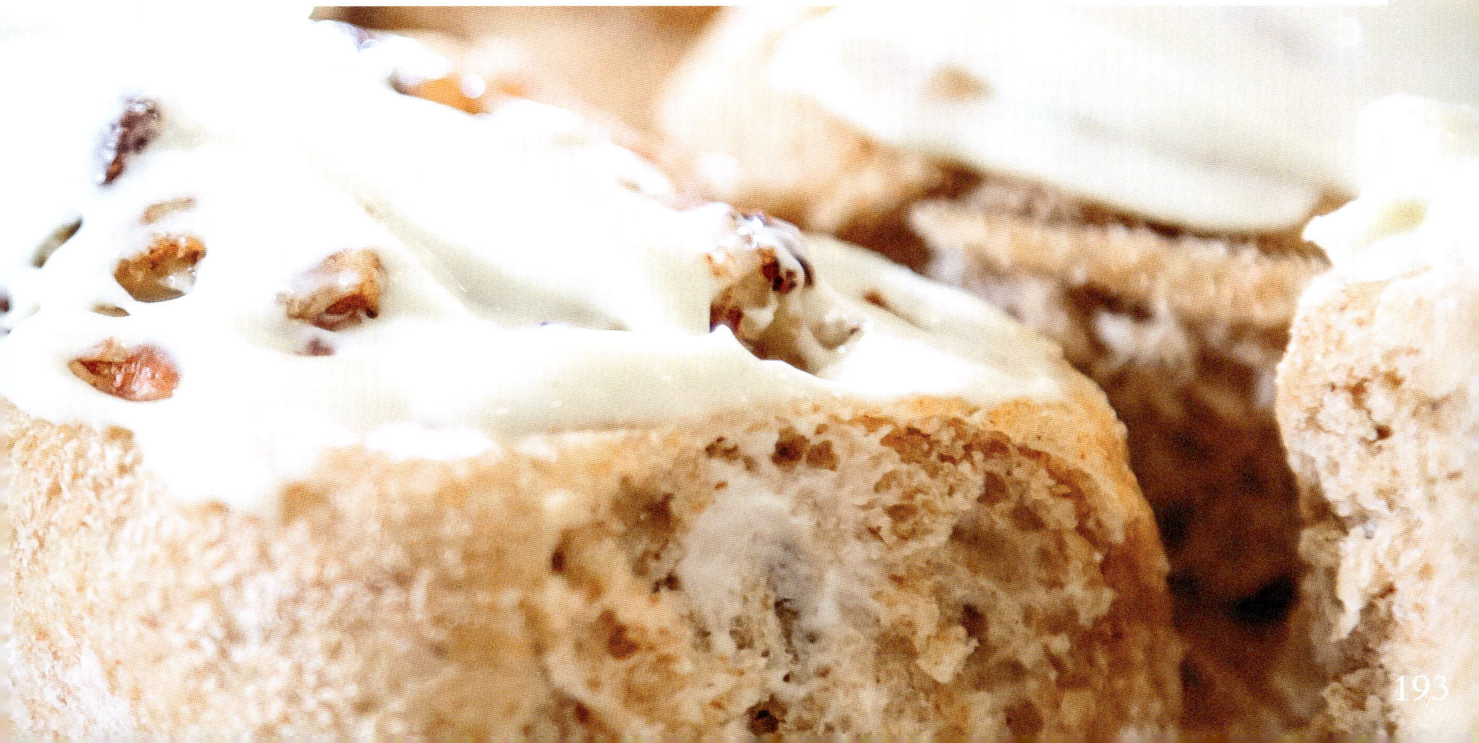

TERI'S FAMOUS CINNAMON ROLLS NUTRITIONAL BENEFITS

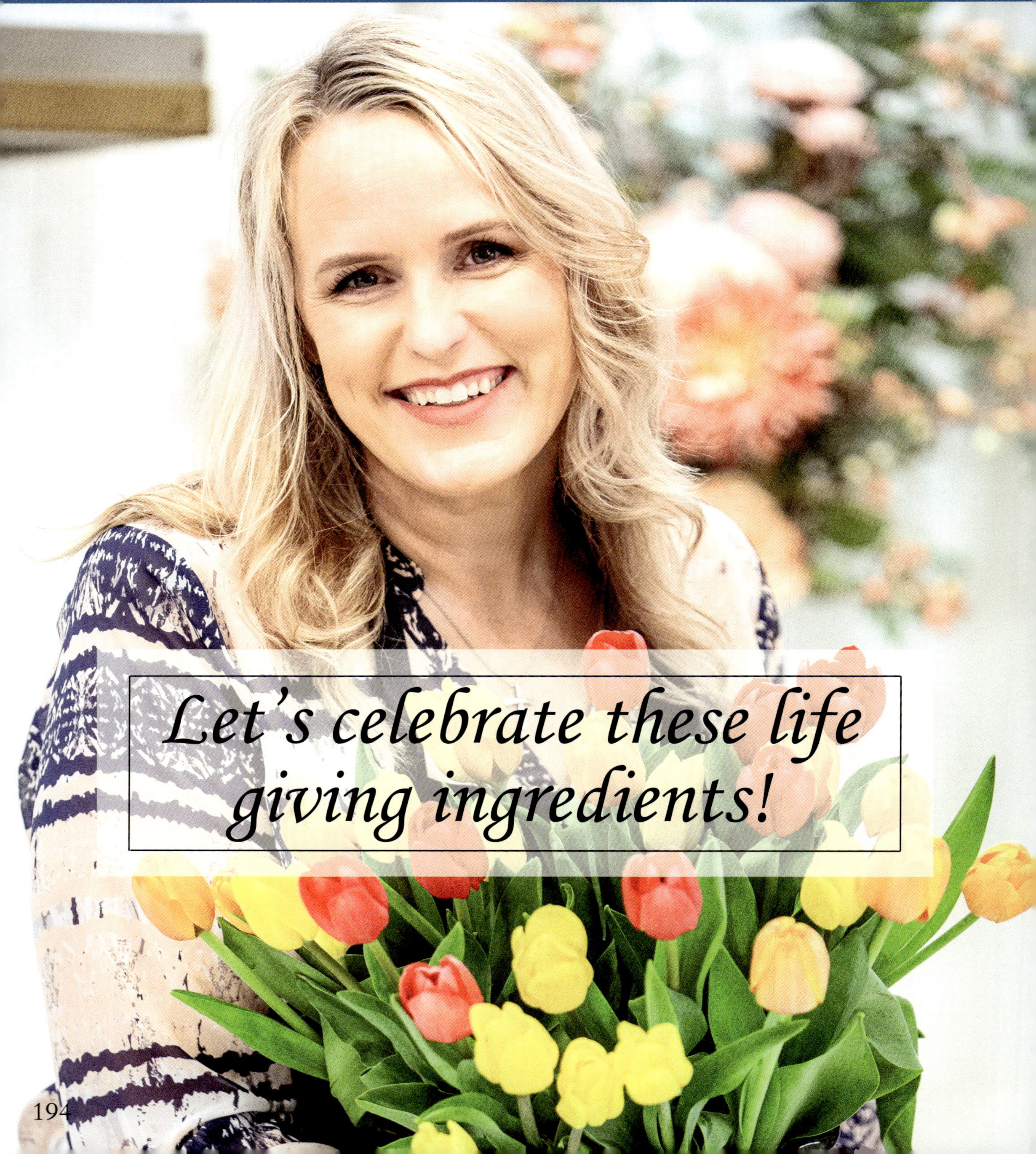

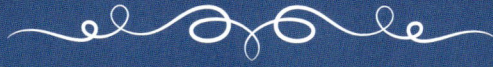

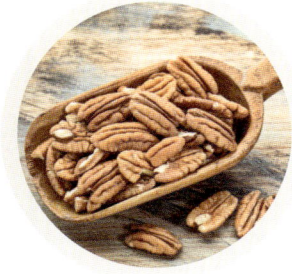

Pecans

- Rich in heart-healthy monounsaturated fats
- Lowers bad cholesterol and reduce heart disease risk
- Good source of protein and fiber
- Aids weight management and promotes satiety
- Contains vitamin E, a powerful antioxidant
- Protects cells from free radical damage
- Provides manganese for metabolism and bone health

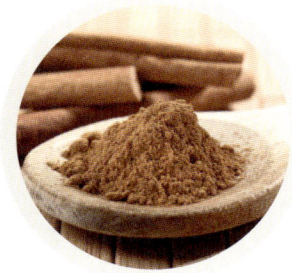

Cinnamon

- Antioxidant-rich
- Helps lower blood sugar levels and improve insulin sensitivity
- Lowers cholesterol, reduces blood pressure, and improves circulation
- Fights bacteria, fungi, and viruses
- Enhances cognitive function and memory

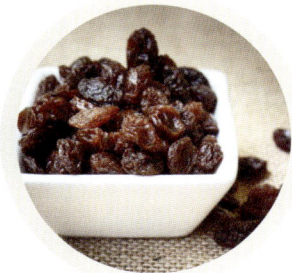

Raisins

- Promots healthy skin.
- Has vitamins K and C
- Contains minerals of potassium, and manganese, supporting bone health, immune function, and electrolyte balance
- Contains antioxidants such as beta-carotene and flavonoids
- High fiber

HONEY CREAM CHEESE FROSTING

Ingredients

1 tsp natural vanilla extract

1/4 cup raw, unfiltered honey
(a light-colored honey
works best for this frosting)

8 oz cream cheese

2 Tbsp softened butter

3 drops YL Vitality Tangerine
or Orange oil
*(Order YL Vitality Essential
Oils on page 39)*

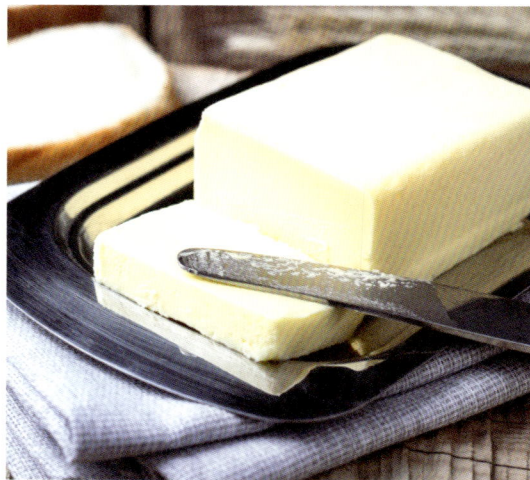

Preparation

1. Whip all ingredients together in a food processor or with a hand mixer until smooth. I usually remove the cream cheese and butter from the refrigerator and hour before.
2. Spread on cooled cinnamon rolls just before serving.

"This Honey Cream Cheese Frosting is your solution to the 'icing on the cake' that will not spike your blood sugar and will not make you tired after eating! Spread it on cinnamon rolls, muffins, cakes and even on toast! Simply to-live-for!"

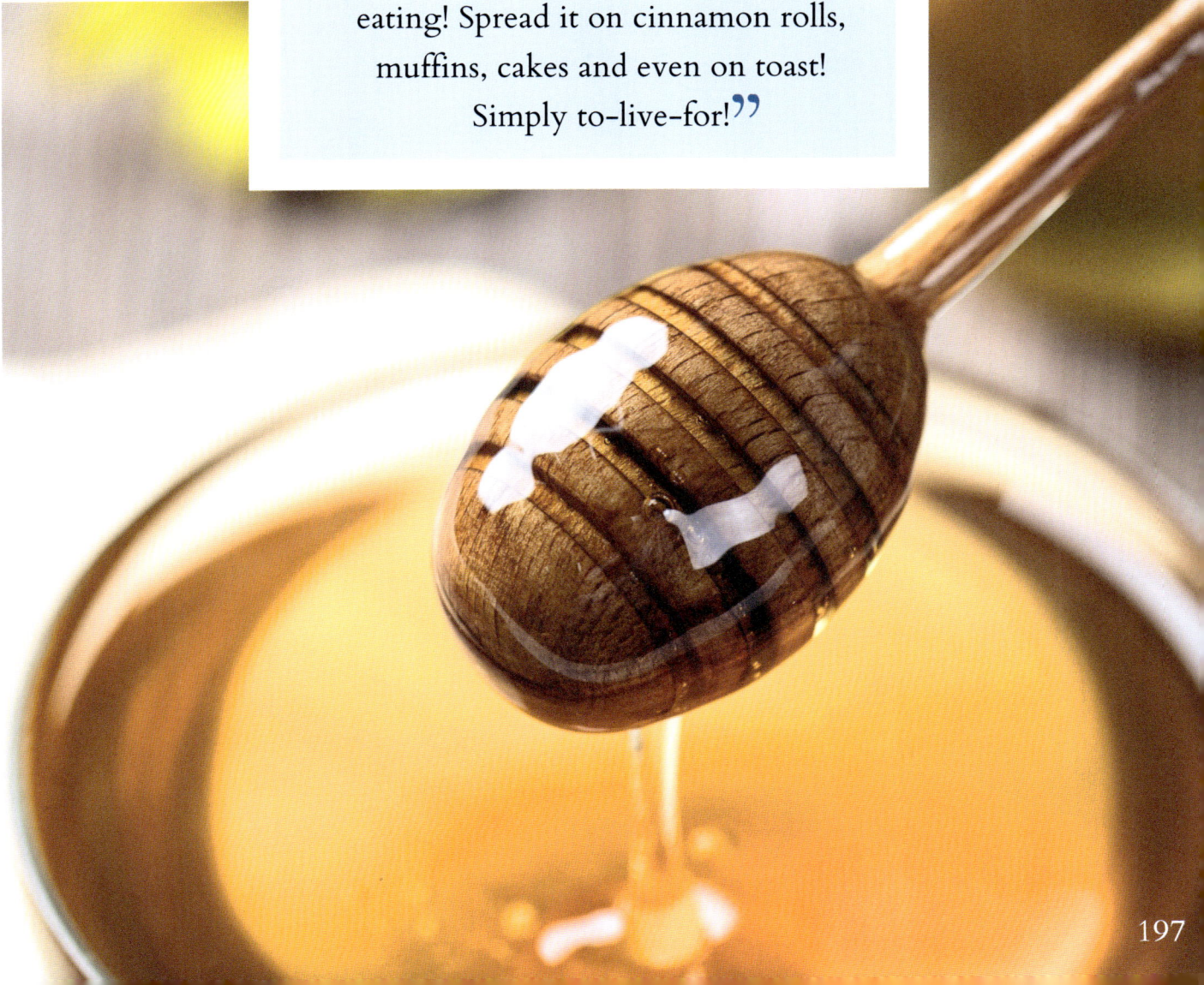

Let's celebrate these life giving ingredients!

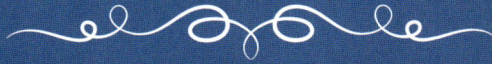

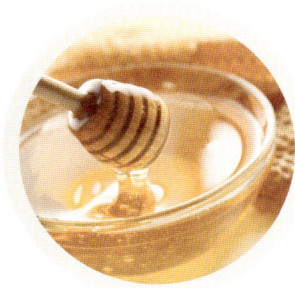

Raw Honey

- Rich in antioxidants, vitamins, and minerals
- Contains flavonoids and phenolic acids
- Has immune-boosting properties
- Used for centuries as a natural remedy for sore throats, coughs, and wounds
- Antimicrobial properties to inhibit the growth of bacteria
- Effective topical treatment for minor cuts and burns
- Natural energy source

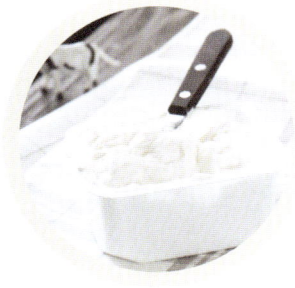

Cream Cheese

- Provides healthy fats that can support brain function and overall cell health, helping you stay energized
- Contains a significant amount of vitamin A, essential for maintaining healthy skin, eyes, and immune function.
- Easier to digest for those with mild lactose intolerance.

Why use raw, organic, unfiltered honey?

- Unfiltered honey contains vitamins, minerals, antioxidants, and amino acids. Refined sugar has no nutritional benefits at all.
- Honey helps combat oxidative stress and inflammation. Sugar causes inflammation.
- Honey causes a slower rise in blood sugar levels than refined sugar which spikes it.
- Honey has other uses like to support wound healing and soothe sore throats.
- Honey undergoes less processing than refined sugar, keeping it closer to its natural state.
- Buying local honey supports local beekeepers and contributes to agricultural sustainability.
- Environmental Benefits: Choosing honey can support bee populations essential for pollinating many crops.
- The rich flavor of honey encourages using less sweetener overall, helping to reduce sugar intake.

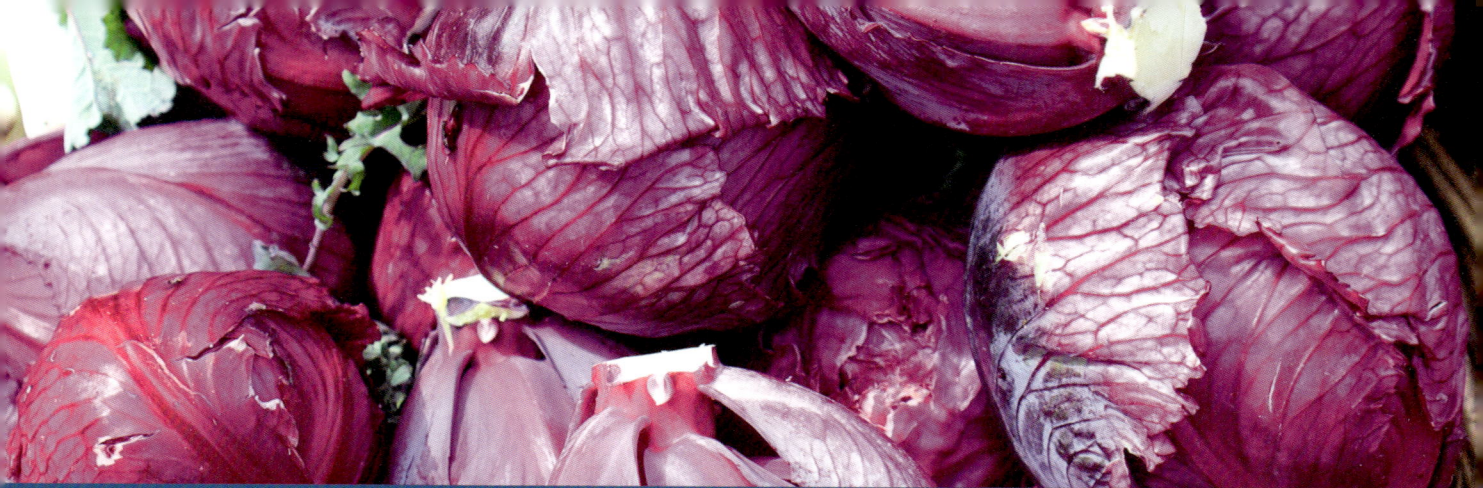

COOL CRUNCHY COLESLAW

Ingredients

3 cups green cabbage, grated

2 cups purple cabbage, grated

1 cup organic carrots, grated

1/2 cup organic mayonnaise

1 Tbsp white vinegar

1/2 Tbsp raw apple cider vinegar

2 tsp monk fruit sweetner

2 drops of YL Vitality Celery Seed oil

(Order YL Vitality Essential Oils page 39)

Salt and pepper to taste

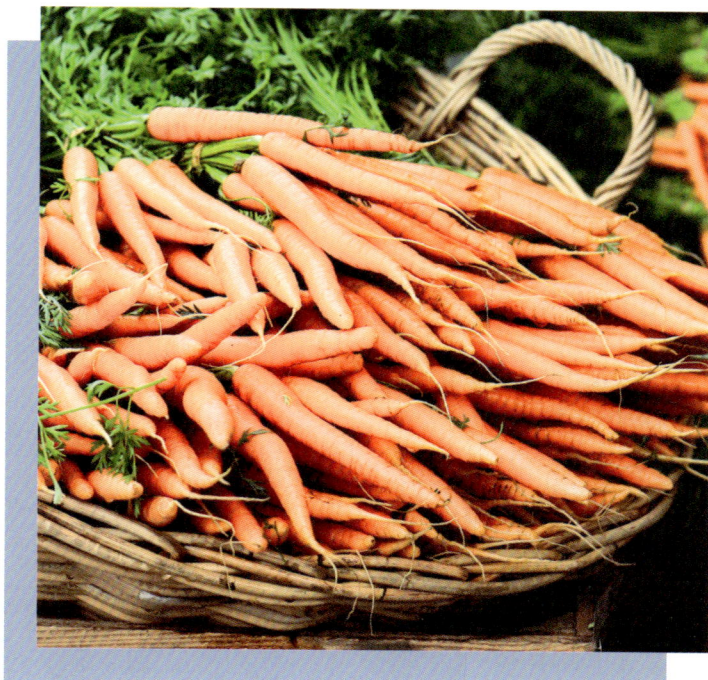

Preparation

1. In a mixing bowl, toss together the green and red cabbage and the grated carrots. Set aside.

2. In a small bowl, whisk together all dressing ingredients until well combined.

3. Pour the dressing over the coleslaw and toss.

4. Cover and refrigerate at least one hour before serving.

5. Place into your favorite salad bowl for a beautiful presentation.

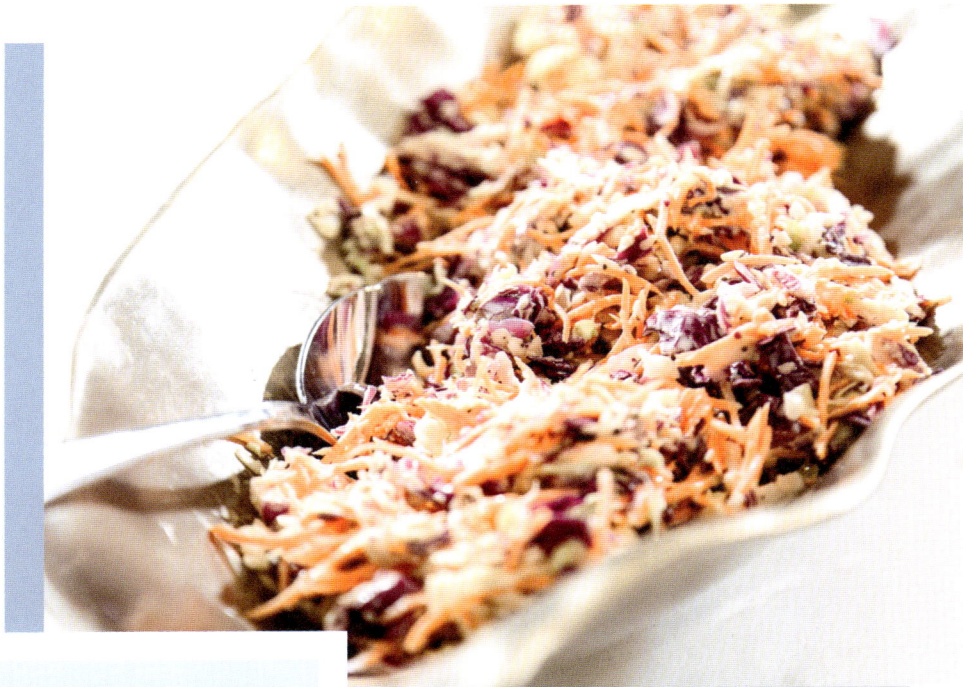

"Eating Cool Crunchy Coleslaw will just make you happy!"

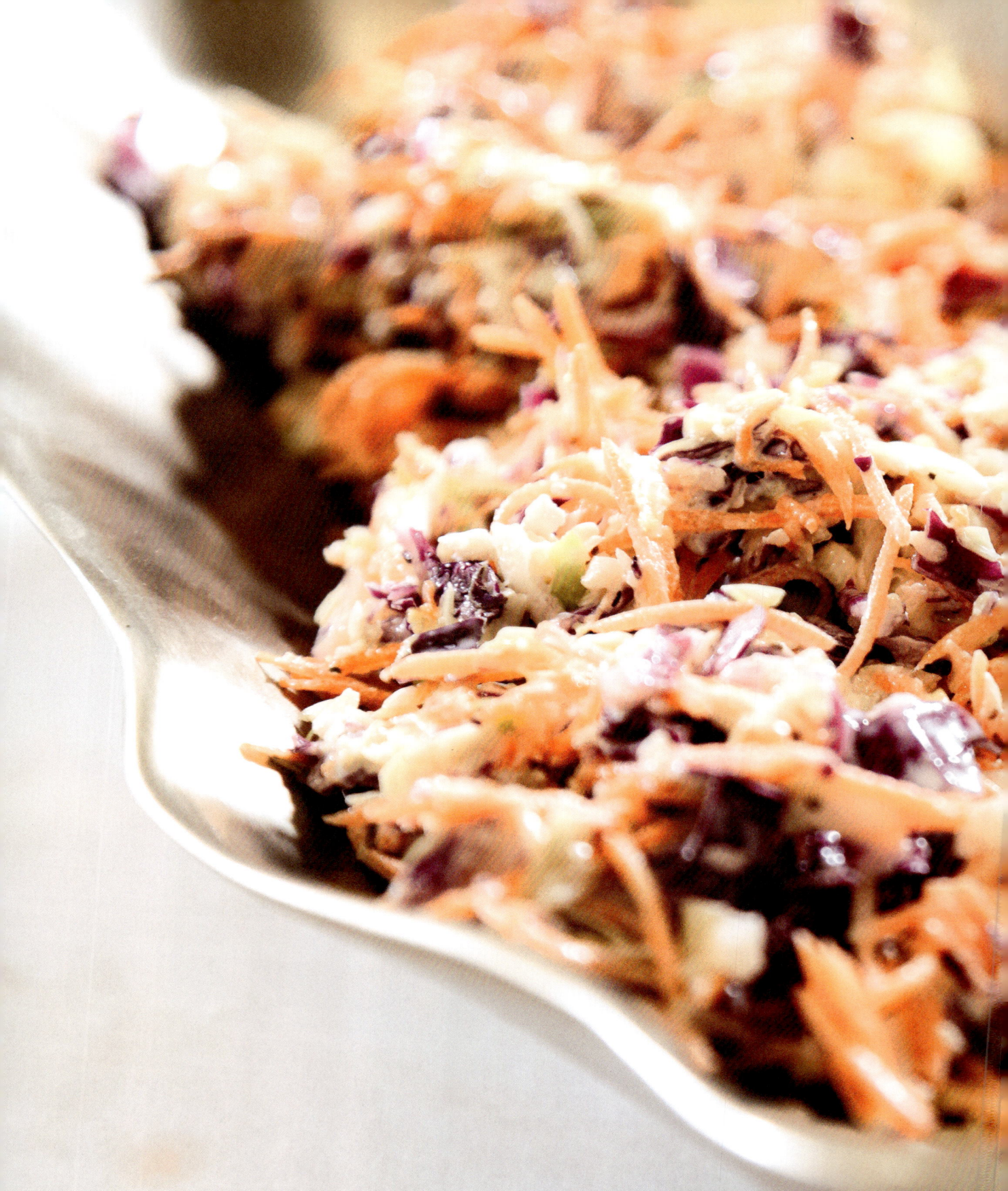

"Let your food be your medicine! Your body loves purple cabbage because it helps protects your cells from inflammation."

Let's celebrate these life giving ingredients!

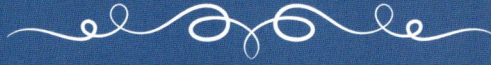

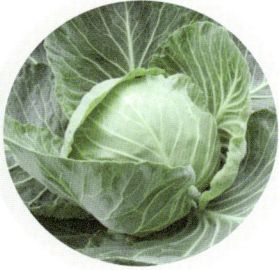

Green Cabbage

- An excellent source of vitamin C, which is crucial for immune function, collagen production, and skin health.
- Contains small amounts of vitamin A and folate
- Rich in fiber, which aids digestion, promotes satiety, and helps regulate blood sugar levels
- Contains important minerals like potassium, manganese, and calcium, which are essential for heart health, muscle function, and bone strength
- Low in calories and carbohydrates

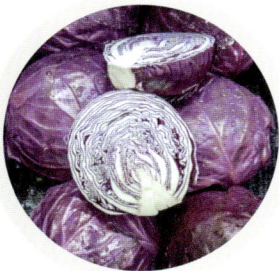

Red Cabbage

- Protects from inflammation
- Antioxidants such as anthocyanins
- Supports heart health
- Promotes digestion and regular bowel movements
- Boosts immunity with vitamin C
- Supports bone health with vitamin K
- Helps prevent osteoporosis

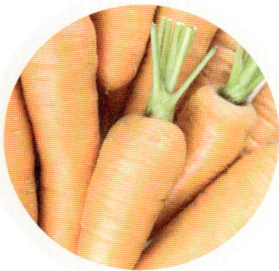

Carrots

- Packed with beta-carotene, a precursor to vitamin A
- Supports vision health
- Immune boosting
- Great for skin health
- Contains antioxidants like vitamin C and lutein
- Helps reduce inflammation
- High fiber supports digestive health
- Promotes feelings of fullness

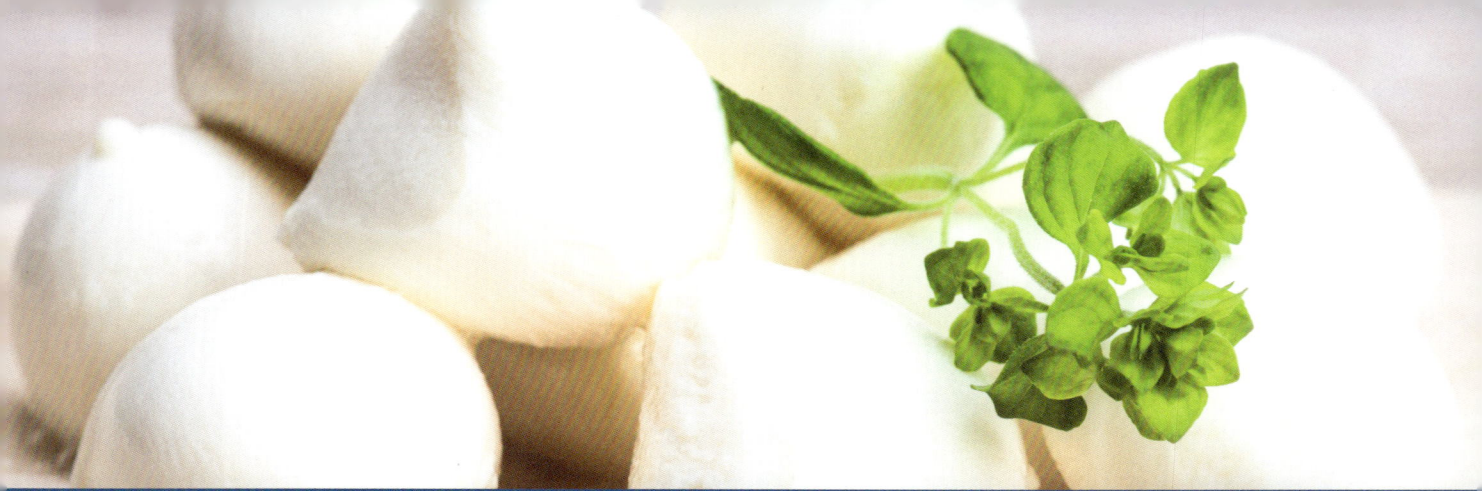

PIZZA WITH PIZZAZZ

Ingredients

1 portion of Fabulous
Five-in-One Dough
1 cup of organic tomato
based pizza sauce
2-3 cups mozzarella
cheese, grated
(see below for additional
pizza topping suggestions)
YL Vitality Oregano oil
YL Vitality Basil oil
*(Order YL Vitality Essential
Oils on page 39)*

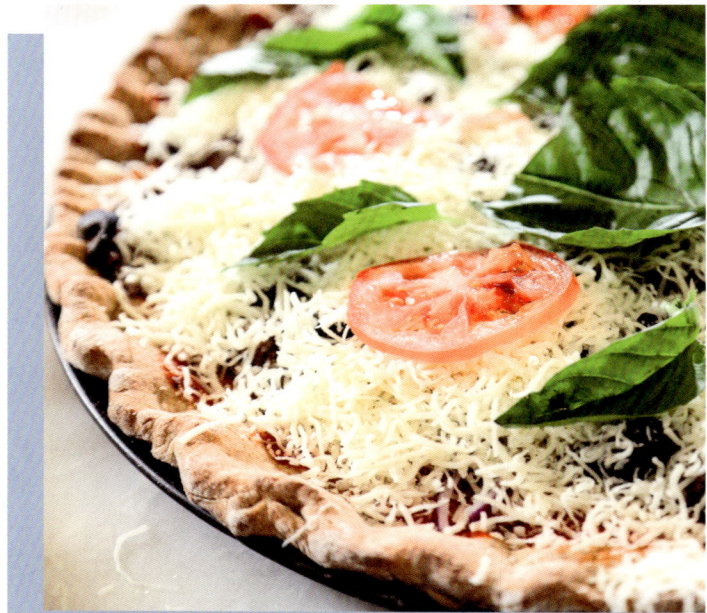

"My absolute favorite toppings over the years
include fresh tomatoes, fresh basil, mushrooms, onions,
black olives, green or red peppers, browned organic
ground sirloin (optional) and mozzarella cheese."

Preparation

1. Preheat your oven to 425°. Oil and lightly flour your pizza pan. I enjoy using a 16" round pan.

2. Place your dough onto the pizza pan. Using your fingers or a small rolling pin, press the dough into the pan all the way to the edge. Create a little lip to hold toppings in place.

3. Using a pastry brush, brush the top of your dough with olive oil. Then, take a fork and prick the dough several times to prevent your dough from bubbling.

4. Pre-bake your crust for 10 minutes. Remove from the oven and set aside while you prepare your toppings.

5. Reduce oven temperature to 375°.

6. In the mood for some real zest in your pizza sauce? Using the toothpick method *(see page 32)* add YL Vitality Basil oil and YL Vitality Oregano oil to your organic tomato based pizza sauce.

7. Sprinkle your favorite ingredients over the pizza crust, according to your taste buds. There is no wrong way to do it.

8. Place the prepared pizza into the oven and bake at 375° for about 15 minutes or until the cheese is bubbly.

"It's really worth investing in a good-quality pizza cutter!"

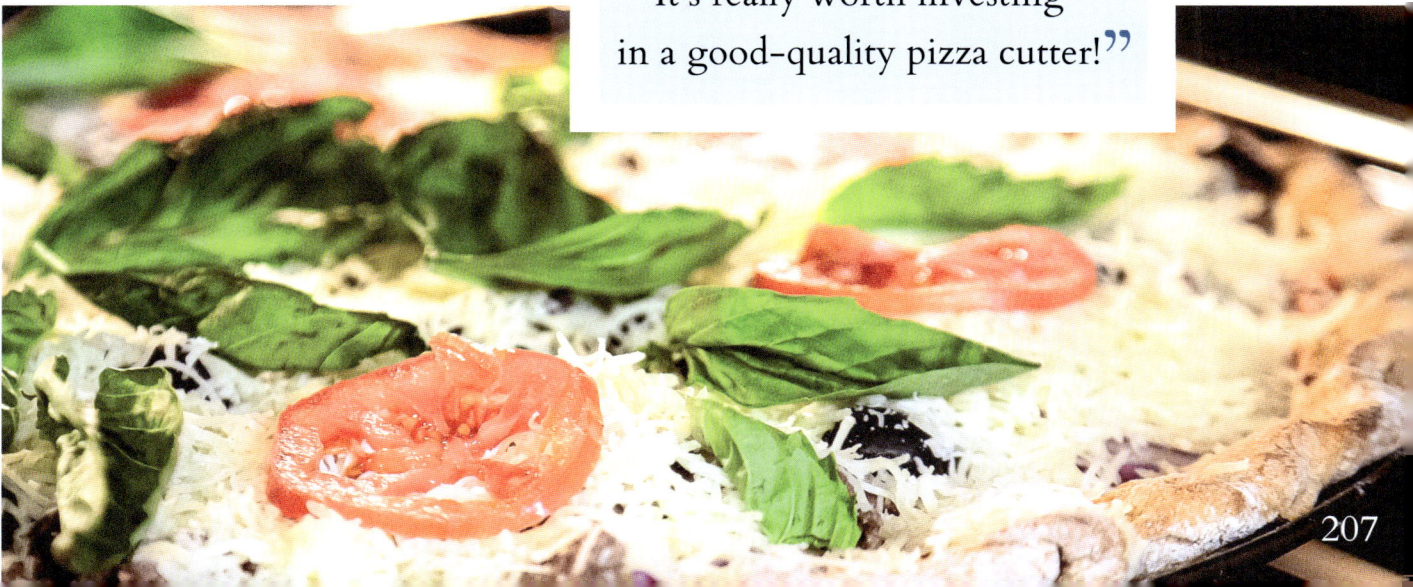

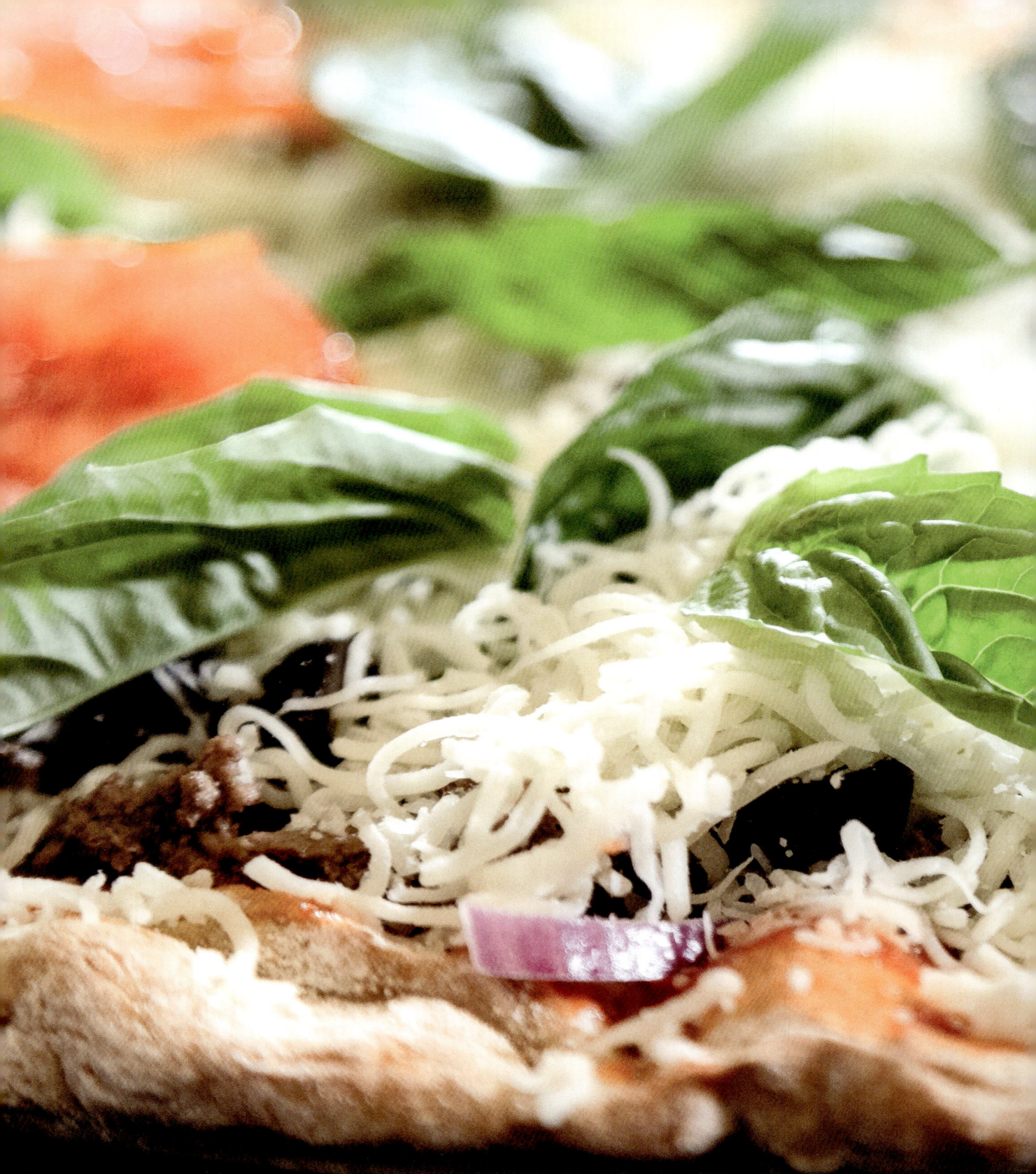

"There is nothing more fun than having a Pizza with Pizzazz party with homemade pizza from scratch! My children learned to think like an artist by creating their own toppings and flavorings. If you desire all your children's friends to come to your home on Friday night, homemade pizza parties are the way to go!"

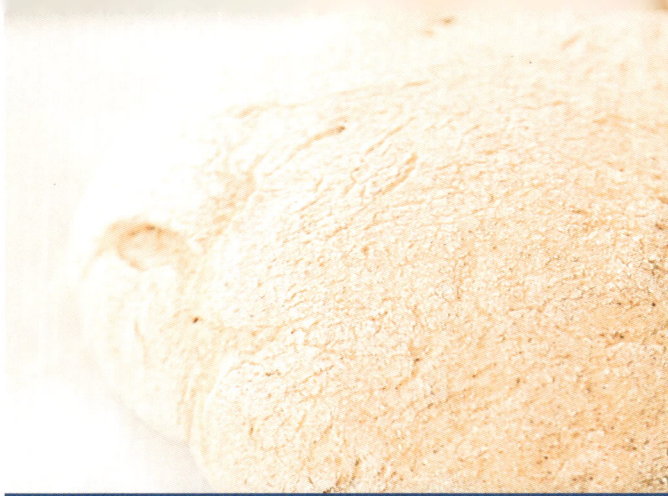

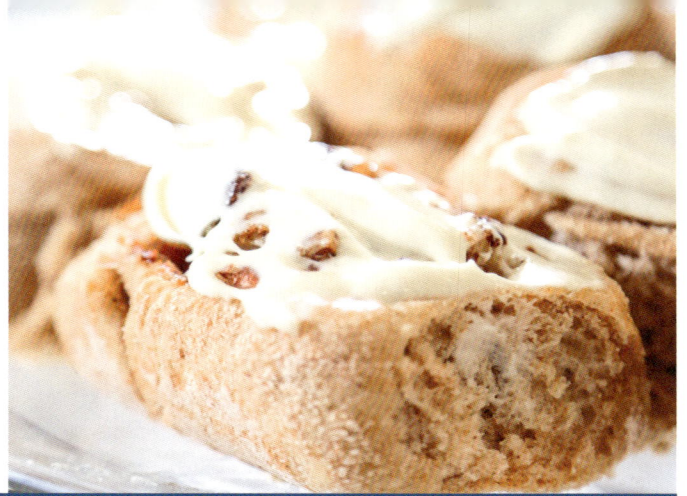

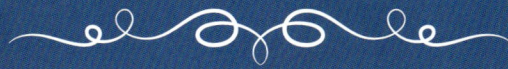

Week 6
Full Menu Shopping List

Baking & Spices

Light raw, unfiltered honey

Olive oil

Dough enhancer (I get mine
from Amazon)

Organic Non-GMO baking flour

Active dry yeast

Organic brown sugar

Raisins

Ground cinnamon

Natural vanilla extract

Monk fruit sweetener

Dairy

Butter

Cream cheese

Mozzarella cheese

From Young Living*

6 cups of Young Living Einkorn Flour
(see page 149 for Einkorn details)

YL Vitality Cinnamon Bark oil

YL Vitality Tangerine or

YL Vitality Orange oil

YL Vitality Celery Seed oil

YL Vitality Oregano oil (optional)

YL Vitality Basil oil (optional)

**SEE PAGE 39 FOR YL VITALITY
ORDERING DETAILS**

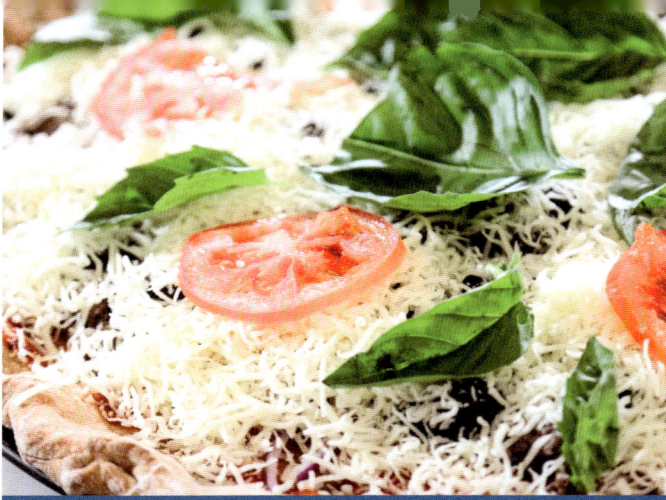

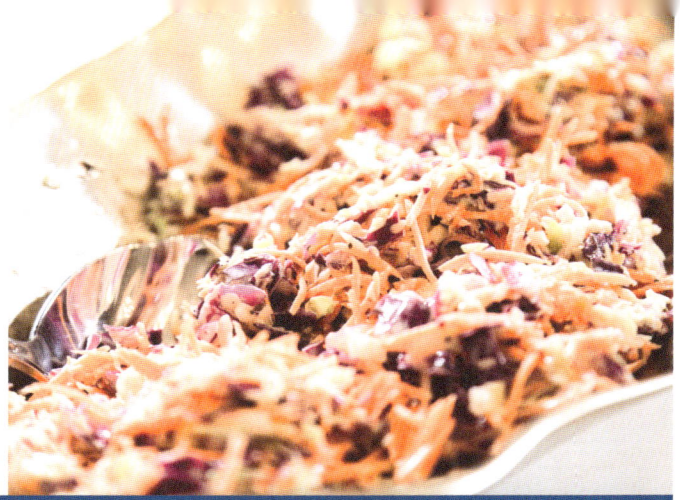

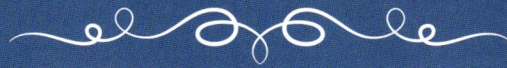

Full Menu Shopping List continued

Produce

Organic green and
purple cabbage

Organic carrots

Fun Pizza Toppings

Fresh tomatoes

Fresh Basil

Red onions

Black olives

Mushrooms

Organic ground beef

Condiments

Organic mayonnaise

White vinegar

Raw apple cider vinegar

Dry Goods

Raw pecans

Pasta

Tomato based pizza sauce

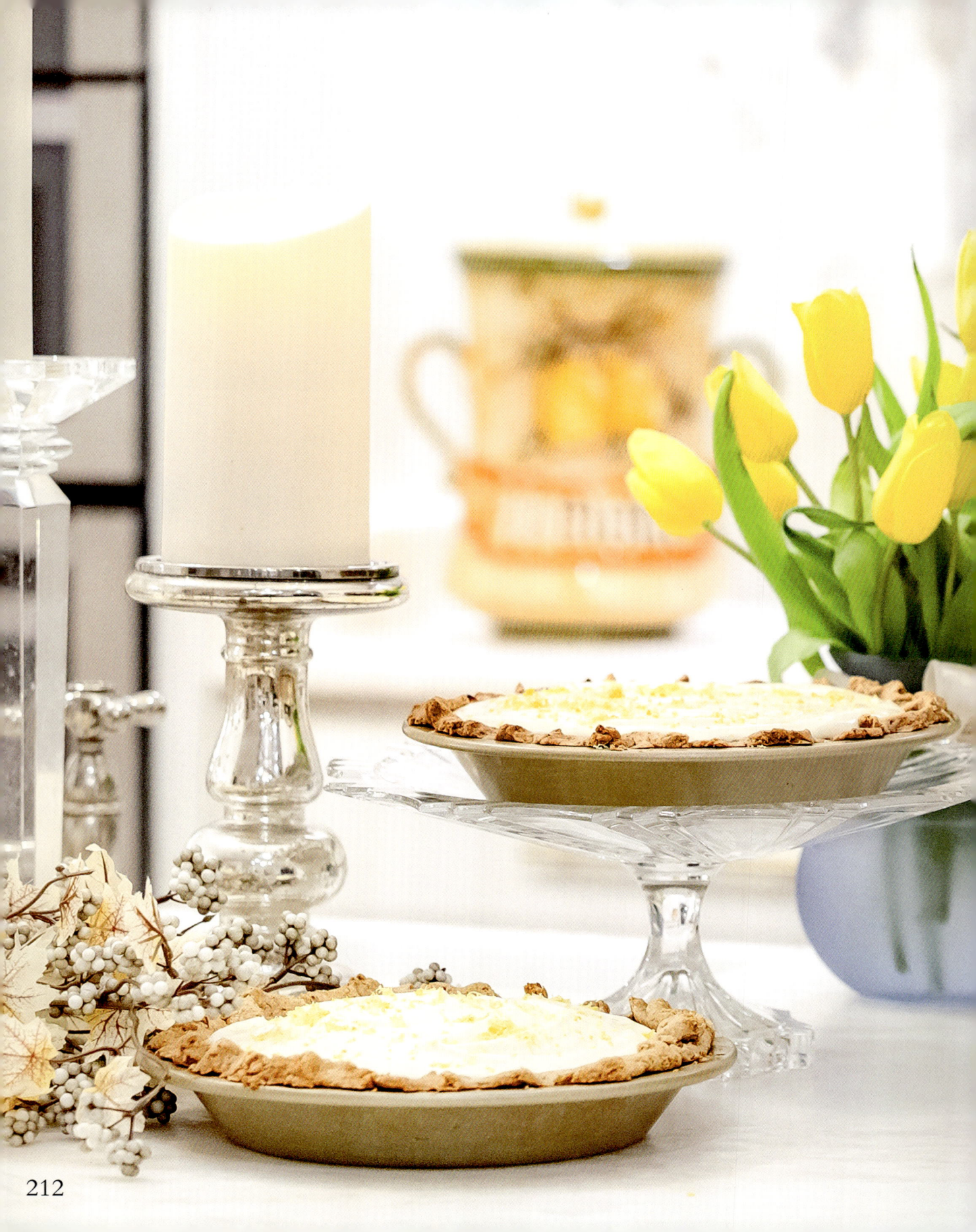

EATING FOR

Life

TERI SECREST

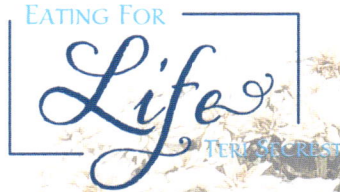

WEEK *Seven* MENU

Adzuki Bean Burrito

❀

Celebration Salad with
Avocado Cilantro Dressing

❀

Heavenly Lemon Cream Pie

❀

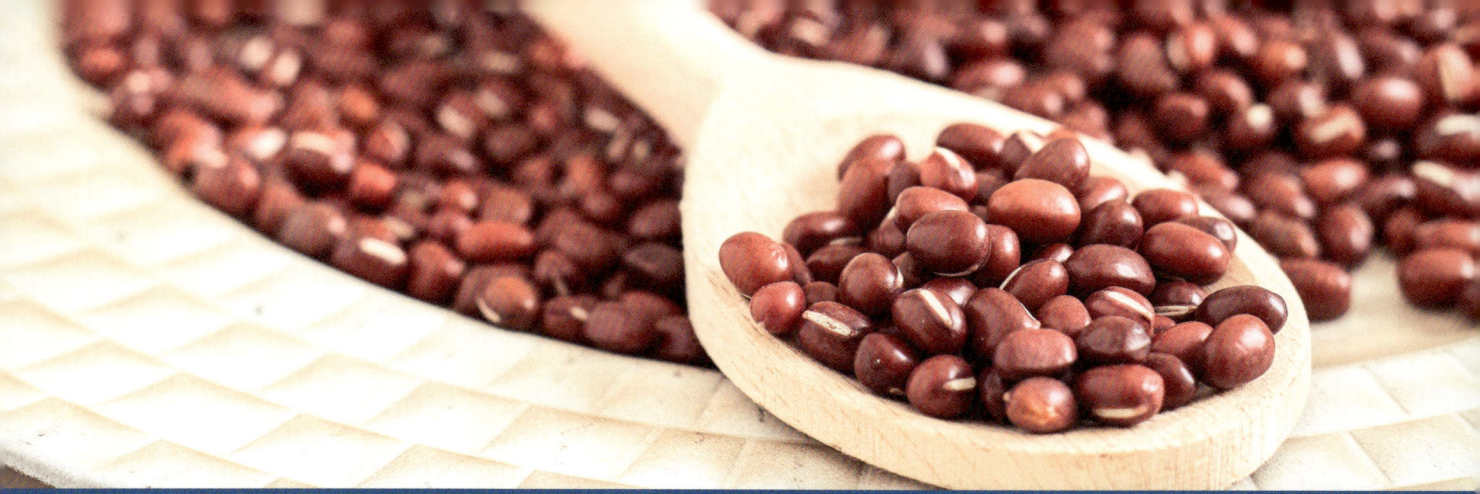

ADZUKI BEAN BURRITO

Ingredients

1 cup dry adzuki beans
(2 cups cooked beans)
3 garlic cloves
1 tsp chili powder
½ tsp paprika
½ white onion
2 cups cheddar cheese,
shredded
8 Tbsp salsa
4 Tbsp olive oil
Pinch of sea salt
1 pkg 8-9 inch diameter tortillas (sprouted grain is best)
1 avocado or black olives and organic sour cream for garnish
1 "toothpick" YL Vitality Oregano oil
1 "toothpick" YL Vitality Thyme oil
1 "toothpick" YL Vitality Black Pepper oil
(Order YL Vitality Essential oils on page 39)

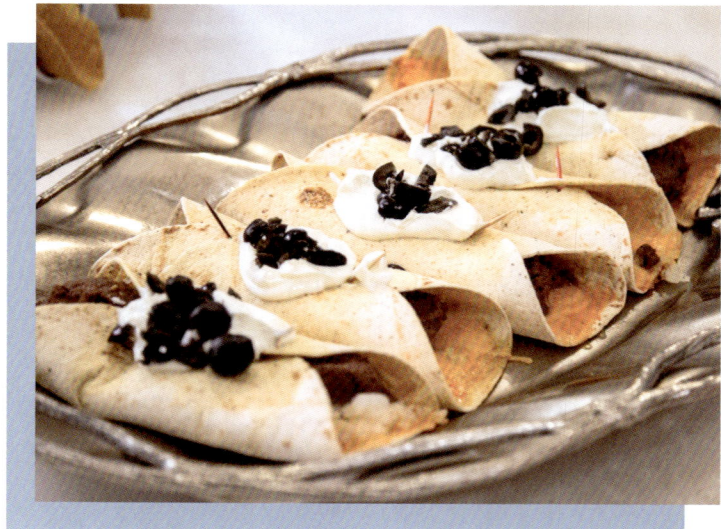

"During four different trips to Japan, I gained a deep love for these adzuki beans. I learned that the smaller the bean, the more nutrition it offers. These have been a family favorite for 20 years!"

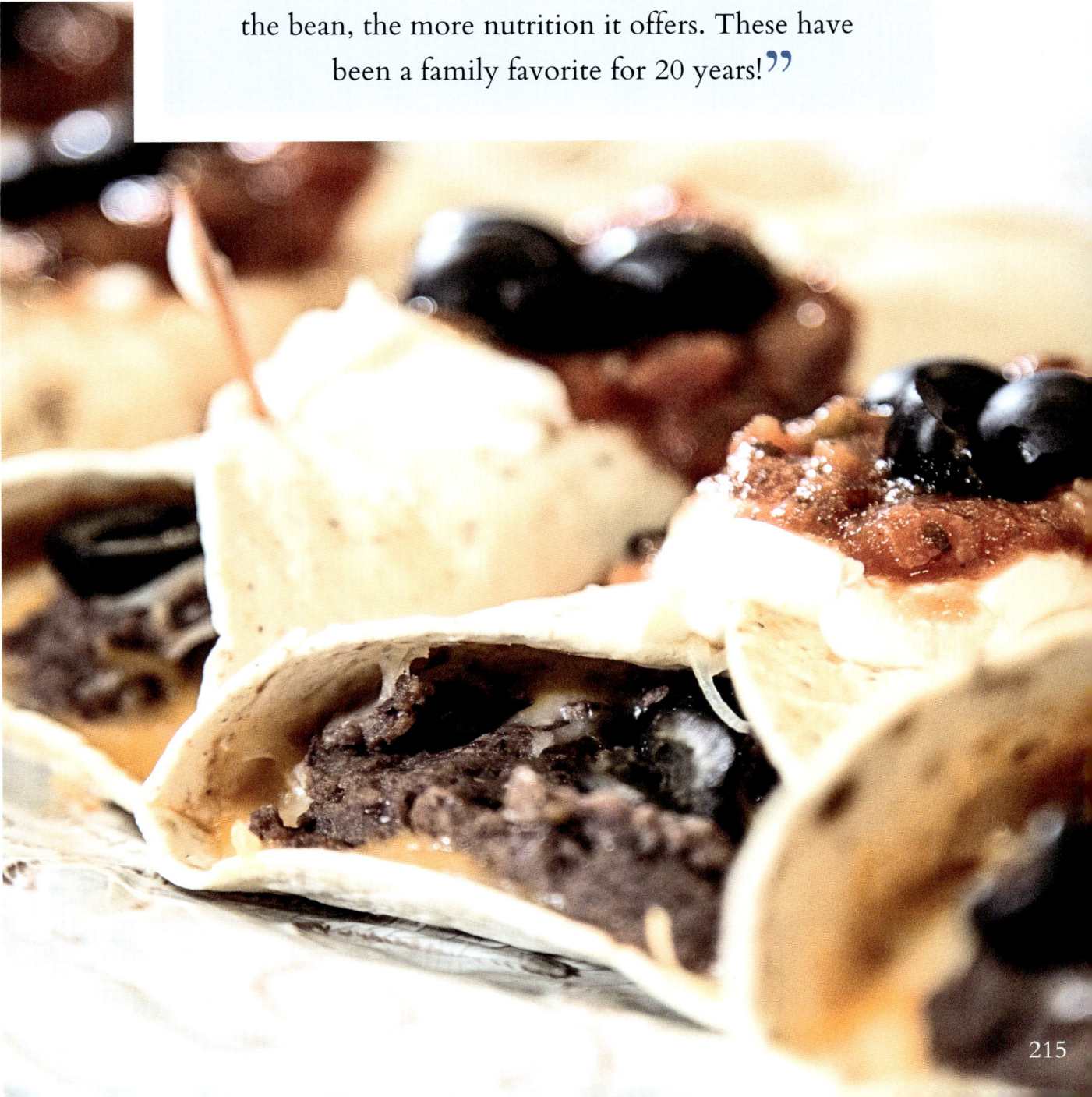

Preparation

If using cooked beans, skip to step 4

1. Put the dry beans in medium-sized pot and cover with water overnight. If you forget to do this, the next best thing is to bring the water to a boil, cover, turn off the heat and let sit for one hour.

2. Drain and rinse the soaked beans in a colander. Return them to the pot with 3 cups of fresh water and a shake of salt.

3. Bring beans to a boil, then reduce heat to a slow simmer. Check to make sure they are not boiling, rather just a slight bubble so you know they are cooking. Cook 20-30 minutes. Check tenderness after 20 minutes. If still hard, continue cooking until they are *al dente* (but not soft.)

4. Meanwhile, sauté the onion in a little butter. Salt lightly to bring out the flavor. Sauté until translucent but not brown. Remove from heat and set aside. Put in a small bowl and set aside.

5. When the beans are done, drain them in a colander over a large mixing bowl to catch the "bean water". Save the bean water!

6. In a food processor, pulse the garlic until fine.

7. Add the beans, chili powder, paprika, and sea salt to the food processor and process on low. Add a very small amount of the "bean water" if needed to thin out the beans so that you end up with a nice, creamy consistency.

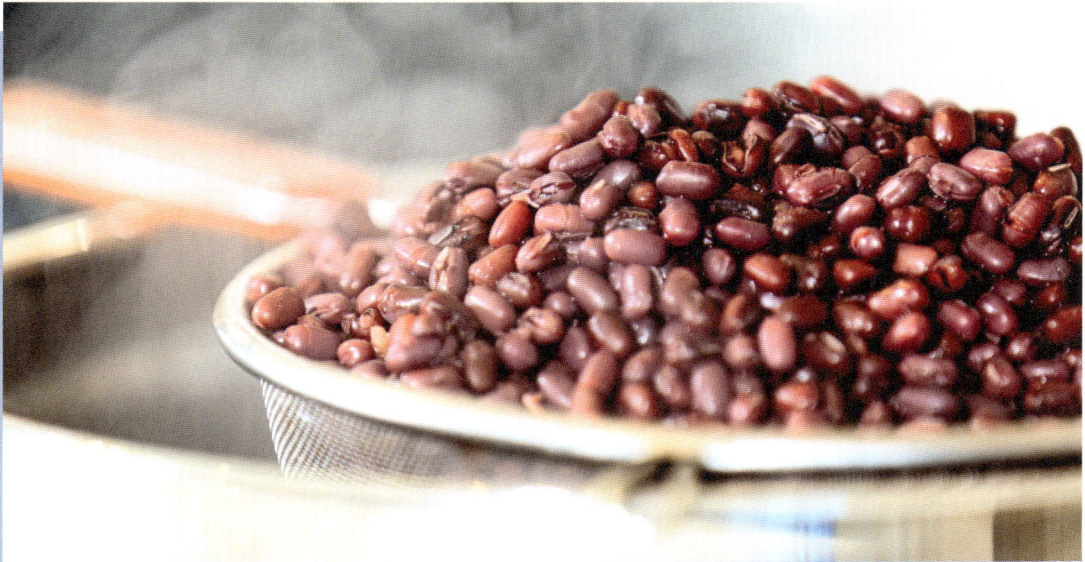

8. Remove bean paste from the food processor and place into mixing bowl. Using the toothpick method *(see page 32)* carefully stir in one toothpick each of YL Vitality Oregano, Thyme and Black Pepper oil and stir (add more YL vitality oil if desired.)

9. Preheat oven to 350° degrees.

10. On a large sheet pan, place your first tortilla and, using a pastry brush, gently brush it with olive oil.

11. Spread one tablespoon of salsa over the tortilla.

12. Take a handful of shredded cheese and liberally distribute on tortilla.

13. Take 3 Tbsp of the adzuki bean paste and gently spread it down the center. Then put a tablespoon of sauteed onions on top.

14. Fold both sides up and put two toothpicks to overlap them together.

15. Brush more of your olive oil on the top and sprinkle with salt.

16. Repeat this with as many burritos as you desire to make.

17. Place in oven for 8–12 minutes, keeping a good watch on it. Let the tops get a little brown but not hard.

18. Remove from oven, place on your plate and garnish.

Let's celebrate these life giving ingredients!

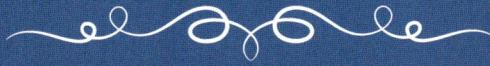

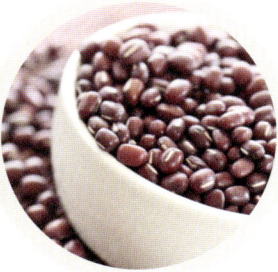

Adzuki Beans

- High in protein, vitamins, and minerals
- Good source of iron, potassium, magnesium, and B vitamins
- Plant-based protein with essential amino acids for muscle repair and growth
- High fiber content aids in digestion
- Great for blood sugar regulation

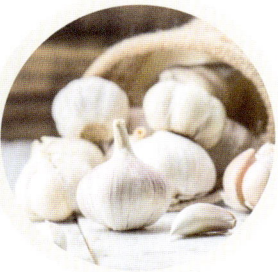

Garlic

- Renowned for natural antibiotic and antimicrobial properties
- Helps combat infections and boost the immune system
- Rich in antioxidants, including allicin
- Well-documented support for heart health
- Lowers blood pressure and improves cholesterol levels
- Reduces the risk of cardiovascular diseases
- Anti-inflammatory properties

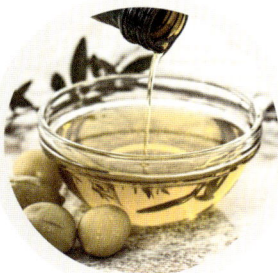

Olive Oil

- Heart-healthy choice
- Lowers bad cholesterol levels and reduces the risk of heart disease
- Packed with antioxidants like vitamin E and polyphenols
- Protects cells from damage caused by free radicals and oxidative stress
- Reduces the risk of Alzheimer's disease

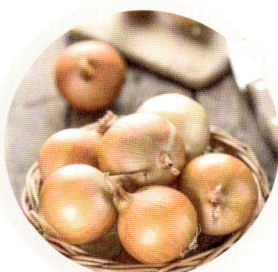

Onions

- Rich in antioxidants, including flavonoids and sulfur compounds
- Anti-inflammatory
- Immune-boosting properties
- Reduce the risk of heart disease and cancer
- High in vitamin C, vitamin B6, and dietary fiber
- Supports brain health

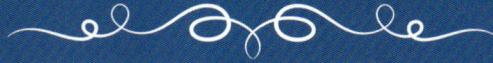

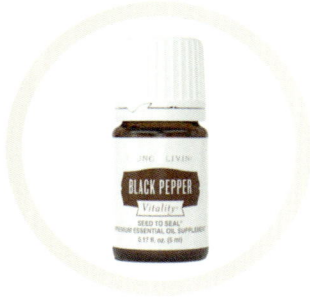

- Aids in digestive health
- Promotes secretion of digestive juices and enzymes
- Helps alleviate digestive discomfort
- Eases muscle tension and discomfort
- Invigorates the mind
- Boosts alertness

YL Vitality
Black Pepper Oil

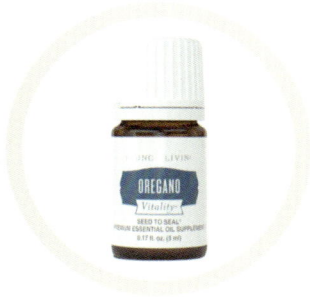

- Rich in antimicrobial compounds like carvacrol and thymol
- High in antioxidants
- Supports digestion
- Provides respiratory support

YL Vitality
Oregano Oil

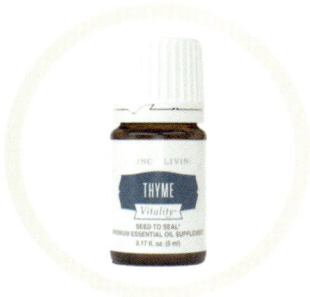

- Rich in thymol which is antimicrobial
- Contains antioxidants
- Supports respiratory health

YL Vitality
Thyme Oil

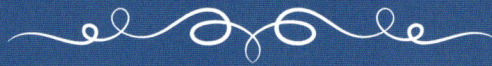

" Once you fold your burritos and put your toothpick in to hold them in place, use a pastry brush to lightly cover the top with olive oil and sprinkle on a little sea salt. As they brown in the oven, something special happens to the flavors that you will only discover when try this recipe for yourself. Happy cooking! "

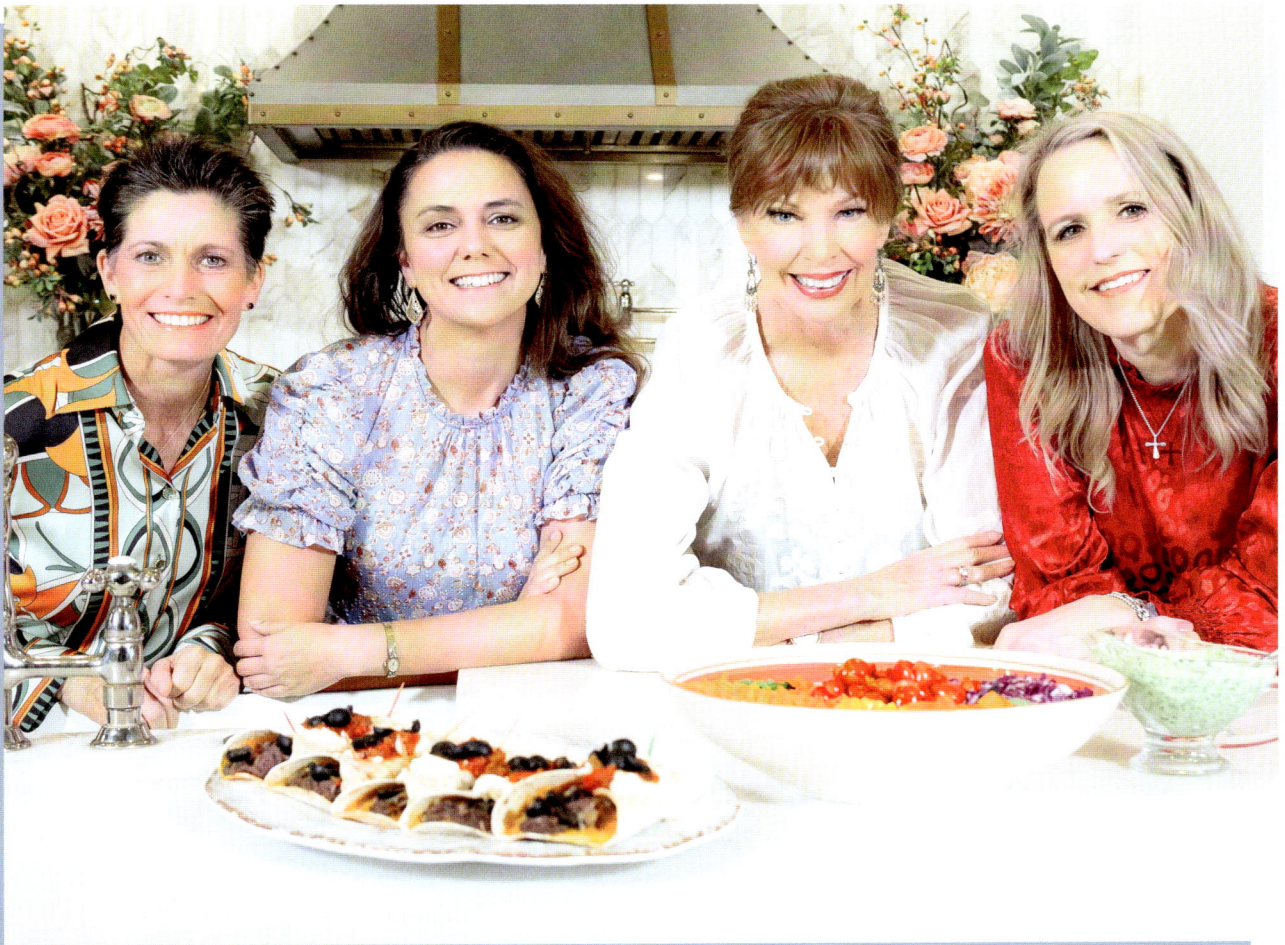

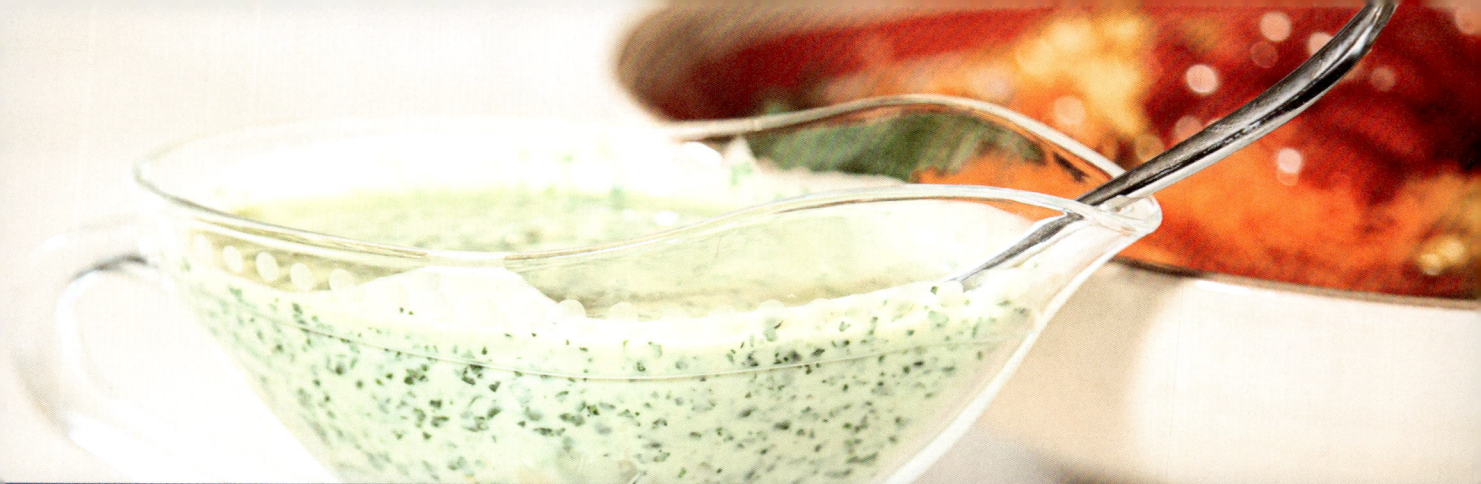

CELEBRATION SALAD
WITH AVOCADO CILANTRO DRESSING

Ingredients

Makes 6 Healthy Portions!

Roasted Sweet Potatoes

2 sweet potatoes

2 garlic cloves, peeled and minced

2 Tbsp olive oil

1 drop YL Vitality Black Pepper oil

1 drop YL Vitality Thyme oil

1 drop YL Vitality Oregano oil

(Order YL Essential oils on page 39)

Salt and pepper to taste

Salad Ingredients

1 cup cooked organic sweet corn

1/2 cup red onion, thinly sliced

1/2 cup carrots, shredded

1 romaine heart, chopped

1/2 cup red cabbage, shredded

1/2 cup sliced black olives

1/2 cup fresh red tomato, diced

Avocado Cilantro Dressing

1/2 of an avocado

1/4 cup Greek yogurt

1/2 cup water

1 cup cilantro, leaves and stems

1 small clove of garlic

1/2 tsp salt

A squeeze of lime juice

Preparation

Roasting the sweet potatoes

1. Preheat the oven to 375°. Prepare a sheet pan by lining with parchment paper.
2. Peel the sweet potatoes, chop into bite-sized pieces, and set aside.
3. Place the olive oil into a small bowl. Add the essential oil to the olive oil and mix. Add the minced garlic and mix.
4. Place the sweet potatoes into a gallon-sized ziplock bag and cover with the oil mixture. Shake vigorously until the potatoes are fully covered.
5. Place potatoes on a cookie sheet and roast for 20 minutes or until desired doneness. Flip halfway through cooking.
6. Season with salt and pepper.

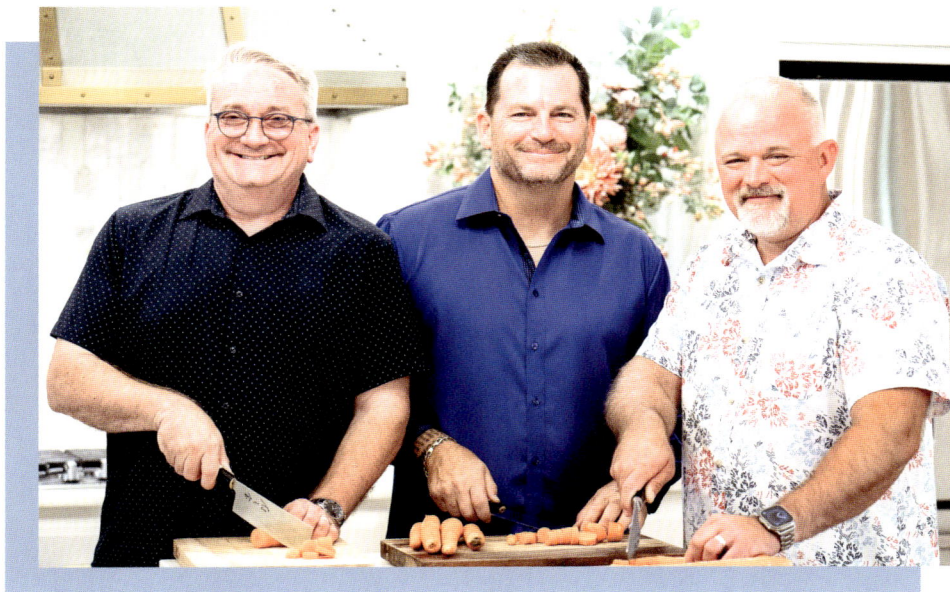

7. Meanwhile, pulse all the Avocado Cilantro Dressing ingredients in a food processor until mostly smooth.
8. Assembling you artwork! Place the romaine on the bottom of your favorite serving bowl. Take each of the other salad ingredients and the roasted sweet potatoes and place them individually like the spokes of a wheel with the exception the tomato. The tomato will be placed at the center for extra color!
9. Slowly drizzle the Avocado Cilantro Dressing over the top.
10. Serve extra dressing using a serving dish.

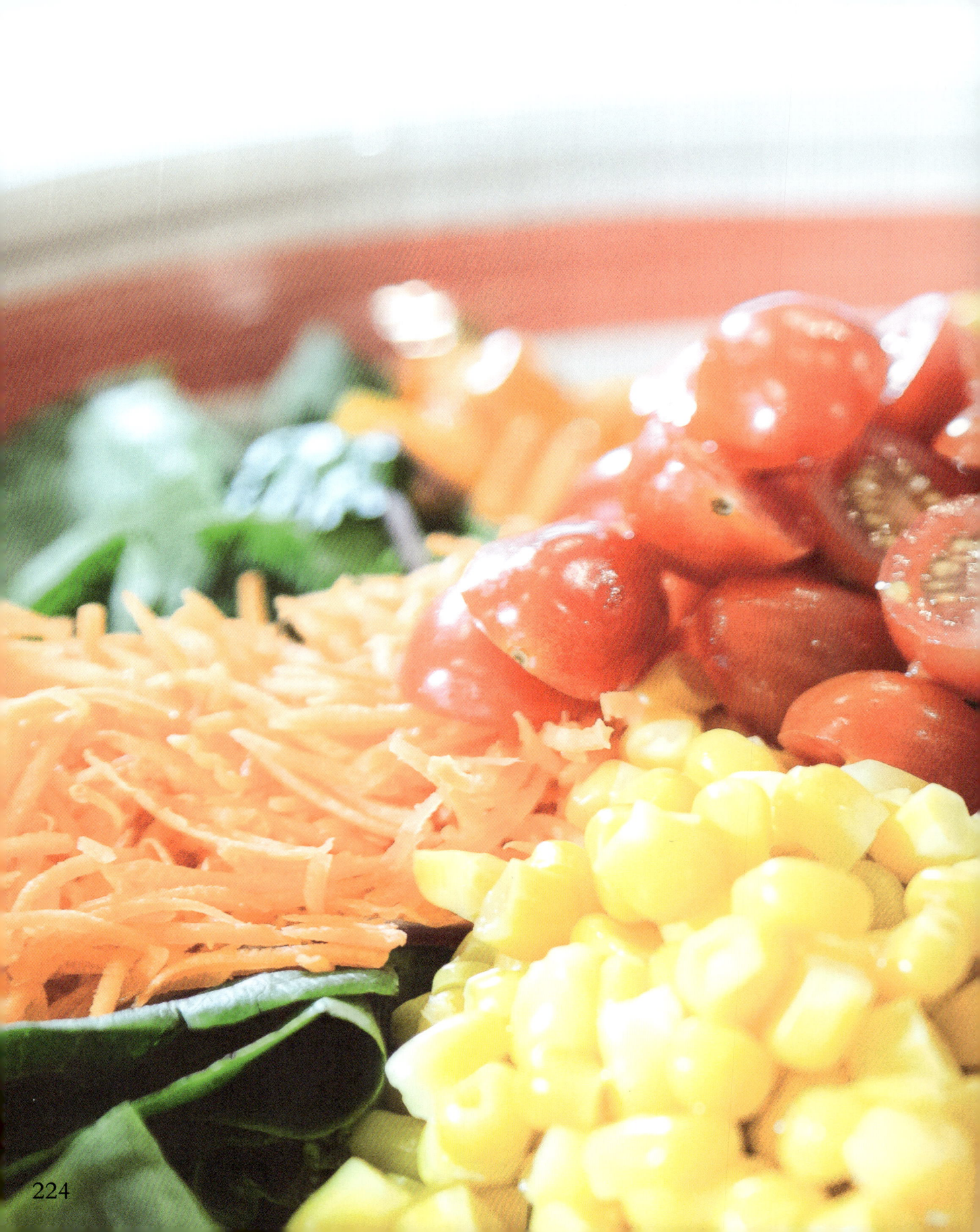

"This salad can be an exquisite main course salad, especially if you add a cup of cooked adzuki beans on top for protein. Imagine how many different farmers it took to grow these vegetables, so let's remember to thank them as we enjoy it."

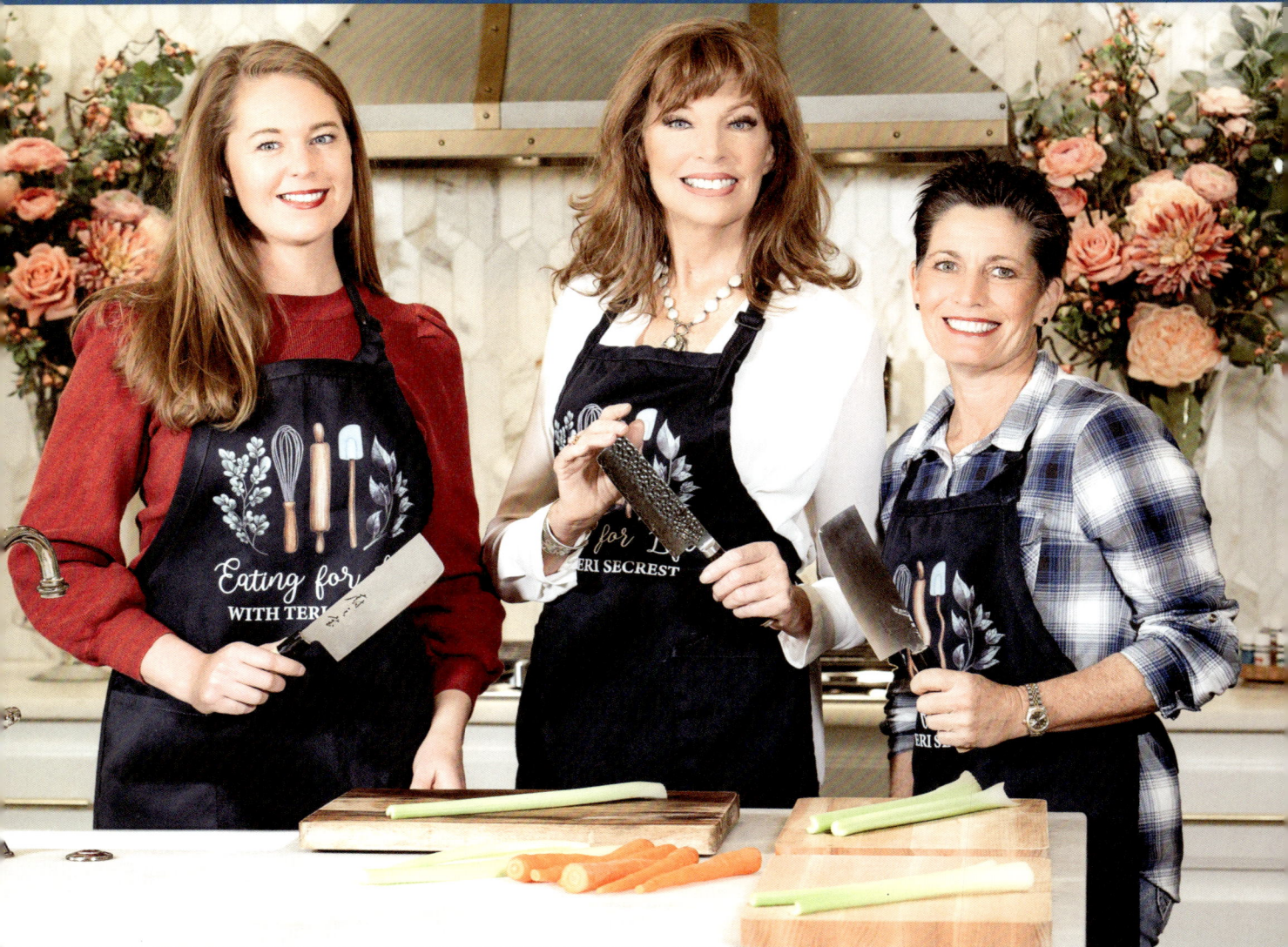

Let's celebrate these life giving ingredients!

Sweet Potatoes

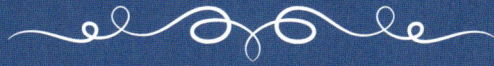

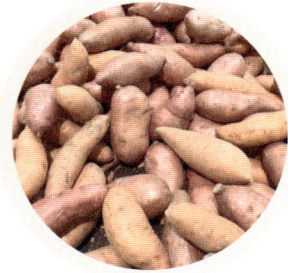

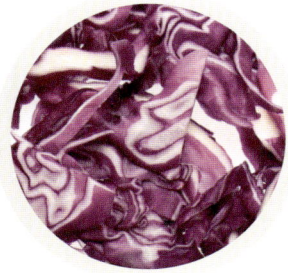

- Rich in beta-carotene which converts to vitamin A, supporting vision, immune function, and skin health
- Complex carbohydrates which provides sustained energy and regulate blood sugar levels
- Vitamins C and B6, potassium, and manganese which contribute to heart health and brain function

Red Cabbage

- Protects the cells from inflammation
- Antioxidants such as anthocyanins
- Supports heart health
- Promotes digestion and regular bowel movements
- Boosts immunity with vitamin C
- Supports bone health with vitamin K
- Helps prevent osteoporosis

Olive Oil

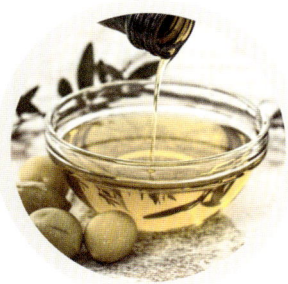

- Rich in monounsaturated fats
- Heart-healthy choice
- Lowers bad cholesterol levels and reduce the risk of heart disease
- Packed with antioxidants like vitamin E and polyphenols
- Cell protection from free radicals and oxidative stress
- Reduces the risk of Alzheimer's disease

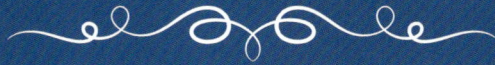

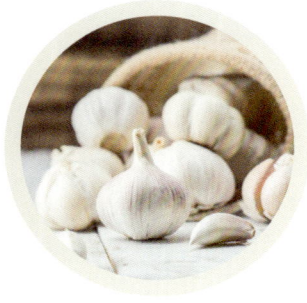

Garlic

- Renowned for natural antibiotic and antimicrobial properties
- Helps combat infections and boost the immune system
- Rich in antioxidants, including allicin
- Well-documented support for heart health
- Lowers blood pressure and improves cholesterol levels
- Reduces the risk of cardiovascular diseases
- Anti-inflammatory properties

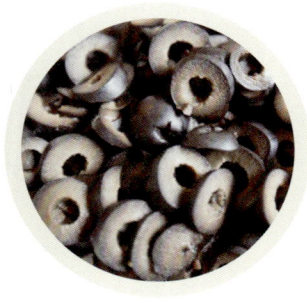

Black Olives

- Rich in monounsaturated fats, which promote heart health and reduce bad cholesterol levels
- Contains antioxidants like vitamin E
- Contains oleic acid, which can reduce blood pressure and improve cardiovascular health
- Rich in vitamin A.
- Contain polyphenols and flavonoids that reduce inflammation
- Provide essential minerals like calcium and iron, which are important for maintaining strong bones

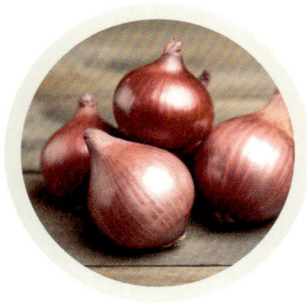

Red Onion

- Antioxidants such as flavonoids and anthocyanins, which help combat oxidative stress and inflammation
- Contains quercetin which is great for lowering inflammation
- Rich in vitamin C

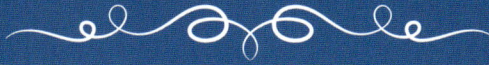

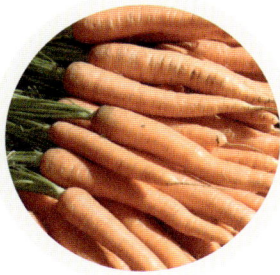

Organic Carrots

- Packed with beta-carotene, a precursor to vitamin A
- Supports vision health
- Immune boosting
- Great for skin health
- Contains antioxidants like vitamin C and lutein
- Helps reduce inflammation
- High fiber supports digestive health
- Promotes feelings of fullness

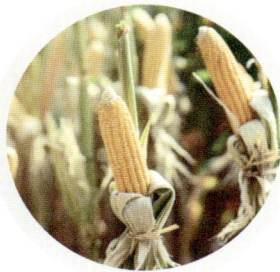

Organic Sweet Corn

- Contains essential vitamins A, B, and C for healthy skin, vision, and immune function
- High fiber content aids in digestion, helps maintain a healthy weight and lowers the risk of heart disease
- Contains lutein and zeaxanthin, protecting eyes from damage and reducing the risk of macular degeneration
- Fiber and phytonutrients help lower cholesterol levels reduce inflammation, and improve blood circulation
- Contains vitamin C to support the immune system

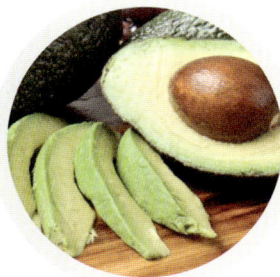

Avocados

- Packed with heart-healthy monounsaturated fats
- Helps lower bad cholesterol and raise good cholesterol levels
- Loaded with fiber for digestion and weight management
- Source of vitamins E and K for skin health, blood clotting, and bone strength
- Provides potassium, folate, and vitamin C

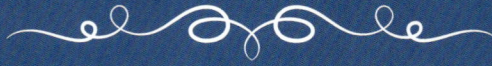

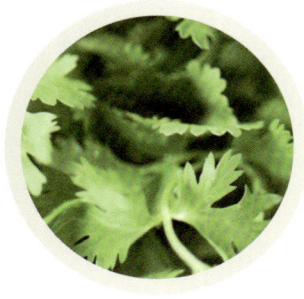

Fresh Cilantro

- Excellent source of vitamin K, which is essential for blood clotting and bone health, and vitamin A, which supports eye health and immune function
- Provides small amounts of vitamin C, an antioxidant that helps protect cells from damage caused by free radicals
- Contains minerals like potassium, manganese, and iron, which play important roles in various bodily functions including muscle function, metabolism, and oxygen transport
- Some studies suggest that cilantro may have antimicrobial properties and could help lower blood sugar levels and reduce inflammation

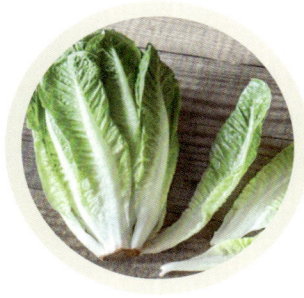

Romaine Lettuce

- High water content keeps you hydrated and promotes a feeling of fullness
- Contains vitamins A, C, and K, which are essential for immune function, skin health, and blood clotting
- High in fiber which aids digestion, promotes a healthy gut, and helps maintain regular bowel movements
- Provides essential minerals like calcium, magnesium, and phosphorus that are important for maintaining strong bones
- Contains beta-carotene and lutein, which help protect cells from damage caused by free radicals.
- Rich in vitamin A and antioxidants that improve skin health and reduce signs of aging
- Contains lutein and zeaxanthin, which are important for maintaining good vision and overall eye health

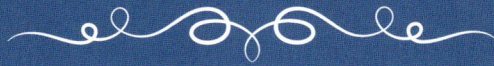

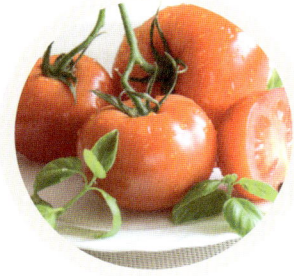

- Includes vitamin C, potassium, and folate
- Supports the immune system
- Rich in antioxidants like lycopene
- Promotes heart health
- Fiber content aids in digestion
- Contributes to weight management

Organic Tomatoes

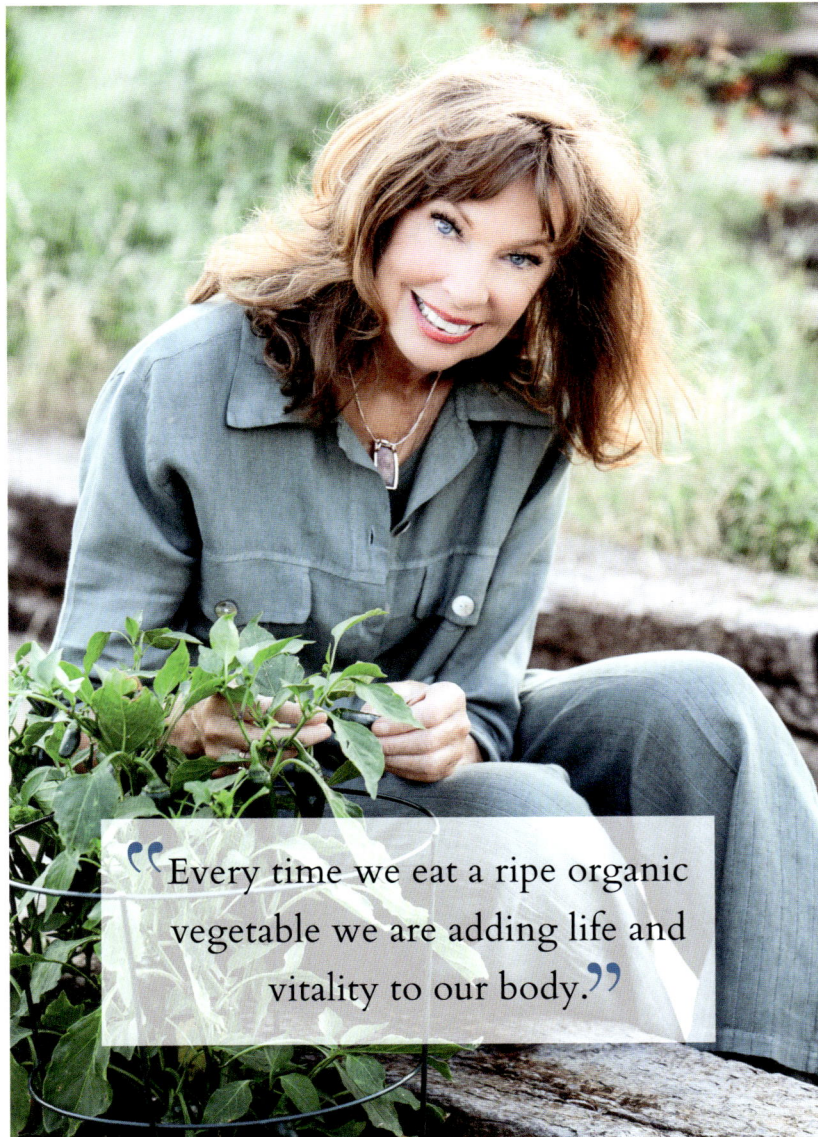

"Every time we eat a ripe organic vegetable we are adding life and vitality to our body."

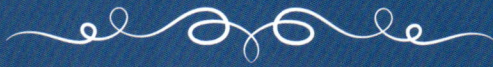

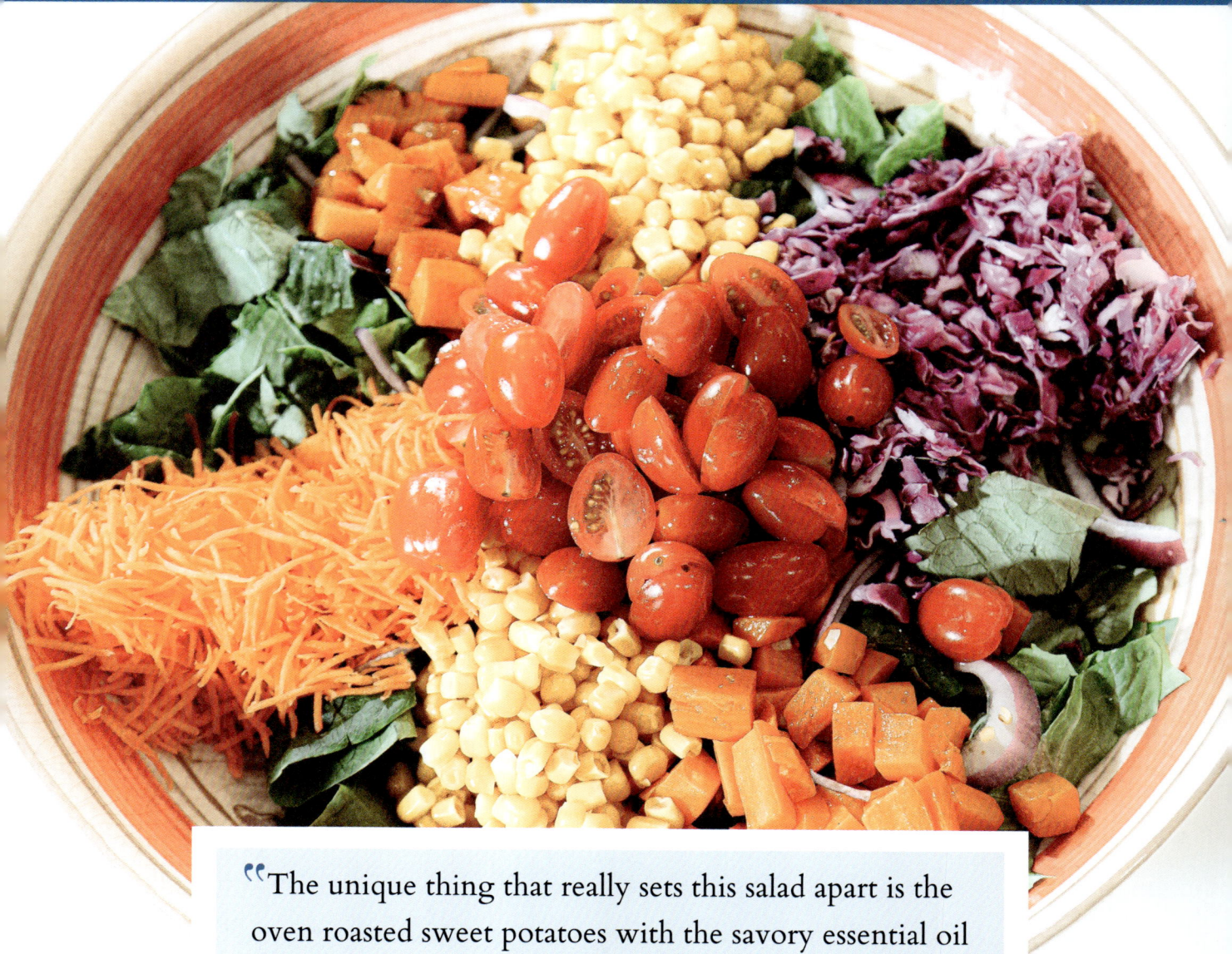

"The unique thing that really sets this salad apart is the oven roasted sweet potatoes with the savory essential oil and olive oil blend. It's an epic autumn salad."

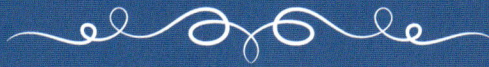

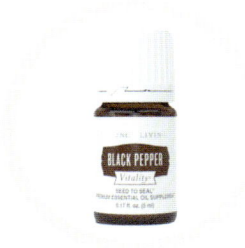

- May aid in digestive health
- Promotes secretion of digestive juices and enzymes
- Eases muscle tension
- Invigorates the mind
- Boosts alertness

YL Vitality Black Pepper Oil

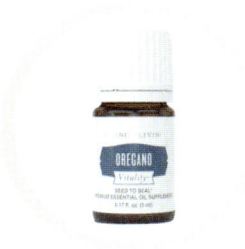

- Rich in antimicrobial compounds like carvacrol and thymol
- High in antioxidants
- Supports digestion
- Provides respiratory support

YL Vitality Oregano Oil

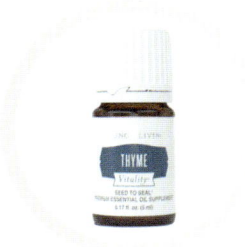

- Rich in thymol which is antimicrobial
- Contains antioxidants
- Supports respiratory health

YL Vitality Thyme Oil

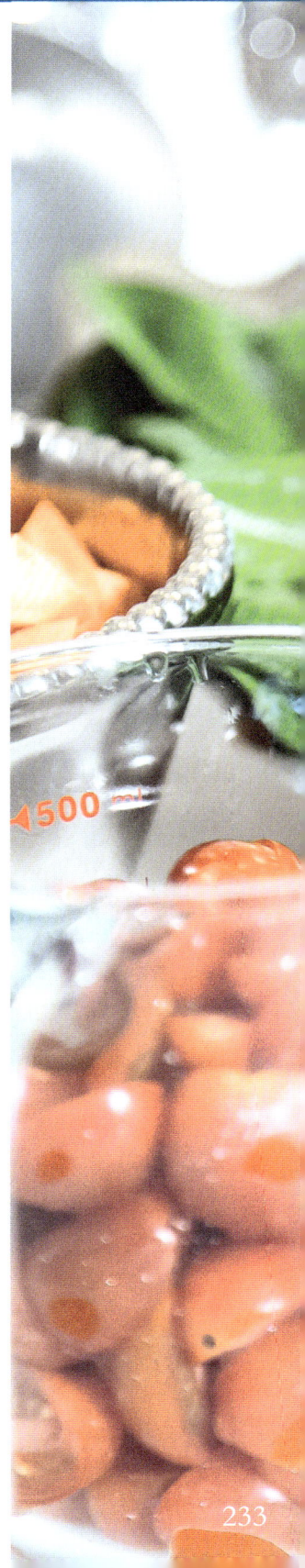

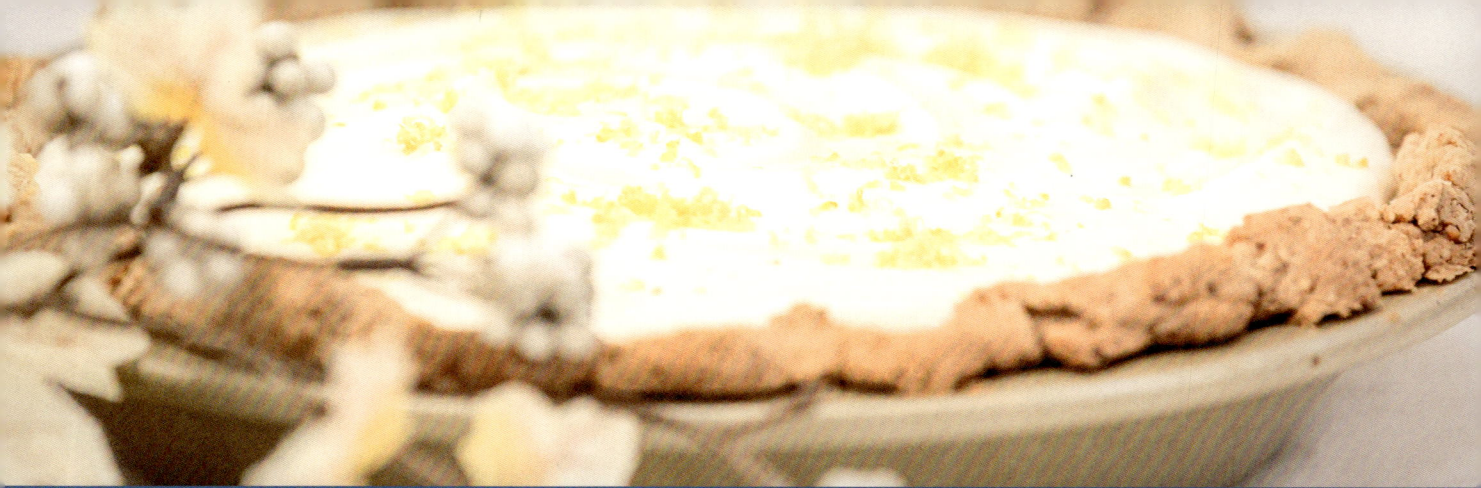

HEAVENLY LEMON CREAM PIE

Ingredients

1 Almond Pecan Pie Crust
(see pag 144)
4 egg yokes
1 cup lemon juice, fresh squeezed
2 cans organic condensed milk
3 drops YL Vitality Lemon oil

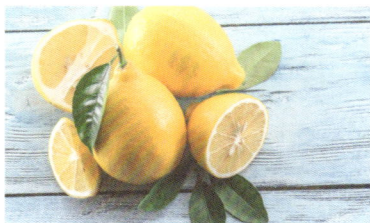

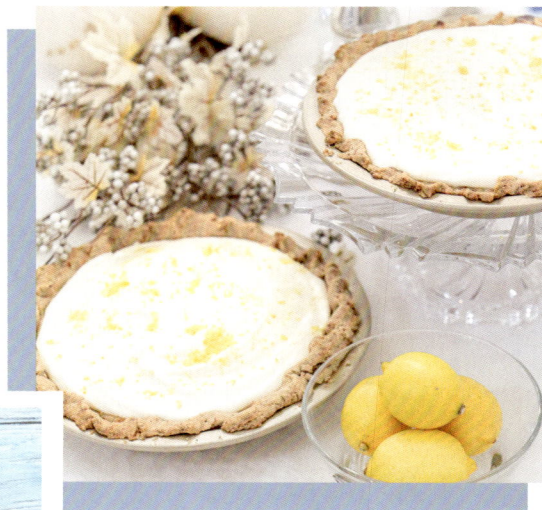

"I like to call this a Heavenly Lemon Cream Pie because the filling has an entire cup of fresh squeezed organic lemon juice... pure fuel for the body! This filling was shared with me by my good friend, Melinda Powers, talented, retired restauranteur from Vashon Island. I love to pair it with my Almond Pecan Pie Crust. It's voted #1 by family and friends!"

Preparation

1. Preheat your oven to 375°.
2. Using a hand mixer or immersion blender, blend all ingredients well.
3. Pour into your Almond Pecan Pie Crust.
4. Bake for 28 minutes.
5. Cool on rack until room temperature and then refrigerate.

"This pie is an explosive sensory experience and you can't just have one piece"

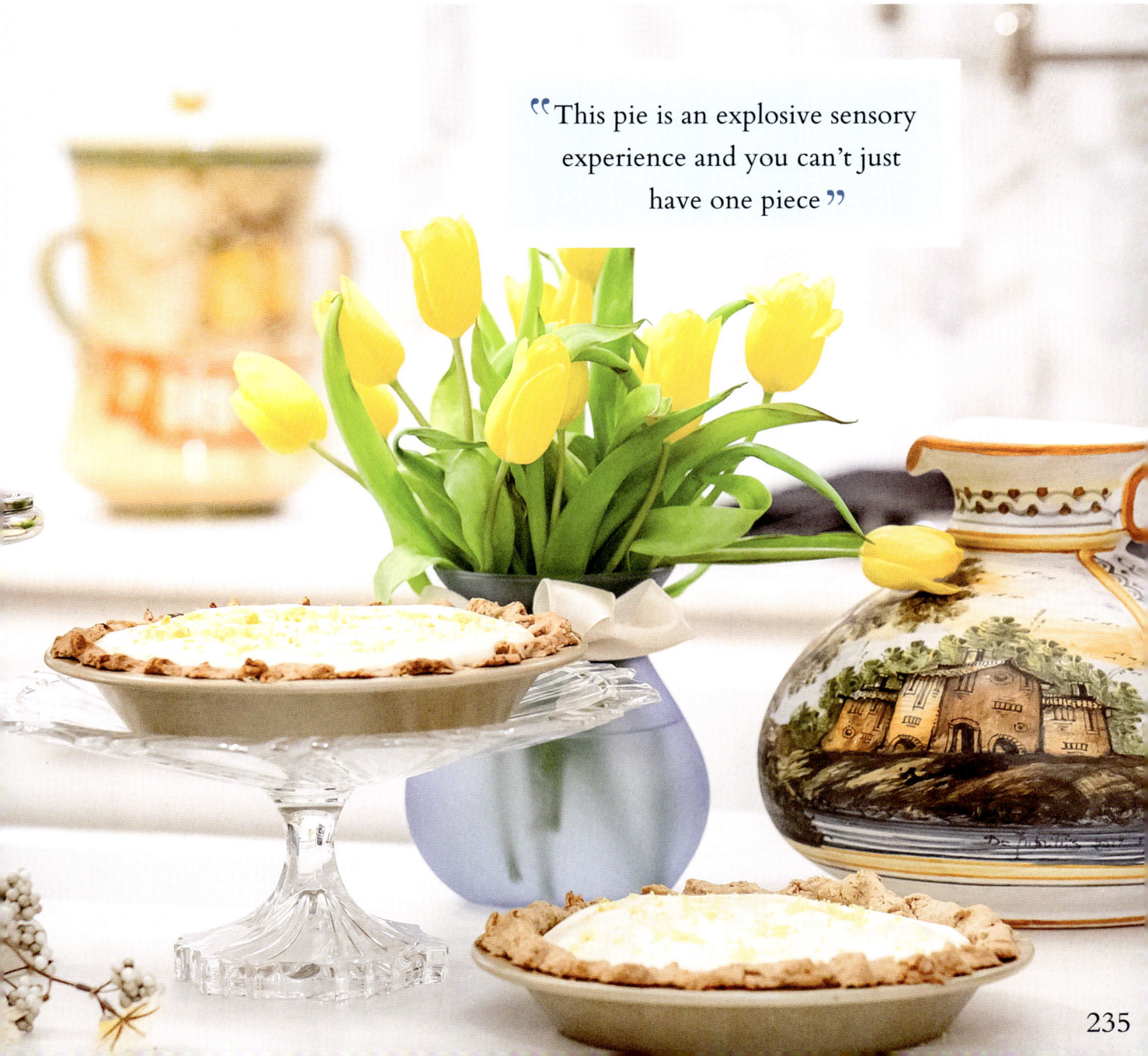

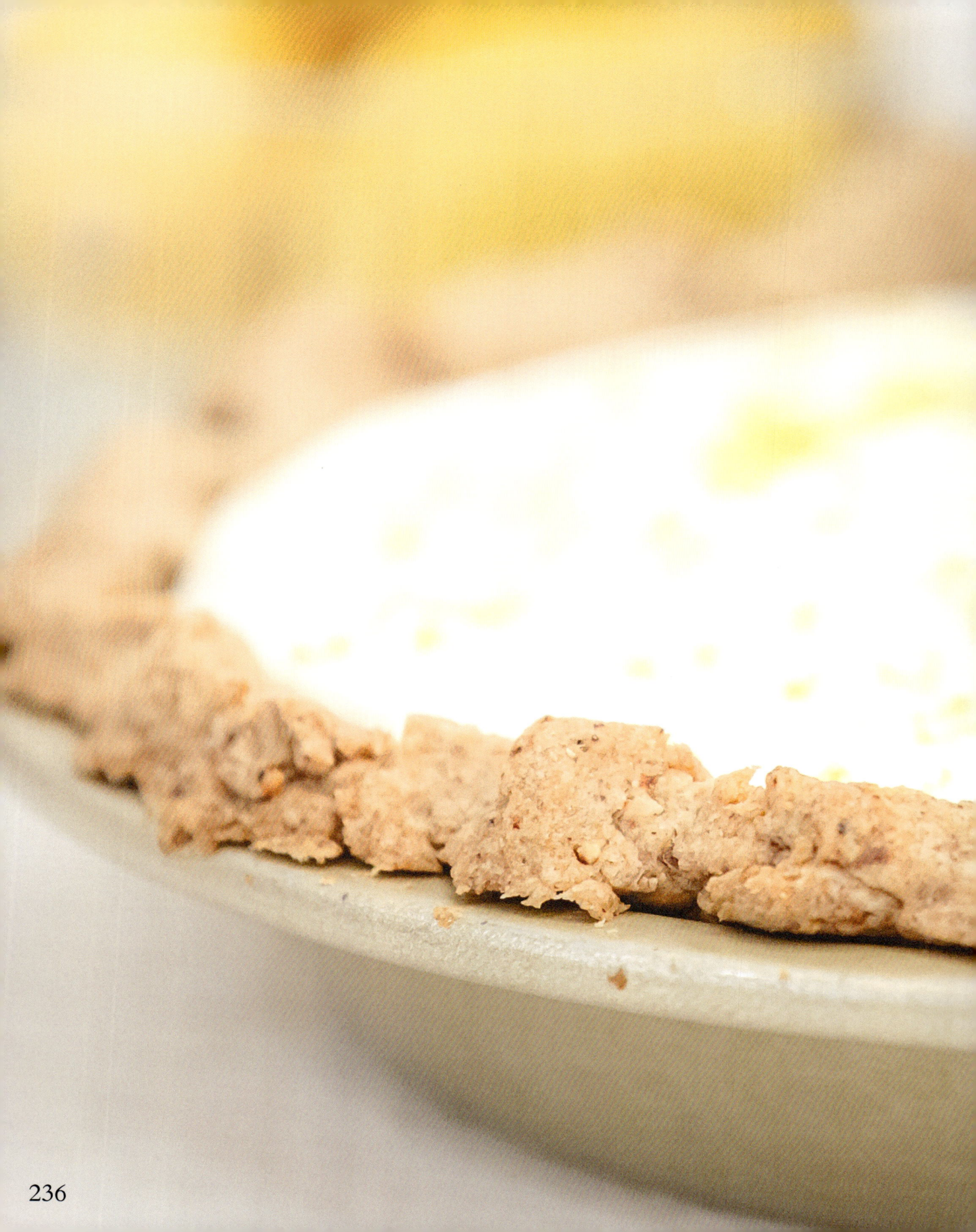

"Eating Teri's Heavenly Lemon Cream Pie is like having a multi-layered experience bursting with flavor! This is the kind of dessert that will make you want to take your plate and sit in a corner all by yourself so you can savor each and every bite without interruption!"

-Lisa Trenary

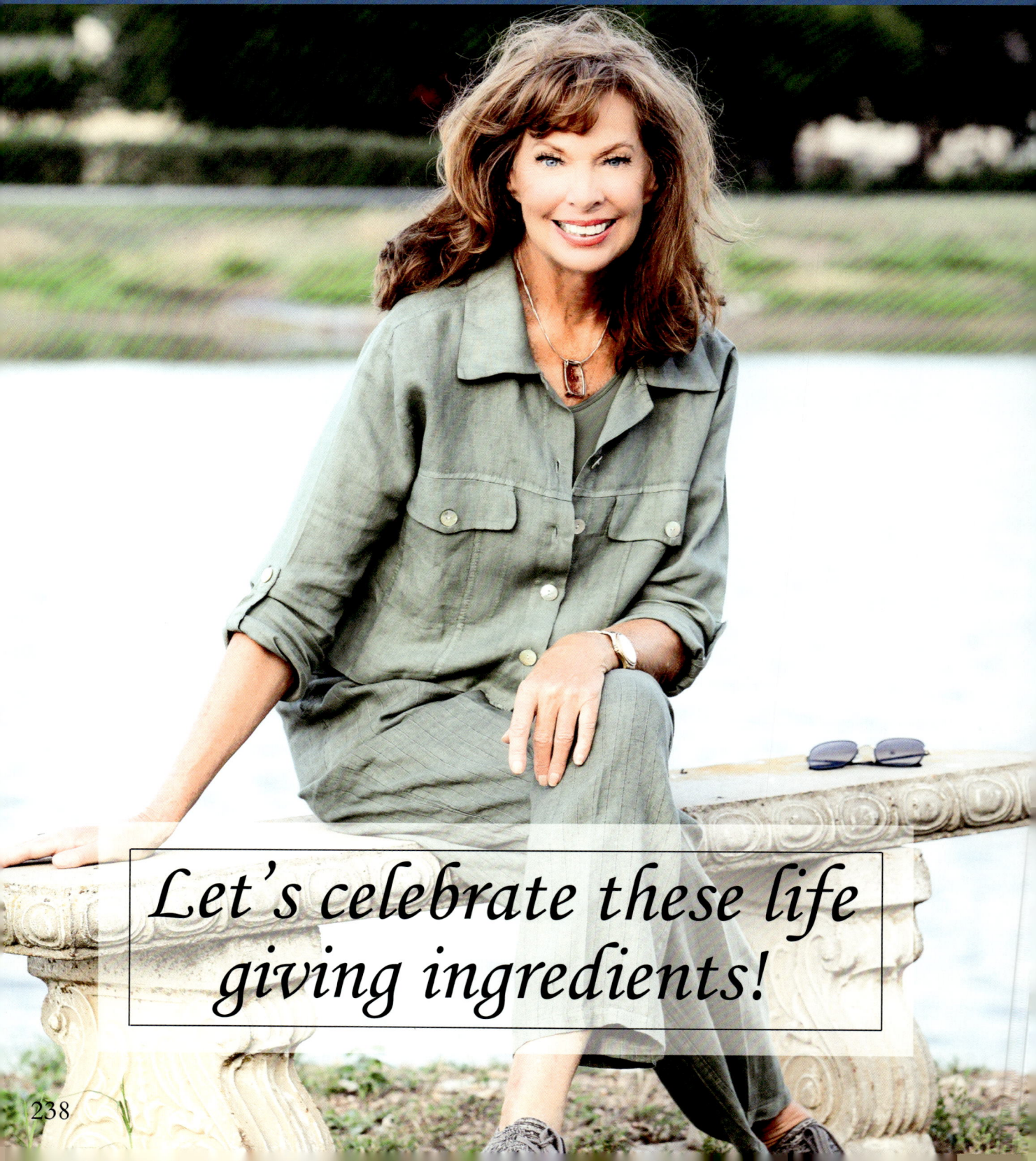

Let's celebrate these life giving ingredients!

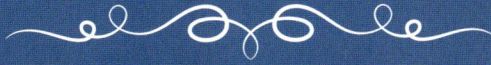

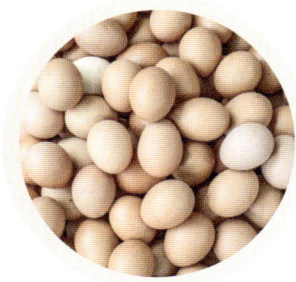

Organic Eggs

- Packed with high-quality protein
- Provides essential amino acids for muscle repair, growth, and overall body function
- Includes vitamin B12, vitamin D, riboflavin, selenium, and choline
- Crucial roles in metabolism, bone health, brain function, and heart health
- Contains lutein and zeaxanthin
- Antioxidants that promote eye health
- May reduce the risk of age-related macular degeneration
- Can improve the balance of HDL (good) to LDL (bad) cholesterol

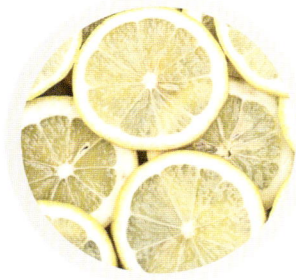

Lemons

- Packed with vitamin C, lemons are a natural immune system booster, helping you fend off colds and infections.
- Despite their acidic taste, lemons have an alkalizing effect on the body, promoting PH balance and overall health.
- Start your day with warm lemon water to kickstart digestion, detoxify the body and support liver function.
- Promotes collagen production

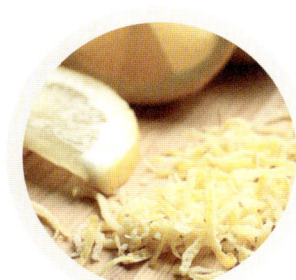

Lemon Zest

- Rich in essential oils and natural compounds
- Vitamin C for immune function and skin health
- Contains antioxidants like limonene and flavonoids
- Helps reduce inflammation and protect cells from oxidative damage

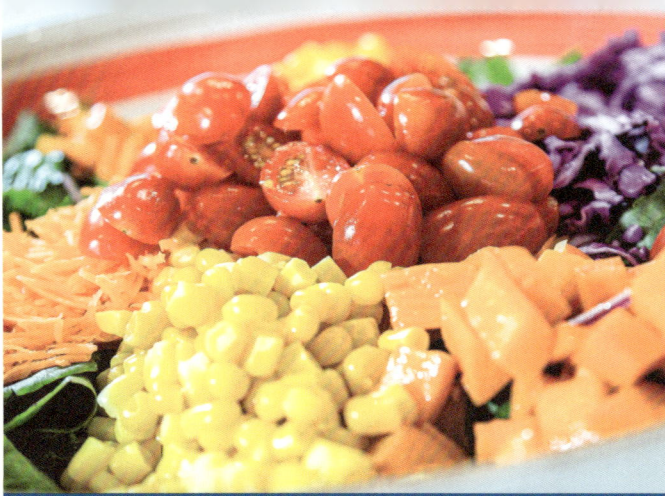

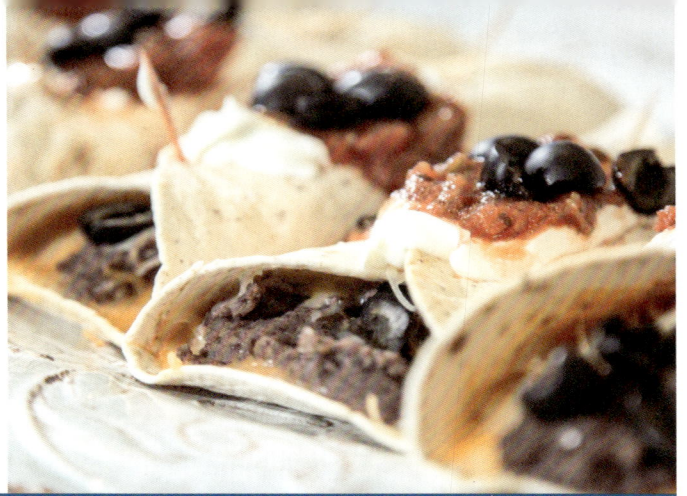

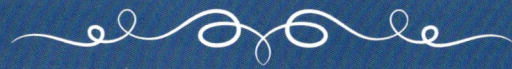

Week 7
Full Menu Shopping List

Produce

6 cloves garlic

1 white onion

2 avocado

2 sweet potatoes

1 lime

4-6 organic lemons

1 med red onion

1 sm beg organic carrots

1 Romaine heart

1 sm head red cabbage

1 med red tomato

1 lg bunch cilantro

Dairy

2 cups organic
shredded cheese

Organic sour cream
for garnish

Plain Greek yogurt

4 eggs

International

Salsa

1 pkg 8-9 inch
diameter tortillas,
(sprouted grain
is best)

Canned Goods

1 can black olives

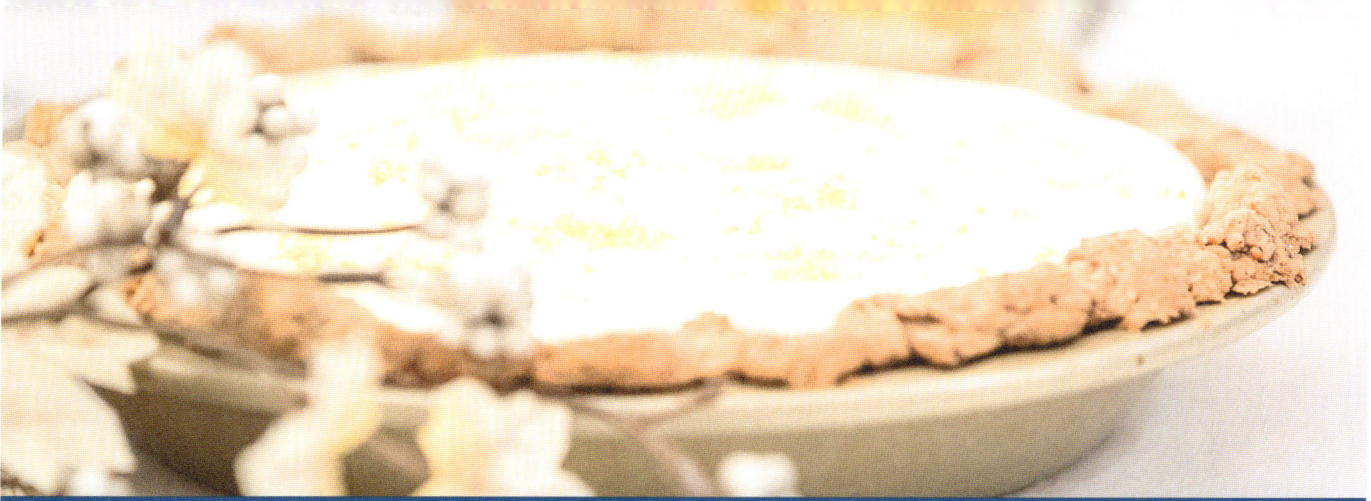

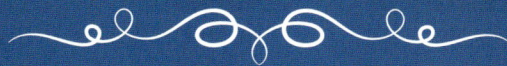

Full Menu Shopping List continued

Baking & Spices

2 cans organic condensed milk

¾ cup raw almond and raw pecan blend (1/2 raw almonds 1/2 raw pecans)

Organic unbleached all-purpose flour

Olive oil

Butter

Chili powder

Paprika

Sea salt

Olive oil

Dry Goods

1 lb adzuki beans

Frozen

1 package organic corn

From Young Living*

YL Vitality Black Pepper oil

YL Vitality Thyme oil

YL Vitality Oregano oil

3 drops YL Vitality Lemon oil

Young Living Einkorn Flour

SEE PAGE 39 FOR ORDERING DETAILS

From my Home to Yours

Thank you for the great honor
to spend this time with you!

My heart is that you are now a more
confident home chef,
filled with the knowledge of
fabulous food and extravagant
hospitality that will bring joy and life
to your loved ones for years to come!

Life is a treasure!
May all who enter our homes feel
loved and cherished!

Happy cooking with love,

Teri Secrest

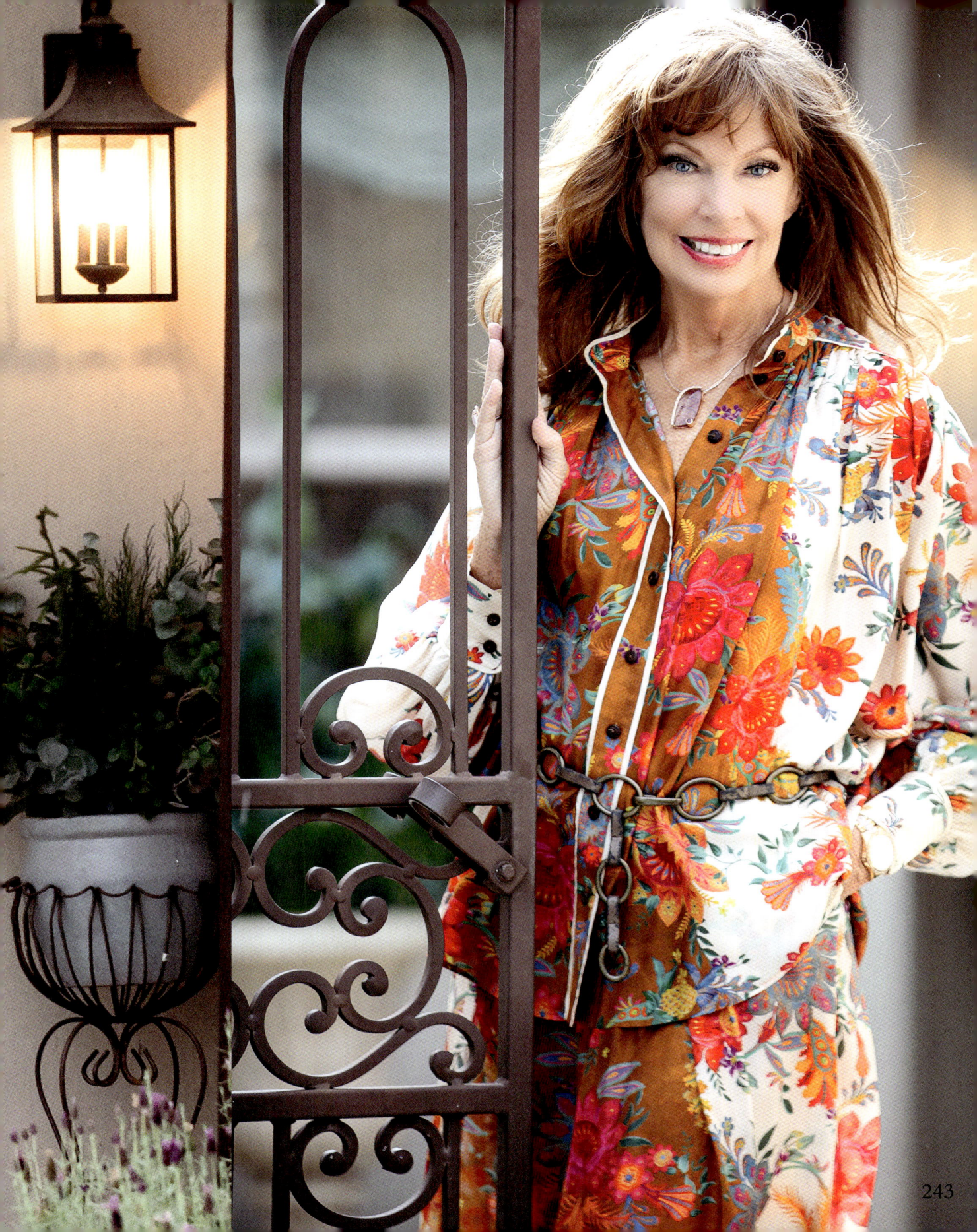

243

You're Invited to join my exclusive 7-Week Digital Healthy Cooking Course!

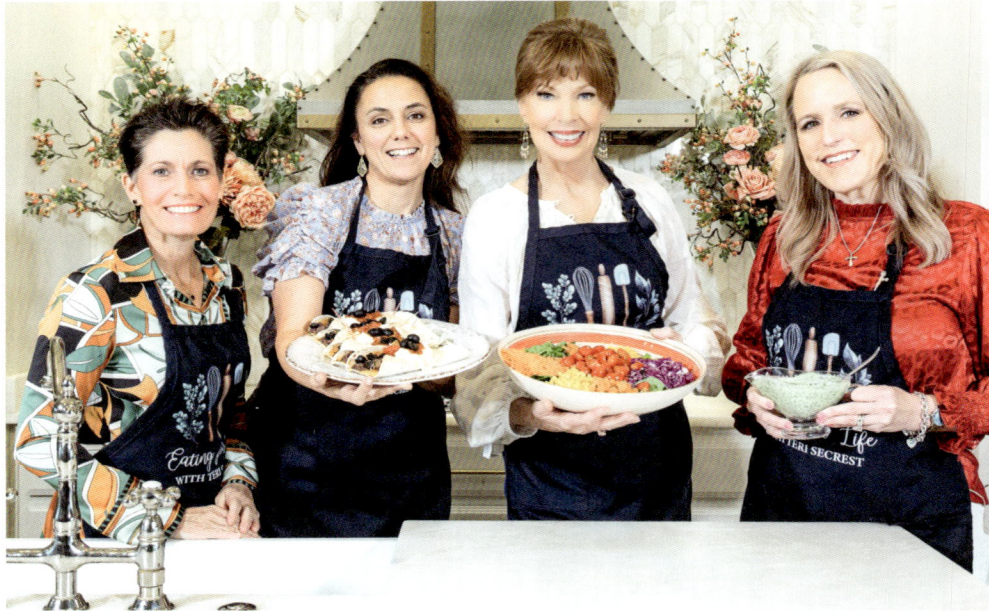

Thank you so much for experiencing Eating For Life with me. If you would like even more support with these recipes, I'd love to invite you to continue this journey with my 7-week digital healthy cooking course. Together, we'll explore these recipes and amazing techniques, cooking side by side to make your kitchen a place of flavor, wellness, and hospitality.

What Makes My Digital Course Unique?

❧ Step-by-Step Video Lessons

We'll cook together as I guide you through techniques that will elevate your skills! You'll learn how to handle a French chef knife with confidence—an essential skill that's easy to learn when you can see it in action.

❧ Cooking with Essential Oils - Made Easy!

In the book, you've already started cooking with essential oils, and now you'll see these techniques come to life! Watch how essential oils can enhance both the flavor and wellness of your meals.

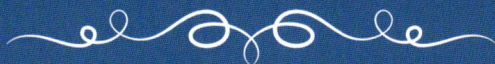

❧ **Interactive Workbook – Track Your Journey**
Our downloadable workbook will help you track your progress, reflect on your learning, and stay inspired. It's designed to support you as you grow in the kitchen.

❧ **Cook with Others in a Supportive Community**
Cooking together is the heart of this course! Join our online community to share successes, ask questions, and celebrate with others as we share the joy of learning.

❧ **Digital Version of the Cookbook**
With your digital Eating for Life cookbook, everything is right at your fingertips. Grab your phone, check your shopping list, and you're ready to go—whether you're at home or away!

❧ **Exclusive Bonuses – Extras to Keep You Going!**
From bonus recipes to spur-of-the-moment live videos, these extras will keep you motivated as we continue this journey together.

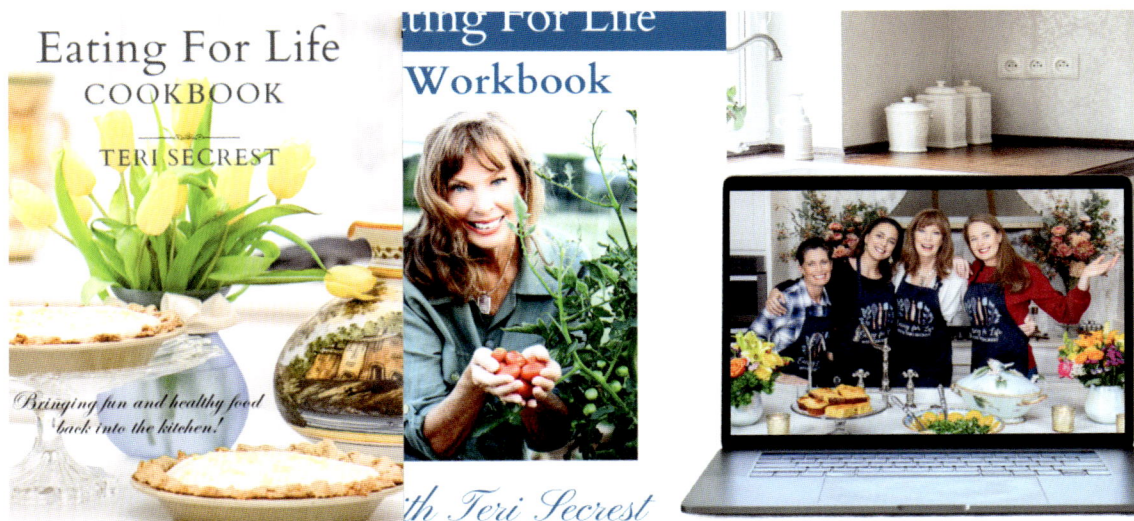

Join me and let's make memories together.
To your health with Love!
Teri Secrest

While a vision may begin with just one person, I believe it takes many hearts and good minds to transform an idea into a beautiful reality. This supportive group of friends helped bring a simple idea to life!

My heart is full of gratitude for each of our "Eating for Life" cooking students and the entire crew who came together cooked, cleaned, danced and laughed... and yes, a few times until 2 AM! Each of you brought your unique spark to this project making it absolutely extraordinary!

With deep love, *Teri Secrest*

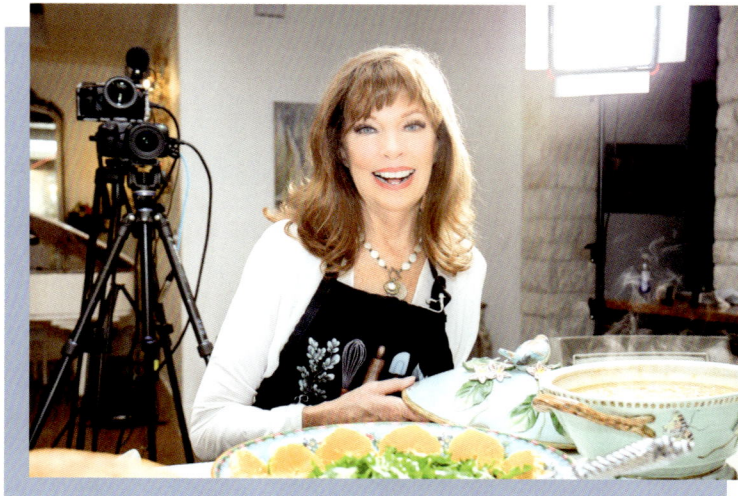

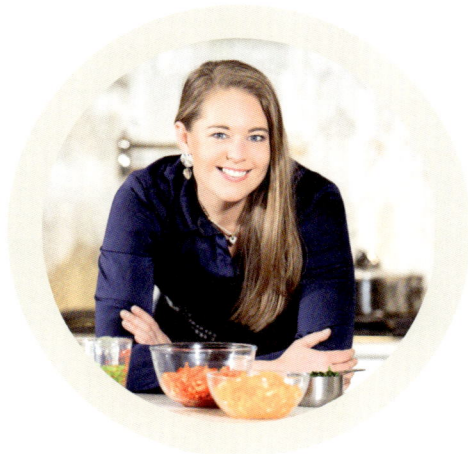

ELIZABETH ROSE
Executive Production Advisor

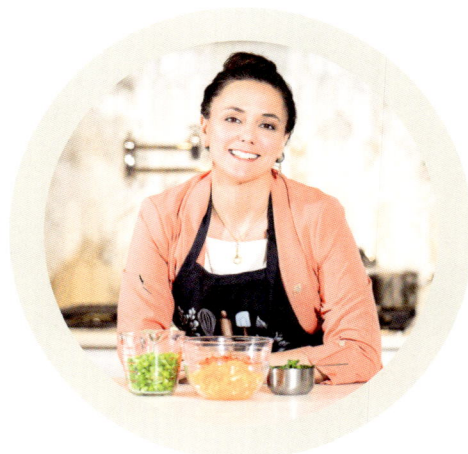

BEVERLY BANKS
Executive Project Director

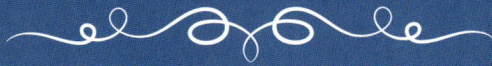

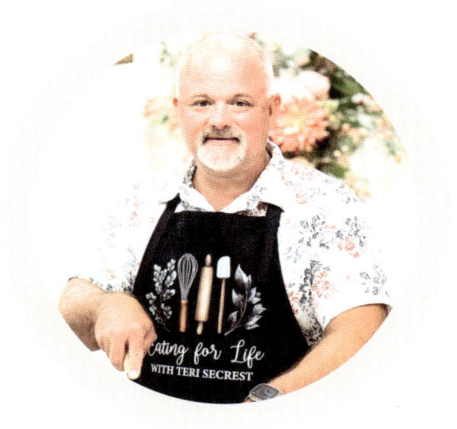

JUSTIN CARPENTER

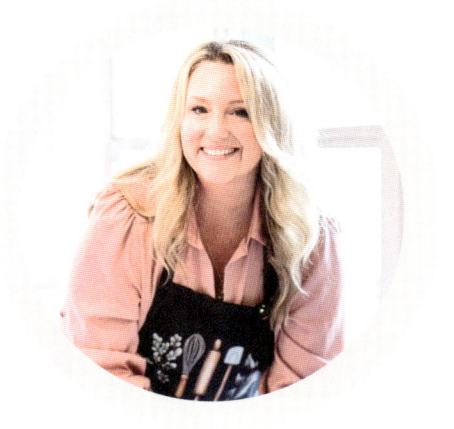

LISA CARPENTER

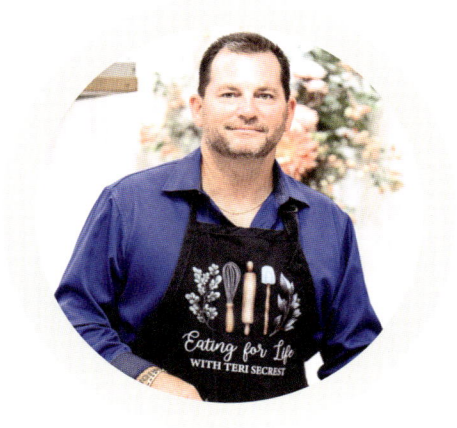

SEAN MCGINNIS

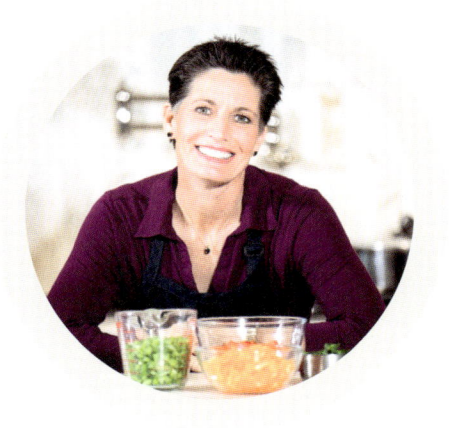

SUSAN MCGINNIS

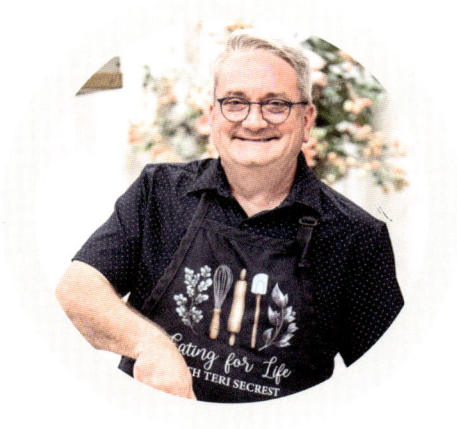

KERRY SUTTON

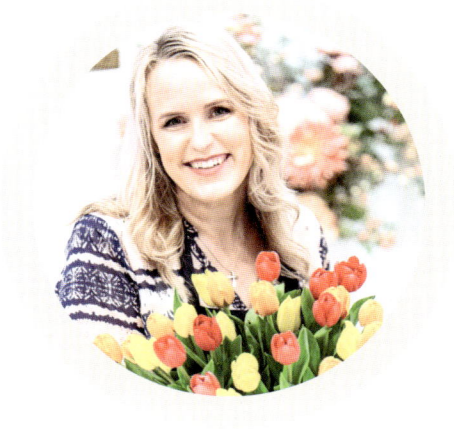

STEPHANIE SUTTON

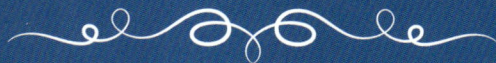

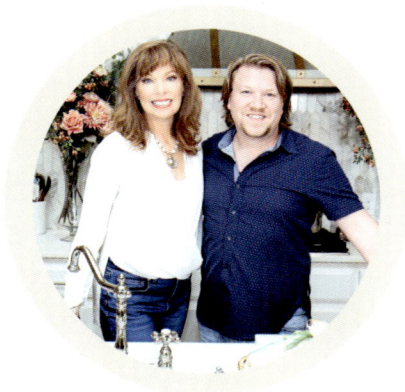

ZAK KINGREA
Chief Videographer

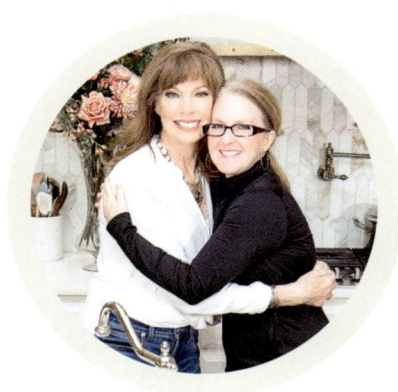

LISA TRENARY
Book Designer and Primary Photographer

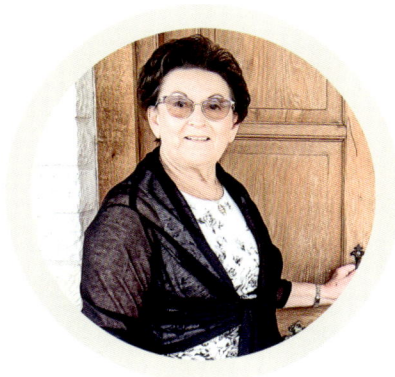

CORY BARKER
Chief Set Coordinator

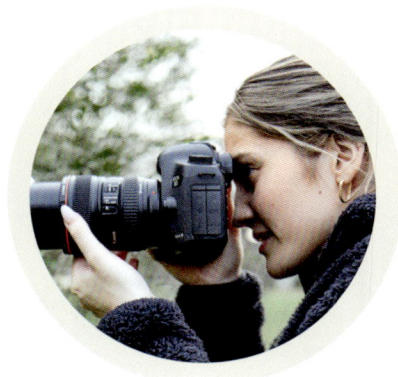

MORGAN MCGINNIS
Support Photographer

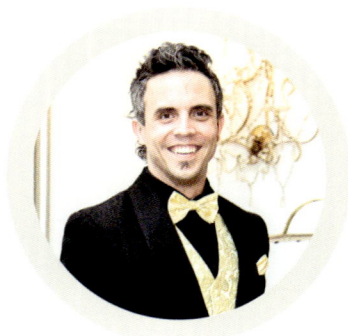

ANTHONEY TEAGUE
Media Team Support

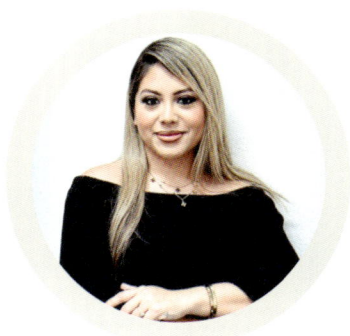

JESSICA MONJARAZ
Jessica's Artistry
Hair Designer and Makeup Artist

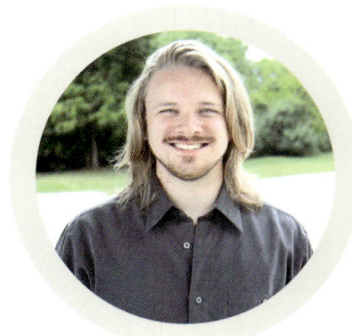

NOAH SHIRLEY
Chief Video Editor

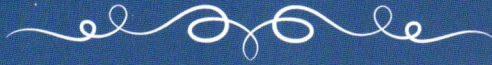

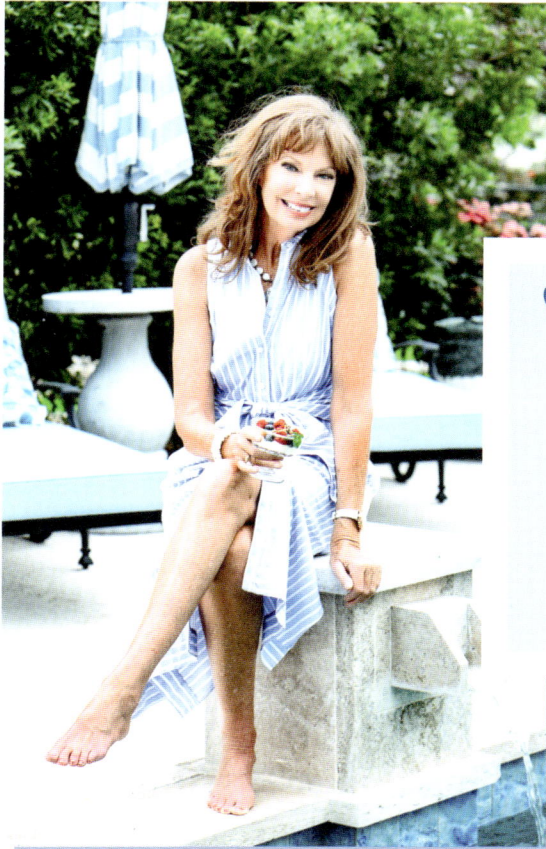

"My hope is that together we can inspire a fast food culture to slow down and enjoy the simple pleasures like dining together with family and friends!"

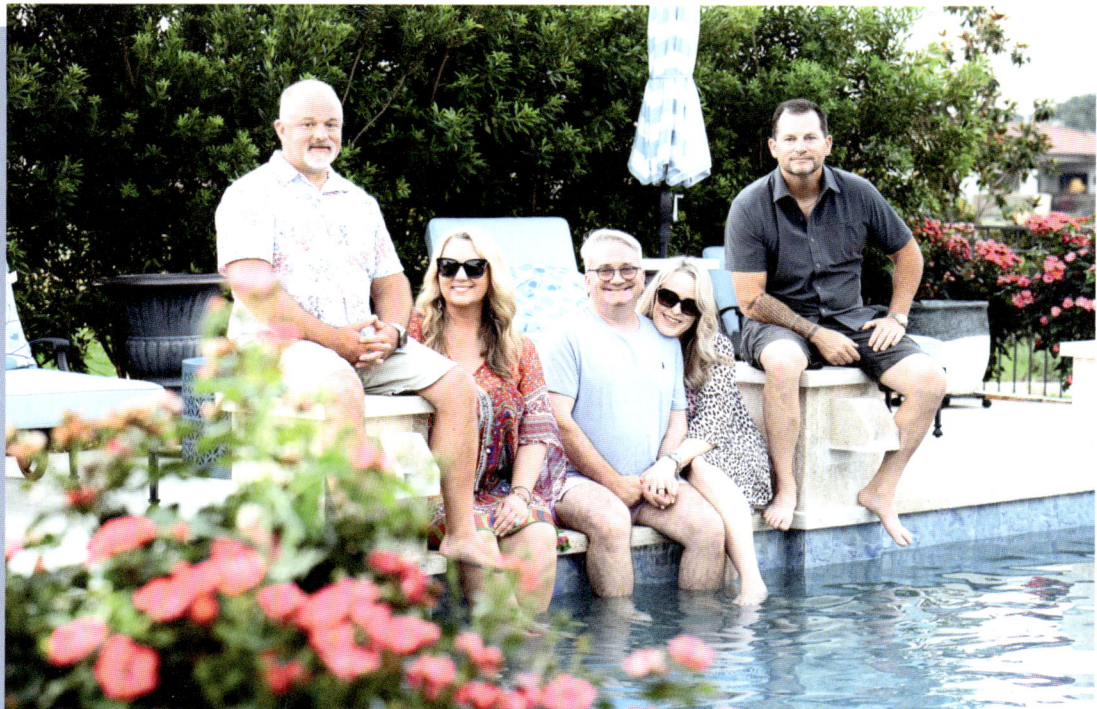

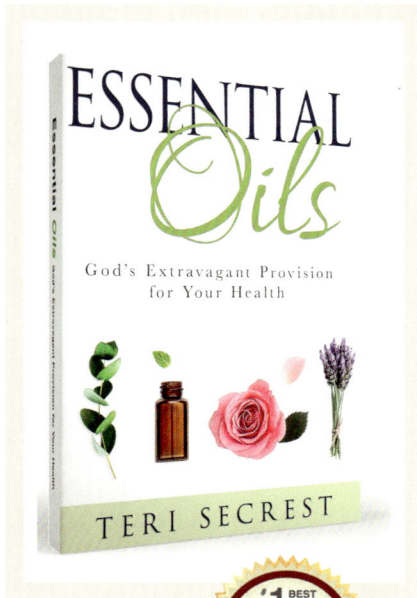

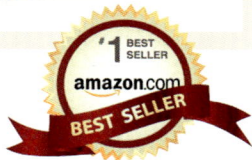

Essential Oils: God's Extravagant Provision For Your Health

Have you ever wondered why the wise men brought frankincense and myrrh to the Christ child? This curiosity ignited Teri Secrest's 28-year journey into the world of essential oils. In Essential Oils: God's Extravagant Provision for Your Health, Teri unveils the mystery and beauty of these biblical oils. Learn practical uses for essential oils in everyday life, from health concerns to creating a peaceful home. Discover the hidden secrets of these ancient oils and pass their benefits on to future generations.

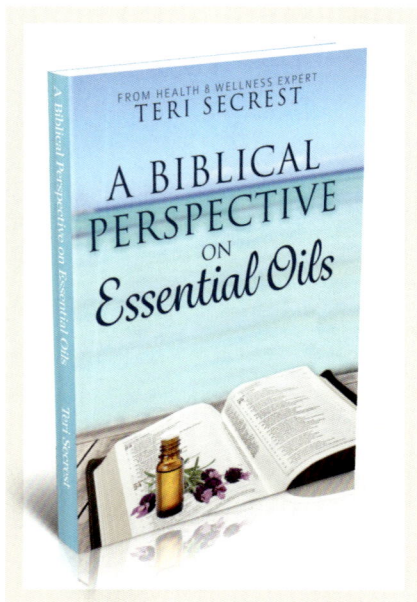

A Biblical Perspective on Essential Oils:

Join Teri Secrest on a journey through the Biblical history of essential oils. Discover the secret to Esther's beauty, why Moses made the Holy Anointing Oil, and how oils were used to sanctify kings and temples. Imagine having access to the same oils used over 2,000 years ago for wellbeing and vitality. This 30-page, full-color booklet is perfect for teaching groups and sharing the timeless wisdom of essential oils.

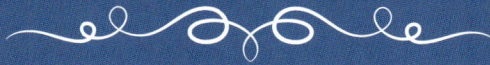

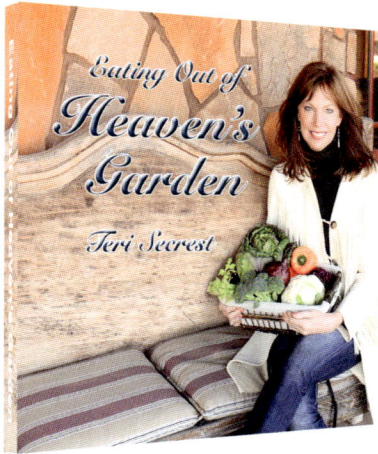

Eating out of Heaven's Garden

Experience vibrant health with Teri Secrest's Eating Out of Heaven's Garden. This beautifully illustrated cookbook offers over 90 pages of simple, whole food recipes designed to nourish both body and soul. With practical steps, stunning full-color photos, and easy instructions, it's your perfect guide for embracing a healthy, joyful lifestyle every day.

Eating For Life!

Eating For Life is more than just a cookbook. It is a way of thinking about food as fuel for life. The life giving health benefits of each ingredient are there to inspire you to live your best life now and also to help you pass this knowledge on to your children and grandchildren. To enjoy the best pricing for multiple books visit Teri's website at TeriSecrest.com.

Visit TeriSecrest.com

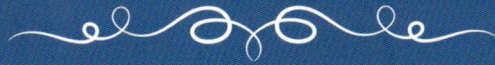

Teri's Recipe Index

Salads

Main Course

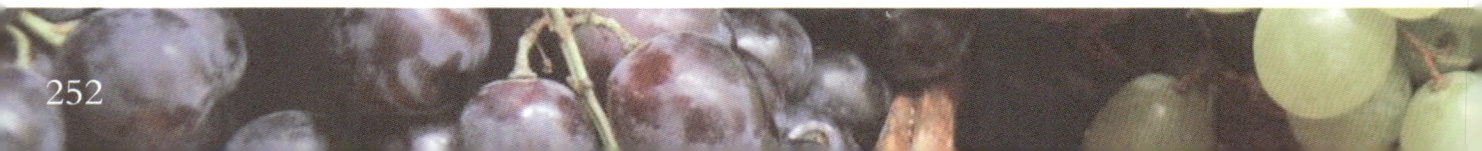

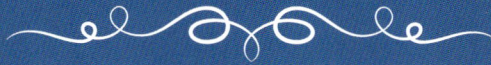

Teri's Recipe Index

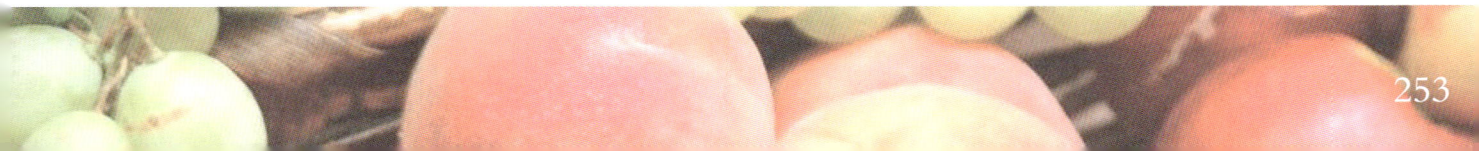